Social Work Practice in the Military

Social Work Practice in the Military

James G. Daley, PhD, ACSW, LCSW
Editor

Routledge
Taylor & Francis Group
NEW YORK AND LONDON

First Published by

The Haworth Press, Inc., 10 Alice Street, Binghamton, NY 13904-1580

Transferred to Digital Printing 2010 by Routledge
270 Madison Ave, New York NY 10016
2 Park Square, Milton Park, Abingdon, Oxon, OX14 4RN

Softcover edition published 2000.

Cover design by Marylouise E. Doyle.

The Library of Congress has cataloged the hardcover edition of this book as:

Daley, James G.
Social work practice in the military / James G. Daley.
p. cm.
Includes bibliographical references and index.
ISBN 0-7890-0625-1 (alk. paper)
1. Military social work—United States. I. Title.
UH755.D35 1999
355.3′4—dc21 98-53340
CIP

ISBN 0-7890-0626-X (pbk.)

Publisher's Note
The publisher has gone to great lengths to ensure the quality of this reprint but points out that some imperfections in the original may be apparent.

CONTENTS

ABOUT THE EDITOR

James G. Daley, PhD, is Assistant Professor in the School of Social Work at Southwest Missouri State University in Springfield. Dr. Daley has published professional articles and four book chapters on such topics as gay and lesbian families, family health, and health care utilization. He is a member of the National Association of Social Workers, the Council on Social Work Education, and the Academy of Certified Social Workers. He is also the guest reviewer for the journal *Research in Social Work Practice.* Dr. Daley is currently working on his second book, *Military Social Work Practice: An International Perspective.*

CONTRIBUTORS

William F. Barko, Colonel (USA), currently serves as Director of the Army Physical Fitness Research Institute at the U.S. Army War College in Carlisle, Pennsylvania.

Steve Bromberek, MSW, is currently stationed at Keflevik, Iceland, and deployed to the Persian Gulf on board ship. Lieutenant Bromberek's first duty station was at the Naval Hospital in Newport, Rhode Island.

Vaughn R. A. Call, PhD, is Professor, Brigham Young University Department of Sociology. He has published extensively on successful human aging issues and the military service context for life cycle transitions.

Spencer J. Campbell, PhD, is chief of the operational stress research unit at the Walter Reed Army Institute of Research in Washington, DC. Major Campbell has served in a variety of key Army social work positions and has been deployed within both combat and humanitarian missions.

Janet Cochran, MSW, is currently stationed at the U.S. Naval Hospital in Yokosuka, Japan. Lieutenant Cochran is on her second assignment with the U.S. Navy. Her first duty assignment was at the Naval Hospital in Charleston, South Carolina.

John Cox, PhD, is Associate Professor, MacMurray College's Department of Social Work in Jacksonville, Illinois. Colonel (retired) Cox had an extensive range of Air Force social work leadership positions during his twenty-plus years of military experience, including his Pentagon position as chief of all Air Force family support centers.

Jesse Harris, PhD, is an icon of military social work. Some of Colonel (retired) Harris's top leadership positions have included social work consultant to the Army Surgeon General, chief of social work at Walter Reed Army Medical Center, commander of the U.S. Army medical research unit at Fort Bragg, North Carolina, and consultant to the U.S. Ambassador to Mozambique on children who were victims of war. He was a primary force in the creation of the annual uniformed services social work conference. He has published extensively on topics of military social work, the mutual impact of the military on soldiers and families, and combat situations. Dr. Harris is dean and professor at the University of Maryland-Baltimore School of Social Work.

Rachel Henry, MSW, is Chief of Social Work Service at the U.S. Army Healthcare Facility in Schweinfurt, Germany. She has worked in both Army and Air Force family advocacy programs and has also worked in Alaska for the U.S. Public Health Services.

James L. Jenkins, PhD, is coordinator for social work education at the Panama City campus of Florida State University's School of Social Work. Colonel (retired) Jenkins oversaw Air Force social work during the most expansive and job redefining time in the history of Air Force social work. He held many key leadership positions including social work consultant to the Air Force Surgeon General and social work consultant to the command surgeon for USAF in Europe. He has published extensively on family advocacy topics.

David Kennedy, MSW, is director of the Navy Family Advocacy Center in San Diego, California, and Southwest regional coordinator for family advocacy programs. He has served as social work speciality leader for the Navy Surgeon General and family advocacy program manager at the U.S. Navy bureau of medicine and surgery in Washington, DC. Captain Kennedy was the first commissioned Navy social worker and has served in a myriad of key leadership positions. Captain Kennedy has played an integral role in coordinating the annual uniformed services social work conference held in conjunction with the NASW national conference.

Griffin David Lockett, DSW, ACSW, LMSW-ACP, is currently social work consultant to the Army Surgeon General and chief of the behavioral health division at Headquarters, U.S. Army Medical Command, Fort Sam Houston, Texas. Colonel Lockett has served in a wide range of positions including chief of the Soldier and Family Support Branch at the U.S. Army Academy of Health Sciences, and chief of the Army Community Service Division and U.S. Army Community and Family Support Center.

James A. Martin, PhD, is Associate Professor, Bryn Mawr College Graduate School of Social Work and Social Research. Dr. Martin has published extensively on military social work topics including his 1996 co-edited book *The Gulf War and Mental Health.* Colonel (retired) Martin's military positions included commander of U.S. Army medical research in Heidelberg, Germany, principal investigator at the soldier and family studies program at Walter Reed Army Institute of Research, and director of Army community services in Baumholder, Germany.

Carla A. Monroe-Posey, PhD, MSHA, is chief of research for Air Force family advocacy at the Air Force Medical Operations Agency at Brooks Air Force Base, Texas. Lieutenant Colonel Monroe-Posey has held several top leadership roles including social work consultant to command surgeon and serving as the first Air Force social worker to work on a TRICARE lead agent program.

John P. Nelson, PhD, is chief of Air Force family advocacy at the Air Force Medical Operations Agency at Brooks Air Force Base, Texas. Colonel Nelson has served a myriad of key leadership positions, including associate director, Office of Family Policy, Office of the Secretary of Defense.

Richard Newsome, PhD, currently serves with the Air Force Inspectors General program at Kirkland Air Force Base, New Mexico. Lieutenant Colonel Newsome has served many key positions including social work consultant to command surgeon, chief of behavioral medicine, and director of three inpatient substance abuse programs (including the tri-service program at Hickam Air Base, Hawaii). He has published on substance abuse treatment issues and developed assessment scales for use with substance abusers.

Mike W. Parker, DSW, BCD, LCSW, is Assistant Professor, School of Social Work, University of Alabama, Tuscaloosa, and Assistant Professor, Department of Geriatrics and Gerontology, University of Alabama, Birmingham. Selected for long-term civilian training, Lieutenant Colonel (retired) Parker completed a National Institute of Aging postdoctoral fellowship at the University of Michigan, and has dedicated his research to honoring aging veterans and their families.

Nancy K. Raiha, PhD, is Chief of Social Work Service at Madigan Army Medical Center in Tacoma, Washington. Colonel Raiha's positions have included chief of social work services in three locations

(Heidelberg and Berlin, Germany; Fort Campbell, Kentucky) and division social worker at Fort Lewis, Washington. She has published extensively on family advocacy and medical social work topics.

Rene J. Robichaux, DSW, is chief of the soldier and family support branch at the Academy of Health Sciences at Fort Sam Houston, Texas. Colonel Robichaux has served in a wide range of positions including Chief of Social Work Service (Landstuhl, Germany; Fort Belvoir) and chief of outpatient social work (Walter Reed Army Medical Center).

Richard A. Ryberg, PhD, is Assistant Professor, Department of Social Work, University of Wisconsin–Eau Claire. Major (retired) Ryberg served in various key positions during his twenty-plus years of military service.

Steven H. Tallant, PhD, is Associate Professor, Department of Social Work, University of Wisconsin–Eau Claire. Lieutenant Colonel (retired) Tallant's twenty-plus years of military service have included director of an inpatient alcoholism treatment program, director of a family support center, and staff member of the Pentagon's family matters office.

Alice A. Tarpley, PhD, is currently social work consultant to the Air Force Surgeon General and chairperson of the department of social work at Malcolm Grow USAF Medical Center at Andrews Air Force Base, Maryland. Colonel Tarpley has served as director of a family support center (Kadena Air Base, Japan and Andersen Air Force Base, Guam), chief of social work services (Shaw Air Force Base and Keesler Air Force Base), and chief of mental health services (Norton Air Force Base). She served on the QREADY task force, which developed Air Force standards for family readiness programs, and was coordinator of the noncombatant evacuation plan and director of the survival and recovery center at Kadena Air Base.

Glenna L. Tinney, MSW, is sexual assault victim intervention program manager at the Bureau of Naval Personnel in Washington, DC, and assistant social work specialty leader for the Navy Surgeon General. Commander Tinney's varied roles have included Navy family advocacy program manager, FAP Regional Coordinator for the Pacific Region vice Hawaii, and head of social work departments at Newport, Rhode Island; Pensacola, Florida; and Yokosuka, Japan.

David J. Westhuis, PhD, is Associate Professor, University of Southern Indiana, School of Social Work. Lieutenant Colonel (retired) Westhuis held many jobs during his military career including chief of family research for the U.S. Army community and family support center, chief of hospital social work services, and chief of a community mental health clinic. He has published extensively and has been involved in research looking at the Army's drug and alcohol program, the impact of Desert Storm on Army spouses, and health care cost analyses.

Lawrence L. Zoeller, MSW, MPA, is the Navy family advocacy regional coordinator in Naples, Italy. Commander Zoeller has been head of social work departments at Bethesda, Maryland; Yokosuka, Japan; Newport, Rhode Island; San Diego, California; and Norfolk, Virginia and head of the Naval community services department in Yokosuka, Japan.

Foreword

In this volume, James Daley provides a much-needed examination of the practice of military social work. His perspective is both wide ranging and specific enough to give a comprehensive view of social work as it is practiced in the three uniformed services (Army, Navy, and Air Force). His vision of what is relevant to understanding military social work comes from having carefully observed his professional peers at work and from personally experiencing the frustrations and joys of doing military social work during his twenty-plus years in the military.

I am especially impressed with the array of talented contributors to this volume. Dr. Daley has called upon, and received, insights from some of the most thoughtful pioneers and current leaders in military social work.

The timing for this volume is right. As the twentieth century draws to a close, it is essential to take a look at where military social work has been, where it presently is, and also to speculate about what the future may hold in the twenty-first century.

This volume is relevant to the entire profession of social work in our country. The subjects covered in this book provide a view of the full potential of social work. The discerning reader will quickly notice that military social work practice, by and large, has moved beyond the divisions of direct practice versus social policy that seem to hinder the development and potential of much of civilian social work practice. "Turf battles" exist in all of social work, but the rich variety of services and conceptual underpinnings in this volume show how diversity may be used for growth rather than stuckness.

I have often been asked the question, "What is the difference between civilian social work practice and military social work practice?" From what is now a combination of twenty years of civilian experience and twenty years of military experience, three differences strike me. First, military social workers are likely to be called upon to perform the full range of professional social work activities. Just some of the range of practice arenas includes direct practice in mental health programs, social work in a medical setting, social work in support of military operations, social work in substance abuse programs, family advocacy programs, program administration, and policy-creating roles. What is the difference between civilian and military social work? Military social workers have more roles. The depth and breath of social work practice in the military provides a picture of the strength of social work as a profession. Second, and important to many people, military social workers perform in a wide range of practice arenas *and* continue to work for the same agency. In other words, the career social worker in the military does not have to change employers to have a diversified professional career. And third, the professional education and competence level of military social workers is high. All military social work officers have at least an MSW. Many have a PhD. The competition to get a commission as a social worker is strong. Military social workers are an outstanding group of professionals.

From the three differences between civilian and military social workers mentioned above, a strong group identity has emerged among the social workers in the three service branches. This group spirit, within diversity, among military social workers is obvious in this book's individual presentations relating to different arenas of social work in the military.

From modest beginnings as social work practice within mental health services, military social work has expanded to a comprehensive span of service, including being policy shapers at the highest levels of command. The sections on the history and role transitions of military social work over the years is instructive for all of us who appreciate the struggles of a profession that practices in various contexts, some of which are not congruent with social work's basic values.

In the section on the unique issues of military social work, the authors address some of the vital ethical concerns that emerge from social work practice in a military context with its own ethical framework. Schools of social work would do well to use the ideas in this section as "points of departure" for seminar discussions about divergent values, beliefs, and priorities that confront social workers, clients, and organizations. In reading this section one sees that the ethical dilemmas which emerge in the military context are not really that different from many of those that show up in civilian life. The content issues may vary between the military and civilian contexts but the *basic* ethical issues are very similar.

Given the downsizing in the military that we hear much about in the news media, the question about the future of military social work in the twenty-first century naturally arises. Will the turn to privatization in other arenas of government spread to the military? Privatization has the potential for creating enormous changes in the delivery of social work services in the military.

What impact will the "lean and mobile" military of the future have on military families? The emotional health of the family has a great influence on the serviceman and servicewoman's readiness to perform his or her duties. Military social work has contributed heavily to services to and research on the military family.

What about research efforts by social workers? The social work perspective has much to offer not only in identifying vital areas of research but in research methodology itself. While the authors in this volume do not claim to predict the future, they provide some insightful "best guesses" about the place for military social workers in the twenty-first century.

This volume is loaded with valuable information drawn from people who have lived the experiences of military social work. We must thank Dr. Daley: he not only lived military social work, he also realized that other social workers such as himself have valuable information to share with the rest of us. As I said at the beginning of this foreword, the timing of this volume is right.

Donald R. Bardill, PhD
School of Social Work
Florida State University

Senior Editor's Comments

As editor of The Haworth Press Social Work Practice in Action Textbook Series, I am pleased to have James Daley's edited volume on military social work published as part of this series. As a former U.S. Coast Guard officer from several decades ago who had the good fortune to do training for the Army in Europe last year, I can attest to the tremendous change in the military over the past three decades. The military changes that have paralleled the changes in the civilian sector have brought about an interconnection between the civilian and military sector that often is unrecognized. Dr. Bardill in his foreword states that this book is relevant to the entire profession of social work. I agree with his observation, and that is why I felt it was a priority to publish this book as part of The Haworth Press Textbook Series: Social Work Practice in Action.

When I visited the Army in Europe, I was impressed with the high level of performance of all the military personnel there, but I was especially impressed by the quality and commitment of military and civilian social workers. At the same time, I was puzzled that in the United States we rarely heard about and knew so little about the work of these dedicated people. I wish the media would give more visibility to the work of the military carrying out these difficult missions far from our shores. I believe that such visibility would provide the public with a better understanding of the role the military plays in our national security in noncombat situations. I hope this book will assist these dedicated professionals as they perform their difficult task as well as enhance the performance of all military and civilian social work professionals where ever they serve.

With the globalization of economies and the increased wars and threat of wars around the world, the role of the military social worker becomes even more critical. The challenge for the military social worker, from my perspective, relates to providing support to our own troops and to assist the victims of aggression and civil strife in their homelands as well as the victims in warring nations. I think it is difficult for civilian social workers to imagine a mission more vast than the global one carried out by military social workers.

In this book, James Daley has captured a comprehensive view of the military social worker that ranges from a historic perspective, to current practice demands and challenges, to a glimpse into the future of military social work. I believe this book will be valuable for career military social workers, contract civilian social workers serving the military, civilian social workers serving military personnel in locales near military installations, and as pointed out by the authors, civilian social workers who have no contact with the military. I salute Dr. Daley and the fine contributors to this impressive volume, and I commend them for a job well done.

Carlton E. Munson, PhD
Professor and Doctoral Program Director
University of Maryland
Senior Editor, The Haworth Press Social Work Practice Textbook Series: Social Work Practice in Action

Preface

Seeking to capture the rich tapestry of military social work, this book is intended for both military and civilian readers. It can be used by military social workers, civilian social workers working with or just curious about this practice arena, or students wanting to explore an excellent example of social work in action.

The military social worker is the consummate social worker in an environment where all aspects of the profession can be demonstrated. In fact, to paraphrase a popular recruiting slogan, military social work is truly the act of social work "being all it can be." I hope, as you read this book, you will agree with me.

Skills such as those of the clinician, advocate, policymaker, resource liaison, organizational consultant occur on a regular basis within the world of the military social worker. While combining generalist practice with micro, mezzo, and macro interventions, the military social worker embraces a lifestyle far beyond any civilian social work job. The impact of some military social workers has been felt at the top levels of the Pentagon. Significant research efforts by military social workers have led to a greater appreciation of the impact of family on military readiness and vice versa, a deeper understanding of life span development of military troops, and a better awareness of clinical strategies with such issues as family violence, occupationally induced family separations, family resilience, fitness for duty, and ameliorating the impact of base closures on the family.

This book seeks to reflect the rich heritage of military social work. The chapters include input from top current and past leadership within the ranks of military social workers. The topics span the wide range of issues being dealt with by military social workers. Each chapter, unless unique to one service, reflects the work occurring in all three services (Army, Navy, Air Force) that employ military social workers.

Social work within the Marines is not separately covered, as their social work services are provided by the Navy, in Family Service

Centers staffed by civilian social workers or Navy active duty social workers. To date, military social workers have not deployed directly with a Marine unit in combat. In fact, the Marines do not have any medical personnel. Rather, they utilize Navy resources or the military medical resource nearest their location.

Likewise, this book does not discuss Public Health Service uniformed social workers, as that uniformed branch is not directly considered military service. Finally, we do not uniquely cover the growing legion of civilian social workers providing contract or civil service to the military. We do, however, discuss the utility of civilian social workers in most chapters. In sum, the primary intent of this chapter is to illuminate one vital component of military social services: the active duty military social worker.

The book has four broad sections: historical context, practice arenas, unique aspects of military social work, and the future of military social work. The historical context section includes a chapter on the history of Army social work (Chapter 1), Navy social work (Chapter 2), and Air Force social work (Chapter 3).

After providing a broad historical perspective, the book offers seven chapters that span the range of service arenas offered by military social workers. Chapter 4 captures the most rapidly expanding arena of practice, family advocacy, which includes a broad array of family violence prevention and intervention services. Chapter 5 illuminates a very complicated topic, TRICARE (the military managed care program), and discusses the impact of TRICARE on military families and social workers. Chapter 6 provides a historical discussion of the changing view of substance abuse treatment within the military and the essential role held by military social workers in providing a multilevel service for clients and the military. Chapter 7 shows the extensive involvement of military social workers in a myriad of medical social work programs serving patients and families. Chapter 8 reviews the traditional mental health provider role held by military social workers and how the role continues as an essential (but not exclusive) skill for every military social work officer. Chapter 9 illustrates another essential skill for military social workers: effective involvement in combat or deployed situations. After an excellent historical review of the issue, this chapter provides an overview of the basic practice principles, case examples of interventions, and concludes with practical guidelines and recommended readings for the social worker preparing for deployment. Chapter 10 advocates the idea that military social workers have served important policymaking positions, increasingly need to assert their expertise in the frequently rapid policy decision-making process within the military, and suggests a framework for policy practice within the military.

The third section includes issues unique to the military setting. Chapter 11 explores the ethical dilemmas inherent in military social work, illustrates some scenarios of ethical awkwardness, and offers a suggested process for making ethical decisions within the military. Chapter 12 reviews the progression of the military social worker's career, and offers some survival strategies for the new military social worker and some insights for our civilian colleagues on how to most effectively collaborate with military social workers. Chapters 13, 14, and 15 are specifically targeted for the reader naive to the military. These chapters offer an overview of each military service (Army in Chapter 13, Navy in Chapter 14, Air Force in Chapter 15) and the unique experiences in each service. The chapters are not on social work practitioners. Instead, each chapter focuses on the social context of each service and offers an insider's view of the world in which the military social worker functions. Chapter 16 blends data and theory to discuss how the life span issues of the military person are impacted by the military career process and suggests a critical primary prevention role for military social workers in facilitating healthy aging as military members and their families navigate retirement and beyond. Chapter 17 explores the impact of deployment on the military person and his or her family and the role of the social worker in enhancing personal and family coping skills. Chapter 18 challenges that being a part of the military can be considered an "ethnic identity," reviews some of the distinctive identity issues inherent in the military lifestyle, and concludes with a suggested "military identity assessment scale" as a focus for basic research.

The final section offers the insights of the current chiefs of military social work on what the future entails for Army social work (Chapter 19), Navy social work (Chapter 20), and Air Force social work (Chapter 21). The book concludes (Chapter 22) with an effort by the editor to coalesce the wide-ranging previous chapters into key issues needing attention to enhance the future resiliency of military social work.

What began as a commitment to capture the essence of military social work has, in this editor's humble opinion, blossomed into an extraordinary collection of insights into an often misunderstood or ignored practice setting. I hope the reader, when finished with this book, is enlightened and proud of what our military colleagues have accomplished. I certainly am!

James G. Daley, PhD

PART I: HISTORICAL CONTEXTS OF PRACTICE

Chapter 1

History of Army Social Work

Jesse Harris

THE CIVILIAN CONNECTION WITH THE ARMY

Any consideration of the history of Army social work must include a discussion of the impact of wars on soldiers and their families. It must also consider the crucial role of the Red Cross and the corps of civilian professional social work organizations that helped to shape what is now Army social work.

Before there were uniformed social workers there were Red Cross social workers. The value of psychiatric social workers to the Army was made known during World War I, as a result of a demonstration project by the Red Cross with the cooperation of the division of neurology and psychiatry of the surgeon general's office.

This project was conducted at the special hospital for neuroses at the U.S. Army General Hospital #30 at Plattsburgh, New York. The first social worker was available for duty on September 1, 1918. The success of the work at Plattsburgh led the Red Cross to increase the number of psychiatric social workers at that hospital from one to three. Later they would assign not only psychiatric but also medical social workers to all hospitals.

American Red Cross social workers continued to work in appropriate Army Hospitals between the two world wars and continued during World War II. Between 1942 and 1945 about 1,000 American Red Cross psychiatric social workers were assigned to named general and regional hospitals, in the United States and overseas (National Association of Social Workers, 1965, p. 15). The Army relied upon the Red Cross throughout two wars.

It was not until June 1945 that an Army social work program was incorporated into the office of the surgeon general. The psychiatric social work branch was established. A full-time position of social work consultant also was created to head that branch. Much of the credit for these events goes to the close coordination of two major professional organizations. The Wartime Committee on Personnel of the American Association of Social Workers (which represented over 14,000 practicing social workers and the forty-two recognized schools of graduate social work) (Anderson, 1944).

Another major organization was the National Committee for Mental Hygiene. This organization interacted with the Surgeon General on social work's behalf during World War I. Finally, there was Elizabeth H. Ross, who, at that time, was the civilian consultant to Brigadier General William Menninger, Chief of the Neuropsychiatry Consultants Division (Ross, 1951).

THE ENLISTED SOCIAL WORK CONTRIBUTIONS

By February 1942, not long after the United States entered World War II, six enlisted men who were professionally qualified psychiatric social workers were assigned to the newly formed Mental Hygiene Consultation Service at Fort Monmouth, New Jersey. This event was the first time that military personnel who were professionally trained social workers were assigned and utilized as psychiatric social workers in a military unit. Myron J. Rockmore, Frank T. Grieving, and Henry Maas were among the first group. They would go on to make significant contributions both in the military and in the civilian sector. All who served in an enlisted status were not trained social workers. By their own initiative many had moved into a working relationship with individual psychiatrists in various Army units and learned their skills at the job site. It should be noted that no official distinction was made between professional and nonprofessional personnel even though a large percentage had advanced degrees or were exceptionally well qualified.

On October 18, 1943, the War Department published the Military Occupational Specialty 263 for Psychiatric Social Work Technicians. The military psychiatric social worker (SSN #263) was defined as follows:

> Under supervision of a psychiatrist, performs psychiatric casework to facilitate diagnoses and treatment of soldiers requiring psychiatrist guidance.
>
> Administers psychiatric intake interviews, and writes case histories emphasizing the factors pertinent to psychiatric diagnoses.
>
> Carries out mental-hygiene prescriptions and records progress to formulate a complete case history.
>
> May obtain additional information on soldier's home environment through Red Cross or other agencies to facilitate in possible discharge planning.
>
> Must have knowledge of dynamics of personality structure and development, and cause of emotional maladjustments. (War, 1943)

Even though there was a need for men and women with social work skills, trained soldiers already on active duty could not expect to automatically be awarded the occupational specialty SSN #263, psychiatric social worker, even if they had social work training. The organization of a social work program in the Army during World War II was in a large measure due to continuing efforts of civilian social workers through the medium of various professional organizations. The American Association of Psychiatric Social Workers established its War Service Office and began to lay the groundwork for a more organized social work structure in the military establishment. In September 1943, in anticipation of the above War Department letter and at the height of World War II, Elizabeth H. Ross, while in the position of secretary of the War Service Office, sent a general memorandum to young men already on active duty. The memorandum stated that a private or noncommissioned man in the Army could apply for reclassification as a psychiatric social worker. Ironically, the memorandum also acknowledged that Army commissioned officers or any person in the Navy, Marines, Coast Guard, Seabees, or Women's Army Corps could not apply to be a psychiatric social worker. Between 1942 and 1945, 711 enlisted men and WACs served in the role of psychiatric social workers. They were assigned to induction centers, named general and regional hospitals, station and evacuation hospitals, and combat divisions.

THE SOCIAL WORK OFFICER

Although social workers served honorably, the war would end before social work was recognized as a discipline of commissioned officers. Those social workers who did have commissions had obtained them through other branches of the service prior to serving as social workers.

Commissioned status for social workers within the Army was finally achieved in 1945, in part because of the continuing efforts of the Wartime Committee on Personnel of the American Association of Social Workers. Major Daniel E. O'Keefe assumed the position as the first Chief of the Army's Psychiatric Social Work Branch on July 1, 1945. During the eight months before his separation from service in February 1946, he was only able to begin a centrally directed social work program. This limited impact was because, with demobilization, almost all trained army social workers were separated. Though a decision was made in June 1945 to grant the military occupational specialty for the professionally trained Psychiatric Social Work Officer (MOS 3506), the decision was not published until February 1946 (after the war was over). February 1946 was the same month that Major O'Keefe returned to civilian life, along with many officers who served during the war. But the creation of the new military occupational specialty assured the continuity of Army social work (Camp, 1951).

With the departure of O'Keefe, the position of Chief of the Psychiatric Social Work Branch was now vacant. However, the Psychiatric Social Work Branch continued with the support of General William Menninger, the Chief of the Neuropsychiatric Consultants division of the OTSG. The Surgeon General called upon Elizabeth H. Ross, who agreed to serve as the civilian Psychiatric Social Work Consultant until such time as a qualified uniformed officer could be recruited and appointed.

There was an urgency to rebuild professional social work in the Army. National advertising occurred with headlines such as "Army Medical Department Seeks Psychiatric Social Workers." One such example is an article in the November 7, 1946, edition of the *Douglas County Legionnaire,* published in Omaha, Nebraska (Army Medical Department, 1946). The article described the need for psychiatric social workers who were officers or former officers to participate in teams with psychiatrists and clinical psychologists providing neuropsychiatric services. The qualifications for the social worker were at least one year of training in an accredited school of social work, a field placement, and one year of social case work experience in a health or welfare agency.

Ironically, the *Douglas County Legionnaire* article helped motivate Harry Adams and Elwood Camp to apply as Army social Workers. Camp had been the director and service officer of the Lincoln and Lancaster County Veterans Service Center (Adams, 1966). Ross served as consultant in a civilian capacity from February 4, 1946, until the appointment of Lieutenant Colonel Elwood W. Camp as the second military Chief of the Psychiatric Social Work Branch and Social Work Consultant to the Surgeon General (Morgan, 1961).

The rebuilding of the program would indeed become a monumental task. In addition to a major drive to encourage master's degree social workers to join the service, the Army adopted the "case aide" plan. This plan is intriguing at this point in time because it proposed to train as paraprofessionals not only enlisted personnel but commissioned officers as well. This latter group was needed to provide leadership until an adequate number of professional social workers could be obtained. This program is discussed later in this chapter.

THE ROLE OF THE PSYCHIATRIC SOCIAL WORKER

The fact that psychiatric social work preceded medical social work in the Army can best be appreciated when one considers the events of World War I. In the thirty-three months from April 1, 1917, to December 31, 1919, 97,650 men with neuropsychiatric disorders were admitted to military hospitals (Freedman, 1944, p. 2). The figures reported for neuropsychiatric problems during the years 1942-1945 (World War II) were equally sobering. One million soldiers were admitted to Army hospitals for neuropsychiatric reasons. These casualties constituted 6 to 7 percent of all admissions. The more than 545,000 troops who were separated from the service for neuropsychiatric disorders accounted for 49 percent of all discharges for either physical or mental defects (Caldwell, 1948).

There was a significant difference in the approach used to deal with inductees of World War I and World War II. The selective service criteria used in the World War I resulted in far greater neuropsychiatric (NP) rejection rates than the criteria used for the 1,850,000 NP rejections for military service during World War II (Caldwell, 1948). Rockmore attributed the difference to the World War II concept of limited service based on differential diagnoses, which eventually supplanted the earlier criteria (Rockmore, 1960).

Another significant factor in the reduced number of psychiatric casualties was the introduction of the Mental Hygiene Units. The mission of a typical Mental Hygiene Unit in the early days of World War II was as follows:

> a. Provide Mental Hygiene facilities to organizations and officers and to assist them with soldiers who present various forms of maladjustment, as inaptitude, unusual behavior, malingering ("goldbricking") recalcitrant, alcoholism and others.
>
> b. Institute such corrective measures as are considered appropriate by the director thereof, to reduce or eliminate the individual's maladjustment and eradicate factors related to incipient issues for mental breakdown to the extent necessary for the soldier to perform military duties. (*Memorandum Number 41,* 1943)

An understanding of the approach used in treating neuropsychiatric casualties can be found elsewhere (Freedman, 1945).

As noted earlier, a soldier diagnosed as a neuropsychiatric case was admitted to the hospital and treated in closed wards. The strategy of early hospitalization in closed wards was replaced by more out-patient strategies with the advent of the Mental Hygiene Units psychiatric compact first aid and the Neuropsychiatric Reconditioning Facility. Mental Hygiene Units in all installations and echelons moved psychiatry out of the protective confines of the mental hospital (Rockmore, 1960).

Based on previous war experience, there was concern that many inductees would experience adjustment problems. Such difficulties were noted and dealt with in the Army Replacement Training Center, where soldiers received their basic and initial specialized training after assignment from the reception centers. Initially, the Mental Hygiene Unit was staffed by one psychiatrist and one social worker. Later the clinical psychologist was included and in time other psychiatric disciplines were included to form the Army's first Mental Hygiene Unit

(American Psychiatric Association, 1944). The concept of a clinical team was later extended to the majority of replacement training centers in this country (Freedman, 1944).

The psychiatric social workers were usually the first to interview the new recruit. It was recognized that a social worker in uniform had increased credibility and was in a better position to identify with his fellow soldier. Freedman noted, "The military psychiatric social worker in the mental-hygiene unit has been trained to understand the nature, varieties and motivation of human behavior. His basic skills in assisting in diagnosis and treatment are here adapted to the needs of the neuropsychiatric casualty . . ." (Freedman, 1944, p. 187).

The Mental Hygiene Consultation Service (MHCS), a successor to the Mental Hygiene Unit, had its birth at Fort Monmouth in 1942. As the concept of consultation spread during World War II, greater emphasis was given to providing on-site consultation to field commanders (Parrish, 1970). Written instructions were often provided for them in layman's language (Freedman, 1944). The MHCS grew out of the efforts of Freedman and others. It became part of the Adjutant's section or what might now be known as G1. When the war ended, the strength of the MHCS movement declined throughout the Army. Not until the Korean War was emphasis again directed to the MHCS. By the Korean War few of the old guard remained and each unit sprang up, run by a two-year reservist who usually had neither knowledge nor identification with the concept of consultation. But they would quickly catch on and make major contributions.

The later Mental Hygiene Consultation Division or Command Consultation Service would reemphasize consultation with the commanders. It often handled the situation as a systems problem. The system of interlocking influences of various roles and personalities within units, families, or cliques may produce a patient as a manifestation of maladjustment within that system. The consultant along with the commander was expected to understand the significant group and the patient's place within the group.

The duties of the MHCS professional staff during peacetime were varied. A typical liaison visit consisted of the psychiatrist and/or social worker or psychologist traveling to dispensaries, military units, or schools, consulting with doctors, commanders, and school counselors or principals, and to a predetermined unit to spend the day in the troop area (Ramer, 1965; Willi, 1968). Dispensary physicians would, in all probability, arrange a staff meeting and problems would be aired and cases presented. The technicians might do preliminary psychiatric workups, such as obtaining historical data and gathering other kinds of background material on newly referred patients. In the afternoon a topic (e.g., "the ineffective soldier") would be presented and a film shown about the function of the Army Mental Hygiene Service with general discussions in the presence of the top noncommissioned officers (NCOs) and officers of the battalion. While workers were in the area, local schools would be visited and consultations with principals and teachers would take place.

MEDICAL SOCIAL WORKERS

The need for social workers in the Army was shown in Army hospitals during World War I, by professionally trained social caseworkers as a demonstration project for the American Red Cross. The success of this project resulted in the acceptance of professionally trained social casework services in other hospitals through the Army (National Association of Social Workers, 1965). The major role that medical social work would enjoy in the Army was due in no small way to significant changes that were about to occur. A pivotal sequence of events was stirred by the Army Surgeon General's publication on January 31, 1951, of *SGO Circular #18, Medical and Psychiatric Social Case Work in Army Hospitals.* This publication prompted a message from the American Red Cross which stated that as of July 1, 1951, the American Red Cross was withdrawing all ARC medical and psychiatric social case functions from Army hospitals. Their rationale was that professionally trained social caseworkers, Army officers or civic service, would pick up the services. The Army's immediate response was to bring Major Barbara B. Hodges on active duty on July 2, 1951, as the first Director of the Army's Medical Social Work Program (B. B. Hodges, personal communication, 1990).

Blue (1966) would later observe that it was not until the early 1950s that the Army recognized and assumed responsibility for providing social work services to nonpsychiatric patients. This decision came over four decades after social work in general hospitals was first established.

Blue also observed instability of the social work organization within the hospital. In the 1950s it vacillated among several different frameworks. In some general hospitals, hospital-wide social work services, which were responsible to the chief of professional services, were established. In other general hospitals, two separate social work programs were established, one program responsible to the chief of the department of psychiatry and neurology and the other responsible to the chief of the department of medicine. In the early 1960s social work in the Army general hospital was suddenly again placed under the chief of the department of psychiatry and neurology (Blue, 1966).

In 1966 the Surgeon General proclaimed that social work should have a separate service with Class II hospitals (Social Work Services, 1966). Fergus T. Monahan, the social work consultant at that time, declared: "Once again we have established social work as a separate service in Class II hospitals. Social Work Service reaffirmed the status of separate service. We see this as an opportunity to demonstrate better the value of social service in a hospital so that the impact of our contribution may be understood more clearly as being unique and in contrast to that offered by other professional disciplines" (Monahan, 1966, p. 2).

Other changes were taking place within the hospital setting that would require social work to play an active role. SGO Circular 119 was published, stating that there would be a Welfare Division in Class II hospitals. The division would be headed by an MSC officer. This circular also described the neuropsychiatry service as having a psychiatric social work section. As a matter of fact, Army Regulation No. 40-605, *Neuropsychiatry* (dated June 20, 1949) had already outlined the policies for this service and provided that the medical department would have a social work section in the department of neuropsychiatry.

The tasks set forth in SGO Circular 119 were specific: to collect, evaluate and record pertinent social and medical data; help patients meet immediate comfort needs, accept hospitalization, and adjust to return to duty or discharge. Social workers were also to perform individual and group therapy as directed by the psychiatrist.

STOCKADES

The military is a microcosm of society and as such often finds that it must mirror the larger society by developing similar institutions. These institutions of confinement for soldiers who become offenders. Similar to its civilian counterpart, the military penal system struggled over the purpose of imprisonment. Was it to punish or was it to rehabilitate?

Colonel William C. Menninger, MC, chief of the department of neuropsychiatry and neurology of the surgeon general's office, stated:

> Rehabilitation should be our first aim in dealing with military offenders, recognizing that some members who are potentially unsalvageable should be separated from the group. The first step on a man's arrival should be psychiatric and social evaluation to determine the nature of the problem and the most promising steps to take in his rehabilitation. To accomplish this mission, every member of the staff from the commandant to guard must know and apply the principles of mental hygiene. (Menninger, 1945, p. 12)

But the treatment orientation was slow to catch on. Colonel Joseph Reeves, former social work consultant, would stress this fact twenty-five years after Menninger. Although the stockades always had some kind of relationship with the mental hygiene consultation service, Bushard noted that "at times various programs were established for short periods, but they rarely included the total prisoner population and never represented a real, co-operative combined effort with both command and psychiatric personnel cooperating" (Bushard, 1957, p. 1619).

In September 1957, AR 210-181 introduced the Army stockade screening program and made provisions for the early identification of maladjusted soldiers and, if possible, the use of remedial efforts to render these individuals useful to the service. It was felt that the objectives of the Stockade Screening Program could best be achieved by the psychiatric evaluation of all prisoners during the first few days of confinement.

Although the stockade screening program used the team approach in the mental hygiene consultation service, examination was most effectively done within the stockade by social work personnel under the supervision of the psychiatrist. Hailed as a major achievement in military corrections, the stockade screening program was part of the organized effort to make the stockade a rehabilitation center rather than what some had believed it had been—a place to isolate offenders and a source of free labor (Gibbs, 1961).

Although there was agreement with Menninger and others of the need to rehabilitate soldiers who were confined, there is evidence that early attempts at treatment did not meet everyone's expectations. Paul D'Oronzio, a social work officer who had been assigned to the stockade, cited surveys which substantiated the fact that social workers played an integral role in nearly all stockades. However, he questioned the models being used. He noted that there were a variety of functions being carried out in the stockades under the rubric of "treatment programs." He observed that most treatment was focused on the classical one-on-one psychotherapeutic relationship or a variety of group treatment approaches. He also noted that many programs rejected the treatment mode and that most social workers were being used to screen new inmates. D'Oronzio argued for a systems approach to treatment (D'Oronzio, 1966).

But according to Major Joseph Reeves (later to be Colonel Reeves, the Social Work Consultant to the Surgeon General), the screening program was viewed as a psychiatric as opposed to a social work function and social workers wanted to get out of it. Reeves posed the question of what social work's point of intervention should be. While individual treatment was being carried out in stockades by social workers, they needed to look at the military community as the point of intervention (Reeves, 1966).

Major Marvin West, a social worker at the Fort Lewis stockade, argued for the model used at Fort Lewis Washington, the community or consultation approach. Major West's command regarded the stockade as a "behavioral reinforcement and ideally we want few rehabilitable soldiers confined there. When a stockade is found to have a large rehabilitation program, group therapy and the like, we feel they *are not* screening their population well enough and *are not* moving their prisoners quickly out of the confinement situation" (West, 1967, p. 4).

While most acknowledged the social work role, there were some who felt that other team members should have been utilized better. For example, a psychiatrist acknowledged the role of social workers in the stockades but questioned the role of the psychiatrist in the stockades. "Regulations for stockade and Mental Hygiene Clinic alike recognize the need for coordination between physician and social worker, and lay 'caretaker,' to achieve these aims. . . . Most programs rely on social casework, the psychiatrist functions largely as a consultant advising on difficult cases and certifying legal sanity . . . the psychiatrist potential is not fully exploited (Simon, 1965).

In 1968, the Correctional Training Facility (CTF) was established at Ft. Riley, Kansas. Its purpose was to provide the training and assistance necessary to return military offenders to duty and hopefully an honorable discharge. Social workers were assigned to the CTF and played a significant role in its development. It should be noted that mental health specialists did not encourage coddling soldiers but did recognize the importance of good leadership in reducing the number of solders who ended up in trouble (Kisel, 1963).

THE ARMY COMMUNITY SERVICE (ACS)

The demographics of the Army changed dramatically during and after the World War II years. In 1940 there were 67,000 families in the Army. By 1965, there were about 450,000 families with over 1,300,000 dependents. In 1940 enlisted men were required to obtain their superior's permission to marry. By 1965, 60 percent of the enlisted men were married and 80 percent of the officers. However, one consequence was that over 100,000 wives were separated from their husbands due to military duties (Krise, 1966).

It was not surprising, therefore, that reports began coming in from major commands about the negative impact on troop morale and retention created by family problems, which ranged from disturbed and retarded children to chronic financial hardship and indebtedness. Lieutenant Colonel Marie Baird, a staff officer in the Department of the Army and the Army social service consultant, and Lieutenant Colonel William Rooney, appointed as the Surgeon General's representative, were assigned to conduct a study based upon these complaints. Their two-year study substantiated the need for the Army to aggressively address these problems. Prototype ACS programs were started at Fort Dix, Fort Benning, and Fort Lewis, installations with high troop and family concentrations.

The mission of the ACS program was to establish at each installation where more than 500 military personnel were assigned "a centrally located responsive and recognizable service to provide information, assistance and guidance to members of the Army community in meeting personal and family problems beyond the scope of their own resources, in order to reduce the man-hours consumed by commanders, staff officers and soldiers in seeking assistance for complex personal problems, and to improve personnel retention by increasing career satisfaction" (Army Community Service Program, 1965, p. 2). Some of the services to be provided included information and referral for financial assistance, availability of housing, transportation, relocation of dependents, medical and dental care, legal assistance, and more complex family and personal issues.

Authorization was approved for forty-two social work officers and nineteen social work specialists to be assigned. This was the first time that social workers, as a group, were called upon to extend their knowledge and skills outside of the Medical Service (Monahan, 1966). By November 1966, over ninety ACS centers had been established worldwide, with over 132,000 individuals having received assistance at these centers (Cocoran, 1966).

In addition to the professional staff the ACS heavily relied on volunteers to carry out its mission. The concept of the ACS program was that its foundation would be a volunteer corps of Army wives who would support a small nucleus of military and civilian supervisors. These supervisors would have direct responsibility for the ACS program. Among the wives who were dedicated to the cause of ACS were Mrs. Harold K. Johnson, wife of the Army Chief of Staff, and Mrs. George S. Patton.

The Surgeon General ordered ACS programs be established at the following major Medical Service Activities (which were known as Class II activities): Walter Reed Army Medical Center, Fitzsimmons General Hospital and Valley Forge General Hospital. Other Class II medical activities were encouraged to be included in programs already in existence at their installations or to initiate their own programs. Social workers played a major role in establishing ACS at Medical Activities (Army Community Service, 1966).

On January 16, 1967, an ACS branch was established within the Personnel Services Division of the Army Deputy Chief of Staff of

Personnel. This was a major milestone in the history of Army Community Service. Lieutenant Colonel Hill became the social work ACS consultant to the new branch.

An innovative and interesting community concept that was monitored by ACS was the Schilling Manor housing, which was located at Shilling Air Force Base in Selena, Kansas. During the height of the Vietnam War, housing was made available to approximately 200 families whose sponsors were serving a tour of duty in Southeast Asia. It soon became clear that, although these families were living in the protective environment of the base, there were problems. Seventy-two percent of the wives were foreign born and a significant number had language difficulties. The average size of the families was 6.8 persons. Colonel Monahan recommended that a civilian social work position be established to assist in the multitude of problems that existed. The request was approved.

One of the less-known facts of the ACS is its symbol, the gyroscope. The idea for what is now the ACS symbol (with minor modifications) originated with certain social work officers at Brook Army Medical Center, with the assistance of the graphic arts section of the Army Medical Service School at Brooke Army Medical Center. The symbol was originally conceived to represent Army social work. The early publications of the *Social Work Proceedings* show the gyroscope on their covers. This symbol was first introduced at the Eighth Annual Army Social Work Conference, held in Chicago on May 10 and 11, 1958 (*Proceedings,* 1958).

EDUCATION AND TRAINING

As noted previously, after World War II there was a major thrust to encourage social workers with a master's degree to join the service. The Army Training Program was initiated for the purpose of procuring psychiatric social workers. Selection would be made from male graduates, students of social casework who were enrolled in graduate schools of social work approved by the Secretary of the Army and who desired a career with the Regular Army Medical Service Corps (Medical Service Corps, 1949).

As a stopgap measure the Army adopted the case aide plan. Under this plan selected officers and enlisted men were trained on a paraprofessional level in a special and intensive course offered by the Army as part of the general training program of the Medical Department. Officers who possessed a college degree and demonstrated an interest in working with people were considered for twenty-six weeks of training in the fundamentals of military psychiatric social work. Applicants were screened for personality strength and potential adjustments to the field.

Enlisted personnel with the minimum of a high school degree were offered a twenty-week course. The first twelve weeks were didactic and the final eight weeks were spent on the wards. These groups were taught by professional social workers, psychiatrists, and psychologists. This emphasis on training would have a lasting effect on the Army's social work program. In discussing the case aides Camp noted: "their valuable service on the assignment is sufficient evidence to the Army to establish the value of the training" (Camp, 1948, p. 877). During the postwar rebuilding period, a course for social work technicians was established at the Medical Field Service School (MFSS). Of the first five trained social workers to enter on active duty during this period, three were immediately assigned the tasks of establishing the program (Morgan, 1961, p. 209). These assignments were a clear indication of the importance placed on social work education.

While the early emphasis on training was due in part to the lack of skilled personnel and the urgent need to rebuild the program, the educational emphasis continued even after the case aide program was terminated. Enlisted personnel continued to be sent to MFSS for intensive training in social work techniques. The sixteen weeks of training required of enlisted personnel to become Army social work paraprofessionals has been described in detail elsewhere (Rooney, 1952). During the Vietnam era, the volume of soldiers going through social work technician training ranged from 300 to 800 solders annually, though a few representatives from other federal agencies (e.g., Indian Health) also attended (Garber and O'Brien, 1974).

Emphasis was also placed on the importance of in-service training. There seemed to be universal agreement that, although the sixteen weeks of training was intensive, the initial training had to be supplemented by continuous education at the soldier's duty station (Spellman, 1952).

Commissioned officers who were social workers also entered MFSS for the Basic Officer's Orientation Course. It was assumed that they were already prepared to assume their professional duties since they had obtained a master's in social work from an institution accredited by the Council on Social Work Education. But these new officers had to be oriented to the Army and the Commissioned Corps. They would be assigned to the Medical Service Corps and attend classes with officers of other disciplines. Within a few years those who chose and were accepted to remain beyond their initial obligation would return to MFSS to attend the Advanced Course.

Selected officers continued to be sent to civilian institutions to receive master's degrees and doctorates in social work. This program was instituted after the end of hostilities of World War II. Consultants continually impressed on the "powers that be" the importance of increasing the number of authorizations for long-term civilian training. In this program officers were selected for two to three years of training in a civilian university in a field deemed necessary to the Army. Tuition and fees were paid and the officer remained on active duty, although not expected to report for duty other than classes.

One of the most innovative and successful educational programs for social work officers has been the two-year Advanced Social Work Program in Family Studies, conducted at the Walter Reed Army Medical Center in Washington, DC. The objective of the program was to meet the recognized need in military communities for social work officers specially trained and highly skilled in techniques designed to promote stability in family life and provide early identification and treatment of military families experiencing stress in coping with emotional and/or situational crises (*Program Instruction,* 1975).

The program was initially agreed upon by the chief of social work service, Lieutenant Colonel Francis Ryan, and the chief of psychiatry and neurology on December 6, 1963. Training spaces for two social work officers each year was approved by the Walter Reed Army Hospital education committee on May 20, 1966.

The program was an immediate success. However, it was recognized that sixteen officers had completed the Advanced Social Work Program in Family Studies in "the last eight years" but received no tangible recognition for the two years of work and study involved.

Lieutenant Colonel Donald Bardill (former dean and currently professor at Florida State University) obtained approval from the medical department to affiliate with the Catholic School of Social Service, Catholic University (NCSSS). This new program would allow officers in the Advanced Social Work Program in Family Studies to pursue and obtain a doctor of social work degree (DSW). Unlike long-term civilian education, students performed service all of the time they were in the program.

Over time, social workers would attend the Army War College, Command and General Staff College, and Armed Forces Staff College. They would obtain faculty positions at West Point and the Uniformed Services School of Health Sciences.

CONCLUSION

This brief summary of Army social work history is only a sketch of an exciting past forged out of the flames of world conflict and nurtured by civilian counterparts. Similar to the rich heritage of the Army social worker of past years, today's social worker-soldier and the many civilian social workers who serve with them are cognizant of current trends in the society at large and its impact on the soldier and the soldier's family. The social worker who practices in the Army setting carries the same values as the social workers of a past generation. They are still dedicated to the mission of the Medical Department and the United States Army. There is a great awareness that the Army social worker still has a wartime mission. Although this chapter does not discuss the social worker in combat, they have served our nation well in past conflicts (see Chapter 9). The social worker and the social work technician have had a presence in most of the major conflicts and peace operations engaged in by the Army (Bourne, 1966; Maillet, 1970; Harris and Segal, 1985).

Sidney Hecter noted that the psychiatric social worker is not only a social worker practicing in a different setting but a soldier who needs to learn the "tricks of the trade" to protect his or her life. He goes on to give an analysis of the functions of the social worker in the division in a combat situation. The psychiatrist and social worker, from an administrative viewpoint, were left relatively free to develop their program and professional function within the limitations operating in any particular division. A team relationship was quickly recognized as the only method of professional operation. The relationship was influenced by factors not usually experienced in a clinical setting. The imminence of combat and the awareness of the dependence of the social worker and the psychiatrist upon one another when faced with the need to develop a new program made for a closeness of relationship that might be considered unnecessary in a civilian clinical setting. He noted that the presence of the clinical team in the division was a novel and unexpected occurrence. During these beginning stages, a significant percentage of time was devoted to administrative reorganization of the clinical setting as well as to problems of orienting key people in the division to the team's function (Hecter, 1951).

REFERENCES

Adams, H.J. (1966). History and development of military social work. *Proceedings of the Sixteenth Annual Military Social Work Conference.* Chicage, May, pp. 1-3.

American Psychiatric Association. (1944). *One hundred years of American psychiatry.* New York: Columbia University Press.

Anderson, J.P. (1944). *Letter to the Honorable Henry L. Stimson, Secretary of War.* Unpublished manuscript.

Army community service. (1966). In *OTSG Regulation 608-2.* Washington, DC: Office of the Surgeon General.

Army community service program. (1965). In *Army Regulation 608-1*. Washington, DC: Department of the Army.

Army medical department seeks psychiatric social workers. (1946). *Douglas County Legionnaire*. Omaha, NE, p. 24.

Blue, J.T. (1966). Social work in the Army general hospital—requirements, realities and appraisals. Proceedings of the Sixteenth Annual Military Social Work Conference, Chicago, May.

Bourne, P.G. (1966). Social science studies in Vietnam. Proceedings of the Sixteenth Annual Military Social Work Conference, Chicago, May.

Bushard, B.A. (1957). A technic for military delinquency management. *U.S. Armed Forces Medical Journal, 8* (November), 1619.

Caldwell, J.M. (1948). The problem soldier and the Army. *The American Journal of Psychiatry, 105*(1), 46-51.

Camp, E.W. (1948). The Army's psychiatric social work program. *The Social Work Journal,* April, 877.

Camp, E.W. (1951). Psychiatric social work in the Army today. In H.S. Maas (Ed.), *Adventures in mental health.* New York: Columbia University Press, pp. 201-212.

Cocoran, C.A. (1966). *Army community service program, CSM 66-479.* Unpublished manuscript.

D'Oronzio, P. (1966). Applications of social work in stockades. Proceedings of the Sixteenth Annual Military Social Work Conference, Chicago, May.

Freedman, H.L. (1944). First aid to mental casualties. *Mental Hygiene, 28*(April), 186-213.

Freedman, H.L. (1945). The mental hygiene unit approach to reconditioning neuropsychiatric casualties. *Mental Hygiene, 29*(2), 275.

Garber, D.H. and O'Brien, L.O. (1974, 26 March). Operationalization of theory in training of paraprofessionals. *Journal of Education for Social Work, 13*(1): 60-67.

Gibbs, J.J. (1961). Psychiatric screening in stockades, *Military Police*, 7(March).

Harris, J. and Segal, D. (1985). Observations from the Sinai: The boredom factor. *Armed Forces and Society, 11,* 235-248.

Hecter, S. (1951). Combat division. In H.S. Maas (Ed.), *Adventures in mental health.* New York: Columbia University Press, p. 44.

Kisel, J.C. (1963). The problem soldier, *Infantry*, March-April, 57-58.

Krise, E.C. (1966). The Army community service program. Proceedings of the Sixteenth Annual Military Social Work Conference, Chicago, May.

Maillet, E.L. (1970). A perspective from Vietnam. Paper presented at The Drug Race—The Counter Culture Conference, Denver, CO.

Medical service corps allied scientist procurement—graduate social work students program. (1949). In *Special Regulations Number 605-60-42.* Washington, DC: Department of the Army, 1-4.

Memorandum Number 41. (1943). Red Bank, NJ: Fort. Monmouth.

Menninger, W. (1945). Psychiatry and the military offender. *Federal Probation, 9*(April-June), 12.

Monahan, F.T. (1966). Annual report of the social service consultant. Proceedings of the Sixteenth Annual Military Social Work Conference, Chicago, May.

Morgan, R. (1961). Clinical social work in the United States Army 1947-1959. Unpublished doctoral dissertation. Washington, DC: Catholic University of America.

National Association of Social Workers (1965). *Mental health and psychiatric services.* New York: National Association of Social Workers.

Parrish, M.D. (1970). *The increasing psychiatric caseload vs. decreasing staff.* Unpublished manuscript.

Proceedings of the eighth annual Army social work conference. (1958). Chicago: Office of the Surgeon General.

Program instruction for advance social work program in family studies (1975). Washington, DC: Walter Reed Army Medical Center.

Ramer, B.S. (1965). The psychiatrist role in school consultation programs. *Medical Bulletin, 22*(November), 426-427.

Reeves, J. (1966). Application of social work in stockades—response. Proceedings of the Sixteenth Annual Military Social Work Conference, Chicago, May.

Rockmore, M.E. (1960). Community planning as a support to treatment. *The American Journal of Psychiatry, 116*(8), 723.

Rooney, W.S. (1952). The psychiatric social work technician, *Journal of Psychiatric Social Work,* June, 181-186.

Ross, E.H. (1943). 263 psychiatric social worker. In *Memorandum 1943.* Washington, DC: War Department, pp. 1-2.

Ross, E.H. (1951). Early efforts of the war service office. In H.S. Maas (Ed.), *Adventures in mental health.* New York: Columbia University Press, pp. 174-175.

Simon, R. (1965). The stockade revisited: Psychiatry in a screening program. *Military Medicine, 5*, 980.

Social work services. (1966). Washington, DC: Surgeon General's Office.

Spellman, S.W. (1952). The utilization and supervision of enlisted technicians in the mental hygiene consultation service. *Proceedings of the Symposium on Military Social Work*, p. 58.

War, D.L. (1943, October 18). Psychiatric social workers, SSN #263. In *War Department Letter, 1943.* Washington, DC: War Department, p. 9.

West, M. (1967). Community approach to the military offender. Paper presented at the Advanced Seminar on the American Family in the Army Community.

Willi, F.J. (1968). The psychiatrist as consultant to a medical service area. *Medical Bulletin, 25*(7), 260.

Chapter 2

History of Navy Social Work

United States Navy Medical Service Corps

Before 1980, a succession of relief and social service agencies, and a variety of medical and administrative personnel provided social work services in naval medical treatment facilities. Founded in 1881, the American Red Cross established its long tradition of providing social services to military families and personnel in medical treatment facilities. Before World War II, the American Red Cross provided a limited number of social workers to assist at naval medical facilities. Beginning in the 1920s, the Navy Relief Society provided a visiting nurse service to assist naval personnel and families with counseling and social service referral. At the end of World War II, the Navy Relief Society employed its first professional social worker to assist Navy members and families with psychosocial problems. However, most professional social work activities were confined to training volunteers to extend social services and assistance to Navy families. A noble effort, the Navy Relief Society's ability to provide services to hospitalized naval personnel and their families was always very limited.

World War II presented a need for social services of epic proportions. American Red Cross and Navy Relief Society volunteers and staff provided extensive social services, with a major assist from physicians, nurses, psychologists, and patient affairs officers.

The American Red Cross ceased their program of psychosocial services in the 1970s. As a consequence, provision of social services

---

This chapter was originally published as Medical Service Corps (1997). The clinicians. In *Many specialties, one corp: A pictorial history of the U.S. Navy, MSC* (pp. 151-153). Washington DC: Department of the Navy. Reproduced with permission of the United States Navy.

declined in naval medical treatment facilities. Other professionals—including physicians, nurses, psychologists, and patient affairs officers—had to share the burden of providing much-needed social work services. The value of professional social work in psychosocial assessment, counseling, discharge planning, social service referral, crisis intervention, and development of treatment modalities was not generally recognized by the naval medical profession. This haphazard approach to social services was only slightly relieved by recruitment of small numbers of civilian social workers under the aegis of psychiatry services.

Civilian psychiatric social workers in the 1950s and 1960s initiated the beginnings of clinical social services at naval hospitals. They provided initial individual psychosocial assessments for psychiatric inpatients, assisted psychiatrists with development of treatment plans, and facilitated group therapy sessions.

The emotional trauma of the Vietnam War further demonstrated the paucity of dedicated social services to render assistance to Navy personnel and their families. The issue was profoundly dramatized by the need to provide counseling and assistance to families of prisoners of war (POWs) and personnel listed as missing in action (MIA). The perceived indifference to families of the POWs/MIAs led to organization of the National League of Families of American Prisoners and Missing in Southeast Asia in 1968. Public awareness of the plight of POW/MIA military families quickened the realization that they had special needs.

A Center for Prisoner of War Studies was established at the Naval Health Research Center in San Diego in 1972. Research with POW families concluded that strong outreach services, collaboration with other agencies, and mental health consultation was necessary to assist returning POWs and their families. When POWs were repatriated in 1973, the Bureau of Medicine and Surgery directed that social workers be employed at hospitals in San Diego, Lemoore, California, Pensacola and Jacksonville, Florida, and Washington, DC, to facilitate a smooth transition for returning POWs and their families, and coordinate community-oriented services. Programs were developed that made family, child, and individual counseling, as well as a wide variety of social services, available. This development heightened the visibility and importance of professional social work in the Navy.

The movement to establish formal social work programs at naval medical treatment facilities, and to commission professional social workers in the Medical Service Corps, continued to gather steam in the 1970s. There was a greater awareness of the importance of healthy Navy families to a strong Navy. The debilitating effects of drug and alcohol abuse in the Navy, and spouse and child abuse among Navy families, were grabbing the attention of policymakers in the military and Congress. Establishment of naval drug rehabilitation centers beginning in 1971, development of family advocacy programs by 1976, and creation of the Navy family service center system in 1978 all generated a dire need for social service providers. Also, Joint Commission on the Accreditation of Hospitals standards on hospital social services revealed a poverty-stricken system barely in place in naval hospitals.

In 1979, only twenty-nine civilian social workers were employed in naval hospitals. The other military services had comparatively robust social work programs, with one military or civilian social worker to every fifteen physicians; the figure in the Navy was one civilian social worker to 170 physicians. Stretched to the limit, this small cadre of social workers was insufficient to satisfy the social service needs of rapidly expanding social service systems.

In the late 1970s, a series of Medical Department mental health conferences attended by physicians, psychologists, nurses, and social workers called for expanded social services in naval medical treatment facilities. A 1979 conference recommended the Bureau of Medicine and Surgery create social work departments staffed and organized consistent with Joint Commission on the Accreditation of Hospitals standards, a social work coordinator on the bureau level, and recruitment of uniformed social workers.

Approved by the Bureau of Medicine and Surgery, a request to recruit and commission thirteen social workers in the Medical Service Corps was submitted to the Chief of Naval Operations, who promptly authorized the bureau to proceed in July 1979. Captain Paul D. Nelson, Chief of the Medical Service Corps, announced plans to recruit accredited social workers. In January 1980, Lieutenant (junior grade) David Kennedy was commissioned as the Navy's first uniformed social worker, and was immediately assigned to Naval Regional Medical

Center, San Diego, to establish a department of social work. Eleven more social workers were on board before the end of the year.

Nineteen seventy-nine was a watershed year for military and civilian social workers in the Navy. The Navy Family Advocacy Program was formally launched, and the first of the Family Service Centers was established. The new, far-reaching family focus of these programs, as well as hospital accreditation standards, generated a critical need for a vitalized social work program in Navy medicine. The next five years witnessed a proliferation of social work services in naval medical treatment facilities, within area Family Advocacy Programs, drug and alcohol rehabilitation centers, and expanded clinical services, including individual, family, and group counseling, crisis intervention, assessment and treatment of family violence, abuse, and neglect, and discharge planning.

By the 1990s, there were approximately thirty social workers in the Medical Department, serving in a variety of roles: family advocacy, medical social work, discharge planning, mental health, crisis intervention, psychosocial assessments, and steering the Exceptional Family Member Program. In addition, social workers serve on Special Psychiatric Rapid Intervention Teams (SPRINT) at Naval Medical Centers in San Diego and Portsmouth, Virginia. During Operation Desert Shield/Storm, social workers were deployed for the first time to a combat zone on board the hospital ships *Comfort* and *Mercy*, and Fleet Hospital Five. They provided counseling and referral services, and mental health support.

Chapter 3

History of Air Force Social Work

James L. Jenkins

INTRODUCTION

When I was asked to author this chapter, my initial thinking was consistent with a traditional historical conceptual framework, a chronological presentation of relevant data such as organizational structure, personnel issues, and job functions. While such data are important to our history, and will be summarized herein, I have concluded that a historical documentation of social work in the Air Force should capture the human drama associated with the evolutionary milestones that shaped our practice. Learning about the personal, professional, organizational, and political events that charted the course of social work delivery in the Air Force should enlighten others who would struggle, as we have, to conceptualize, design, and develop innovative practice models to meet the changing needs of clients while responding to imposing forces within our society.

This historical presentation will focus on the process, rather than the outcome, of the evolution of social work practice in the Air Force. I write as the representative of all the social workers who have participated in our past and invite you to incorporate what you desire from our experience in developing strategies for the design and implementation of effective social work delivery systems.

ORGANIZATIONAL STRUCTURE

The United States Air Force was established as a separate military department in 1947. At that time, many of the organizational characteristics of the Army were carried over into the Air Force. Accordingly, social work was included as a specialization within the Air Force Medical Service and was located within the Medical Service Corps in the office of the psychiatric consultant. In 1965, a new corps was formed within the Medical Service and social work was transferred from the Medical Service Corps to the Biomedical Sciences Corps.

> This corps was composed of allied science disciplines such as social work, psychology, optometrist, laboratory officers, pharmacists and other medically related professions. An Associate Chief was appointed for each discipline. It is his duty to advise on policy formulation regarding members of his specialty and to make recommendations regarding assignments. This arrangement has afforded a more personalized approach to handle the needs and desires of professionals within each discipline. (Jenkins, 1974)

Colonel Jack Davis was designated as the first Associate Chief of the BSC for Social Work in 1967. Successors in order of appointment have been Colonel John McNeil, Colonel Hugh Ferrell, Colonel Stewart Myers, Lieutenant Colonel Louis Rosato, Colonel James Jenkins, Colonel Louis Rosato, Colonel Jack Butler, and Colonel Alice Tarpley.

Initially, social workers were assigned to larger medical facilities with the senior social worker being designated as the Chief of Social Work Service. However, by the early 1970s, it was common for a single social worker to be assigned to a small medical facility, sometimes as a member of a multidisciplinary mental health team or, on occasion, as the only mental health provider.

PERSONNEL

The following data summarizes personnel factors including our numbers, education, gender, race, rank and tenure, and assignment locations.

Number of Active Duty Social Workers

- 1947: unknown number, enlisted personnel supporting psychiatry
- 1952: 6 initial commissioned social work officers
- 1955: 20, response to psychiatric casualties during Korean conflict
- 1966: 42, gradual increase based on local initiatives
- 1973: 90, response to Vietnam war
- 1975: 120, requirements for substance abuse programs
- 1980: 173, requirements for child abuse programs
- 1984: 205, expanding roles
- 1988: 225, peak of expansion
- 2003: 180, projected drawdown

Number of Civilian Social Workers

- Mid-1950s: Few, supporting Family Services and special needs children
- Mid-1980s: 90, GS-11 temporary position for child abuse prevention
- Mid-1990s: Several hundred, contracted family advocacy services
- Future: Projected increase to support family programs

Educational Level

A master's in social work degree was the standard established for social work practice in the Air Force. A lack of quality control in the 1950s and 1960s resulted in some individuals with a master's degree in fields such as counseling occupying social work positions. However, by the early 1970s, all social workers had an MSW and many earned a PhD through Air Force Institute of Technology assignments to civilian graduate social work programs.

Gender

Historically, Air Force social work has been male dominated. The first female social worker was commissioned in the late 1960s, followed by a gradual increase in female social workers to 10 percent by 1979. Females currently compose 50 percent of social work officers and clearly dominate the ranks of civilian social workers.

Race

Air Force social work has been, and continues to be, racially imbalanced with an estimated 90 percent Caucasian presence. Black social workers have had ongoing representation in small numbers while there has been a limited representation from other races.

Rank and Tenure

In the 1950s and 1960s, the rank structure among social work officers was predominately company grade officers (lieutenants and captains). Prior to 1968, social workers were commissioned as second lieutenants and were promoted to first lieutenant with two years of service and then to captain with four years of service. In 1968, social work officers were given two years' constructive credit toward promotion for their graduate education and, thereafter, were commissioned in the grade of first lieutenant and promoted to captain after three years in grade. In the 1950s and 1960s, less than 10 percent of social work officers achieved the rank of field grade officer (major, lieutenant colonel, or colonel). It was uncommon to have more than one social work officer in the grade of colonel within the whole Air Force prior to the 1980s.

By the 1980s, most social work officers had remained on active duty long enough to be eligible for promotion to higher ranks. By the mid-1980s, over 40 percent of active duty social workers were field grade officers and seven were promoted to the rank of colonel in the late 1980s. Since 1994, a majority of the field grade social work officers have retired. Consequently, the rank structure has shifted back to a composition of predominantly company grade officers.

Assignment Location

In the 1950s and 1960s, social work officers were assigned almost exclusively to large medical centers with a staff of two or more social workers. In the 1970s and 1980s, as social work assumed positions that were required at every Air Force installation, they were then assigned to almost every medical treatment facility. Most of the small medical clinics had only one social worker assigned. These assignments were dubbed "Lone Ranger slots" and were often filled by less experienced officers because they had a company grade rank designation. These assignment factors were important determinants for practice and have significant implication for later discussions about determinants for practice.

EVOLUTION OF PRACTICE

The increasing number of social workers in the Air Force, as well as the expanding assignment locations, were a result of practice requirements levied on social workers. As the Air Force responded to requirements to establish new services, social work was identified as the specialty to assume primary responsibility for many programs. The expanding practice functions of social work in the Air Force will be presented next. The events serving as catalysts for new practice requirements will be discussed in the final section of this chapter.

Mental Health Services

During the first twenty years of the program, Air Force social work remained predominantly psychiatric in nature. Between 1947 and 1952, enlisted social work technicians may have provided paraprofessional support to neuropsychiatric services. When social work officers were commissioned in 1952, they began the task of establishing a professional social work practice role. Often, they were restricted to a variety of administrative tasks in support of psychiatry and the medical service. The number of psychiatric casualties during the Korean War solidified this practice role and increased requirements. Over time, social workers became contributing members of multidisciplinary mental health teams composed of psychiatrists, psychologists, social workers, psychiatric nurses, and enlisted mental health technicians. Social workers assumed assessment and treatment functions in both inpatient and outpatient mental health units. The mental health function has remained a primary practice function for clinical social workers in the Air Force to the present time.

Provider-Specific Programs and Services

During the 1950s and 1960s, psychiatric social work practice was influenced by a number of social workers who developed expertise in practice areas outside of traditional assessment and treatment functions. Davis (1973) described that many military social workers created programs that, originally, were temporary and at a specific base. These programs focused on issues such as mental hygiene, alcohol abuse, prisoner rehabilitation, child guidance, or patient education. Ironically, many superb programs perished when the creator or advocate transferred to his or her next assignment. By the late 1960s and early 1970s, most programs of this nature had been established as social work practice requirements throughout the Air Force Medical Service.

Social Welfare Services

During the 1950s, the Air Force developed programs to provide social welfare services for its members and their families. However, it failed to utilize its professional social work officers in these programs. An example of this is the Family Services Program:

> The Family Services Program is a welfare function that provides a wide range of services extending from welcoming new arrivals at an Air Force base to "counseling." . . . This program is a social welfare project that was conceived and developed by interested laymen, is administered by non-professional social workers, and is implemented primarily by volunteers. (McNeil, 1966)

Programs Addressing the Special Medical and Educational Requirements of Family Members

In the mid-1960s the Air Force Personnel Office established an assignment assistance program known as Project Children Have a Potential (CHAP) to assure that active duty personnel with family members having special medical or educational needs were assigned to installations where the required services were available. Initially, the CHAP Program provided an administrative response to the special needs of family members. This approach by the military was characterized as ". . . a self-contained social institution, realizing its needs, trying to solve its problems within itself" (Jenkins, 1974). However, after approximately five years under this arrangement, the need for professional intervention was recognized and the CHAP Program was transferred from the Personnel Office to the Office of the Surgeon General. Since that time, professional social workers have been designated as CHAP Officers. The CHAP Program was expanded to include assistance with securing required services and support services.

In the mid-1980s, the CHAP Program was redesignated as the Exceptional Family Member Program (EFMP) when the Department of Defense, Office of Health Affairs, assumed a more active role in standardizing these services among all military departments and increased quality control to ensure compliance with federal legislation.

Substance Abuse Programs

In the early 1970s, a major expansion of the practice role of social work outside of mental health followed a recognition of a significant substance abuse problem among Vietnam veterans. Social workers made a significant contribution to the development and implementation of treatment services. A Special Treatment Center was established at Lowry Air Force Base in Colorado and social work was included as part of the treatment team. The first Air Force inpatient alcohol treatment center opened at USAF Medical Center Wright-Patterson (Dayton, Ohio) in 1966, with nine more inpatient programs established between 1971 and 1976. These programs have been directed almost exclusively by social workers from their inception to the present.

In the early 1970s, the Air Force established a substance abuse awareness program to combat substance abuse in the military utilizing nonmedical military personnel who were provided special training. This program was an element of the Social Actions Program operated by the Personnel Office. Social workers provided consultation and coordinated the medical component of this program. In the mid-1990s, responsibility for all chemical dependency programs was transferred to the medical service and social workers were again called upon to utilize their practice skills to manage the new Drug Demand Reduction Program.

Family Maltreatment Programs

In 1975, the Air Force Child Advocacy Program was established in response to a growing national awareness of child abuse coupled with congressional pressure for the military to address child abuse issues within its ranks. Social workers were assigned primary responsibility for developing and implementing this program. A comprehensive multidisciplinary/interagency program was established to address the legal, medical, and social dimensions of child abuse. In 1980, the Child Advocacy Program was expanded to address spouse abuse and was redesignated as the Family Advocacy Program.

Family maltreatment intervention programs have had the single greatest impact on the expansion of social work practice in the Air Force. The scope and magnitude of the program requirements resulted in large numbers of social workers being assigned to the Family Advocacy Program as a full-time primary duty at almost every Air Force installation. Since psychiatry had been limited to specifically designated medical facilities, social workers were now organizationally located outside of psychiatry. In addition, specific funds appropriated by Congress assured the development and expansion of the Family Advocacy Program. Limited authorizations for uniformed officers resulted in a significant expansion of civilian social workers to support the program.

Occupational Social Work

By its very nature as an organizationally based practice, military social work has had an occupational focus. Employees manifesting maladaptive behavior have been evaluated for their fitness for duty by social workers. During the mid-1980s, social workers assumed leadership in designing and implementing outreach and early intervention services at technical training centers. The Human Development Program was designed to meet the psychosocial needs of young airmen during their technical training assignment. A practice objective was the reduction of attrition from technical training through prevention and the early intervention in crisis situations among trainees. A community outreach and consultation model provided visibility and rapid access to services for trainees as well as problem management strategies through consultation to instructors and supervisors and policy impact awareness for managers.

Hospital Social Work

Although social workers were assigned to major medical centers from the outset, establishing a practice role in the provision of hospital social work services was a long and difficult achievement. Initially, social work practice was established in support of mental health services. There was considerable resistance on the part of psychiatry for a social work practice role outside of mental health. Also, psychiatric social workers often lacked training or motivation to explore hospital social work as a practice opportunity. The first initiative to establish a Department of Social Work occurred at Wilford Hall USAF Medical Center in the early 1970s:

> It is recognized that the Air Force remains one of the few medical care systems without established and operating Departments of Social Work providing social services to patients accepted for care, as well as to their families. (Jenkins, 1974)

During the 1970s, social workers became increasingly involved in providing hospital social work services, which resulted in full-time hospital social work positions being established at a number of Air Force medical centers in the 1980s.

Corrections

During the 1960s, social work positions were established in military corrections programs at Fort Leavenworth, Kansas, and Lowry Air Force Base, Colorado. Social workers assumed primary responsibility for prisoner treatment and rehabilitation programs as well as family liaison and aftercare arrangements.

Family Support Centers

The historical roots of social work practice are founded in the neighborhood house concept of providing services in the environment of the client. The Family Service program, established as a grassroots attempt to provide services to Air Force families in the 1950s, was expanded in the 1970s with Family Support Centers, a neighborhood house approach to practice. An increasing appreciation of the value of supporting the family as a condition for achieving the organizational mission of operational readiness resulted in a visible effort on the part of Air Force leaders to provide a variety of social services. The Family Support Center is a base agency developed outside of Air Force social work channels designed to provide traditional social work services.

Psychological Operations

A limited number of social work officers were recruited from the medical service into the arena of psychological operations because of their effectiveness in bringing social work practice to highly specialized military operations. Their understanding of human responses in the unique environment of combat operations provided a major contribution to planning and executing a wide range of military operations.

Critical Incidence Response

Air Force social workers have provide valuable practice functions as practitioners and consultants in political and humanitarian incidents in Cuba, Africa, Bosnia, Southwest Asia, and Guam as well as in response to disasters such as Hurricane Andrew, the 1993 Midwest flooding, and the Oklahoma City federal building bombing.

Policy and Research

Air Force social workers have increasingly demonstrated their practice power in the areas of policy and research. The first significant opportunity for social work to have representation in the highest policymaking levels came in the 1970s when a social work officer was assigned to the staff of the Air Force Surgeon General to manage family violence and substance abuse programs. Social workers became program managers and consultants in mental health, family support, substance abuse, family maltreatment, and special medical and education needs programs addressing psychosocial issues within the military community. In the 1990s, social work officers were appointed to command positions where they demonstrated their practice skills in managing people and administering programs. Some social workers surfaced as extremely competent researchers and made valuable contributions to the development of social work programs during the 1980s and 1990s.

Overview

In a recent presentation at the October 1997 Uniformed Services Social Work Conference, Colonel Alice Tarpley, the current Associate Chief for Social Work, highlighted the evolution of Air Force social work. She described the corps of Air Force social workers as transcending the view by some as "baby" psychiatrists to become a profession respected in its own right. From a relatively inexperienced small group of professionals peering into the unknown of military social work, Air Force social workers have emerged with a wide range of expertise including PhD training (fourteen in 1997) and a myriad of specialized expertise. They have excelled in mental health and family advocacy clinics, Air Force and Major Command-level staff jobs, research positions, faculty positions at the Air Force Academy and numerous Family Practice Residencies, directorship of substance abuse programs, directorships of Family Support Centers, and leader positions on disaster preparedness teams. Further, they have been on the Inspector General's team, have been senior BSC advisors at bases, clinical experts in corrections facilities, and served quite well when deployed during Operation Desert Shield/Storm and humanitarian missions. In sum, she emphasized that Air Force social work has a rich heritage of functioning quite well in the military environment and making significant contributions to the betterment of military service members and their families. She encouraged continued vigilance about our gains and determination to pave new ground for social work contributions to the Air Force.

CATALYSTS FOR PRACTICE

The preceding discussion describes the composition and practice functions of the Air Force social work corps. This concluding section will present a series of vignettes intended to illustrate situations and events that served as catalysts for the determination of our practice functions as they have expanded over the course of our history.

"I'm a Psychiatric Social Worker"

During the early years of Air Force social work, it was prestigious among social workers nationally to achieve a job classification as a psychiatric social worker. Accordingly, two primary factors operating simultaneously served as catalysts for a strong foundation in mental health practice for Air Force social work. The predominant factor was the placement of social work organizationally within the office of the psychiatric consultant to the Air Force Surgeon General. Social workers were, in fact, hired to provide psychiatric social work services. Secondary to structure, there was a functional issue: the national trend in the profession to assign status to those providing psychiatric social work services. Consequently, not only did psychiatry achieve a sense of ownership for Air Force social workers, social workers themselves desired employment in the mental health arena.

"Patients Sleep Better with Dr. Deutch"

The expansion of social work practice beyond traditional assessment and treatment roles was accomplished by individual social workers based on their own specialized training and initiative. Services incorporated into social work practice through individual initiative included group therapy, stress and pain management, weight reduction, substance abuse intervention, medical social work, and family therapy. An example of such initiative is illustrated by a needlepoint completed by a client, which hung in the biofeedback/hypnosis lab where a PhD social worker conducted his specialized services. The artwork read "Patients sleep better with Dr. Deutch." Biofeedback, hypnosis, relaxation therapy, and stress management were the hallmark of Dr. James Deutch. Over time, many of these functions became formalized as practice responsibilities of social work.

"Only Physicians Can Use the Word Prognosis"

This vignette illustrates numerous incidents that occurred in the life of Air Force social workers which served to motivate them to expand their scope of practice. In 1968, I had conducted a fitness for duty evaluation and written a letter to the commander who had referred the client, reporting the evaluation findings and my recommendations. It was administrative policy that correspondence required review and approval by the Chief of Hospital Services prior to distribution. Upon reviewing the letter I had written, the Chief of Hospital Services took exception to my use of the word "prognosis" and returned the letter to me with "Only physicians can use the word prognosis" written in bold red ink across the letter. This incident had a profound impact on me, contributing to my becoming obsessed with a gaining increased decisional participation in the determination of social work practice in the Air Force.

Advanced Education and Training

The Air Force has maintained a very aggressive education and training program that provided opportunities for social work officers to earn doctoral degrees and specialized training. Many social workers were selected for training programs at civilian institutions where they engaged in studies and conducted research in a variety of practice areas. Upon their return to clinical practice in the Air Force, their specialized knowledge served as an important catalyst for the development of social work practice in the Air Force.

I was fortunate enough to return to graduate school, where I conducted research on the concept of organizational professionalism, "the utilization of professional manpower in bureaucratic organizations and the impact of the organization upon the professional employee" (Jenkins, 1974). My research findings revealed that a participatory organizational climate in which individuals are provided an opportunity to achieve their desired level of participation in decision making about their practice functions resulted in higher levels of job satisfaction and more productive work centers. The conceptual framework associated with this study would be operationalized ten years later when I would spearhead the first long-range planning initiative to determine the future of social work practice in the Air Force.

National Events

The social unrest of the late 1960s and the 1970s shifted the focus of social work away from psychiatric social work toward issues of diversity and equality. Racial tensions, the Vietnam War, and drug abuse all influenced the future of social work practice in our nation. Increased public awareness and concern about chemical dependency and child abuse served as significant catalysts for social work practice in the Air Force as large numbers of social workers were recruited to develop and implement substance abuse and family maltreatment programs.

"Do Your Social Work After Your Mental Health Responsibilities"

The transition from mental health clinician to other practice functions was not smooth. Social workers with mental health experience were suddenly required to develop and administer new programs. While they were struggling to incorporate new roles into their scope of practice, their supervisors were often less than supportive in providing time and resources. Psychiatry viewed this role expansion as inappropriate and a threat to mental health resources. It was not uncommon for social workers assigned to child advocacy duties to be told to take care of their social work after their mental health responsibilities were accomplished.

In Turn

Learning how to hurdle supervisors who blocked practice development was a milestone in the evolution of social work practice. In the military, as in most bureaucracies, loyalty to your supervisor and utilization of the chain of command are fundamental principles. Becoming armed with an administrative tool for going through blockading supervisors served social workers well when submitting practice proposals. By addressing the proposal "in turn" to each desired level up the chain of command, each person addressed was obliged to review the proposal, comment if they desired, and forward it, in turn, to the next level. Thus, while a supervisor could recommend disapproval, the option to kill the proposal at his or her level was eliminated and the originator could gain access to higher levels. This strategy was utilized effectively by many social workers to gain access to and support from decision makers on their installations.

Empowerment Through Collective Action

A basic social work principle, generally associated with community organization, addresses the power of collective action. The Child Advocacy Program required the development of a multidisciplinary Medical Child Protection Team and a base-level interagency Child Advocacy Committee. Social workers who had previously functioned as mental health clinicians suddenly had a team of very influential people supporting them. The collective utilization of these people was a source of empowerment for social workers assigned as Child Advocacy Officers.

When I was designated as the first Child Advocacy Officer at an Air Force Medical Center, I was initially unsuccessful in having my mental health responsibilities reduced so I could have time to develop child abuse services. I solicited the collective support of the Medical Child Protection Team and a document emphasizing the critical nature of my new practice role was drafted, signed by all members of the team, and sent in turn through the Chairman of the Department of Psychiatry to the medical center commander. The outcome of that collective action was that I was reassigned by the medical center commander from the mental health service to work for the Chief of Hospital Services as a full-time Child Advocacy Officer.

"Partners for Practice"

The probability that you will win a dance contest is determined not only by your skill, but also by the skill of your partner and how well you can execute your routine together. Air Force social workers have learned the power of effective partnerships in their pursuit of practice opportunities. When I was assigned to work with the Chief of Hospital Services, I joined a partnership that would influence the development of social work practice for years. My new boss, Colonel Sloan, had a vested interest in bed utilization throughout the medical center and was very supportive of introducing hospital work services. Colonel Sloan's career path led to positions as a Medical Center Commander, the Deputy Surgeon General, and eventually, the Surgeon General of the Air Force. He was a great partner who understood the value of social work practice. As social workers demonstrated the value of practice functions such as hospital social work at individual medical facilities, they laid the groundwork for the formal establishment of these functions in the future. Many Air Force social workers engaged in partnerships that paid solid dividends for social work practice in the future.

Restrictive Policies

In the early 1980s, the Director of Health Affairs in the Department of Defense established a policy that excluded social workers from participating in occupational practice where recommendations were made concerning fitness for duty based on personality disorders. Only psychiatrists and psychologists were authorized to render professional opinions, which were based on the very essence of social work practice, an understanding of the capacity of an individual to function in his or her environment.

In response to this policy, many psychiatrists recommended that social workers continue conducting these evaluations, which would then be countersigned by a psychiatrist or psychologist. Social workers responded to this restrictive policy, and to the suggestion of countersignatures, with a position of, "If I can't sign it, I'm not doing it." When organizations impose restrictive policies, the consequence of a strict compliance with the policy may be just what is required to cause the organization to reverse the policy.

Fenced Funding

A fundamental principle of social work that was played out in the evolution of practice in the Air Force involves both the access to and the opportunity for resource utilization. Access to financial resources for social work practice was made possible through the appropriation of "fenced funding" for military family advocacy programs by the U.S. Congress. Funds appropriated for military child abuse programs could only be used for that purpose. Since a senior social work officer was assigned as the Family Advocacy Program Manager in the Office of the Air Force Surgeon General, the incumbent was responsible for managing a substantial budget that could not be diverted for other expenditures. This provided access to financial resources for implementing practice initiatives.

"You Have a Job to Do—Go Do It"

As the professionalism of social work gained acceptance, policymakers became eager to utilize social work as social issues overwhelmed them and they needed to find solutions. Further, as social workers demonstrated their ability to address these issues, their practice roles were expanded. When I reported for my initial assignment to the Office of the Air Force Surgeon General as the consultant for Health Promotion, my new boss said, "You have a job to do—go do it."

Participative Management Within an Autocratic Organization

In 1985, I was selected for assignment to the Office of the Surgeon General as the Consultant for Social Work. This assignment included the responsibility for managing the Air Force Family Advocacy Program. Thus, as the designated leader for Air Force social work, I was armed with the authority and the financial resources to implement the concept of decisional participation I had researched during my doctoral studies.

An advisory group composed of the senior social work officers was formed to identify and prioritize critical issues that would influence the future of social work practice in the Air Force. A broad range of practice issues were identified and a member of the advisory group was designated as the action officer to be responsible for each critical issue.

An invitation was extended to every Air Force social worker to participate in an initiative to design the future of social work practice in the Air Force. Social workers were asked to complete a survey in which they prioritized the top three critical issues with which they desired to be involved. Fifty percent of the 220 social workers in the Air Force responded to this invitation to have decisional participation in determining the future of social work practice. A working group, led by the designated action officer, was established for each of the critical issues based on the preferences of each participant. This initiative was launched at Little Rock, Arkansas on March 3, 1986, with a working group conference. Over a period of several months, each of the working groups developed and submitted a proposal for the design of future social work practice in response to their designated critical issue. A list of the critical issues and the working group members are provided in an addendum. These social workers are the heroes of their time in that they chose to participate and gained recognition for their level of competence and expertise in determining their own practice functions.

Prevention: A Practice Dilemma

In the mid-1980s, limitations on the number of officers on active duty placed restrictions on the expansion of social work practice. In response, a decision was made to utilize the fenced funds for child abuse programs to hire civilian social workers as "outreach workers" to establish child abuse prevention programs. Approximately 100 outreach workers were hired to provide prevention services at most Air Force installations. The educational activities of the outreach workers increased public awareness and reporting, which overwhelmed the already overextended Family Advocacy Officer.

An important lesson learned from this initiative was that resource requirements must be anticipated and provided as practice functions are expanded. Subsequently, civilian social workers and support staff were hired and a Family Advocacy Team composed of prevention, treatment, research, and administrative specialists was added to the Family Advocacy Program at most installations.

Standards of Practice

A milestone in the evolution of social work practice in the Air Force was the development of standards of practice for family maltreatment intervention. A Family Advocacy Task Force, utilizing a series of working groups, designed and published a manual providing Family Advocacy Officers throughout the Air Force with clear standards of practice and supplemental guidance for a unified approach to family maltreatment. Practice requirements were specified and procedures for implementing them were established. All required documents were developed and provided on computer disks, along with the computers and funding for a position to accomplish the administrative functions. Considerable praise was given to Air Force social workers by managers at all levels of the organization for this systematic approach for assuring a uniform standard for quality practice.

SUMMARY

This chapter has presented an overview of the historical evolution of social work practice in the United States Air Force, beginning with an exclusive mental health function and expanding over a period of fifty years to include a broad range of programs and services. During the past twenty years, the social workers employed within the Air Force have been a major force in shaping their own practice. A series of vignettes highlighted the process of designing and implementing social work practice in the Air Force.

ADDENDUM—SOCIAL WORK TASK FORCE INITIATIVE TO ADDRESS CRITICAL ISSUES FOR SOCIAL WORK PRACTICE

Consultant for Social Work

Lieutenant Colonel James L. Jenkins

Policy

*Colonel Eugene Pletcher
Major Mark Juhas
Major Bill York
Captain Debra Morrison-Orton
Captain Virginia McKinley

Wartime Mission

*Lieutenant Colonel Frank Goldstein
Major Royetta Marconi-Dooley
Major Tony Anthony
Captain John Civitello
Captain Linda Jenkins
Captain Jim Retzlaff
Captain Jack Smith

Quality Assurance

*Lieutenant Colonel Jerry Tuttle
Major Claudette Bohanon
Major Bob Ferguson
Major Jim Parker
Captain Mike Haynes
Captain Carla Monroe-Posey

Organizational Structure

*Lieutenant Colonel John Steele
Major Melinda Mitchell
Lieutenant Ciro Olivares

Role Function

*Lieutenant Colonel Louis Rosato
Lieutenant Colonel Doreen Hall
Captain Leo Ward
Captain Dave Wolpert

Education and Training

*Lieutenant Colonel Tom Cleary
Captain John Adkins
Captain Roy Franklin
Captain Mel Meldrim
Captain Ren Perillo
Captain Margaret Ronan

Family Support Center/Family Advocacy Interface

*Lieutenant Colonel John Cox
Major Jerry Murray
Captain Bill Ashley
Captain Jan Gilliard
Captain Carl Rohbock
Captain Alan Snyder

Hospital Social Work

*Lieutenant Colonel Ron Tenaglia
Major Lynnette Jung
Major Don Tartasky
Major Jim Rosenfield
Major Nelson Smith
Captain Rose Mary Hendler
Lieutenant Alan Brankline

Family Practice Residency

*Lieutenant Colonel John Stokes
Major Jack Butler
Major Jim Cheatham
Major Gary Larson
Major John Nelson
Major Doug Posey

Interagency/Interservice Networking

*Lieutenant Colonel Lou Pagliuca
Captain Marsha Headstream
Captain Marlina Hidalgo
Captain Lynn Lowry

Family Advocacy Program

*Lieutenant Colonel Jim Larison
Major Hank Vader

Child Abuse Committee

*Major John Dehler
Major Terry Sybrant
Major Raleigh Riggs
Lieutenant Yvonne Jones

Spouse Abuse Committee

*Captain Neil Brennecke
Captain John Dillon
Captain Bob Winchell
Captain Gail Wiggins

Sex Abuse Committee

*Major Rose Mary Conde
Major Richard Pugh
Major Larry Warren
Captain Alice Tarpley
Captain Tom Ziemann

Family Outreach Committee

*Lieutenant Dari Tritt
Major John Charles
Major Charles Daud-Weiss
Major Bernie Duncan
Major Dave Moyer

Communication/Information

*Major Bob Anderson
Major John Cassidy
Major Rob Hight
Captain Jim Daley
Captain Dave Schwalson
Captain Julia Clancy-Stokes

Clinical Mental Health

*Major Bob Kreager
Major Dale Whitney
Captain Deborah Garrett
Captain Joe Maiden
Captain Leonard Penkowski
Captain Beth Thompson
Lieutenant Brian Squires

Corrections

*Major Bill Black
Major Randall Peacock
Captain Martha Davis
Captain Cynthia Steffey
Captain Robert Zazula

Drug and Alcohol Rehabilitation

*Major Phil Moser
Major Chris Brown
Major Rick Siefke
Major Bill Zahler
Captain Al Brewster
Captain Rich Greenlee
Captain Richard Newsome

Research

*Major Suzanne Awalt
Captain John Long
Captain Steve Tallant
Captain Bill Keiffer

AIDS, Psychosocial Factors

*Major Terry Cowles
Major Harry Harshbarger
Lieutenant Jim Coffidis
Lieutenant Develin Jones
Lieutenant Roger Sullivan

CHAP Program and Medically Related Services for Handicapped DODDS Students

*GS-12 Al McClure	Captain John Acker
GS-12 Adorine Maloy Holloman	Captain Mike Clawson

Nonuniformed Social Workers

*GS-12 John Waltz	GS-11 Jimmie Womack
GS-12 Deborah Bell	Captain Mark Johnson
GS-12 Norma Harrera	Captain Bill Martin

*Task Force Action Officer(s)

REFERENCES

Davis, J. A. (1973). Personal letter written to the author. San Antonio, TX.

Jenkins, J. L. (1974). *The effects of decisional participation upon organizational effectiveness: A study of social work officers in the United States Air Force.* Unpublished doctoral dissertation, University of Denver, Denver.

McNeil, J. S. (1966). *The United States Air Force Family Services Program.* Unpublished paper presented at the Military Social Work Program held in conjunction with the National Conference on Social Welfare, Chicago, IL.

Tarpley, A. C. (1997). *History of Air Force social work.* Unpublished paper presented at the Uniformed Services Social Work Conference, Baltimore, MD.

PART II: PRACTICE ARENAS

Chapter 4

Development and Evolution of the Family Advocacy Program in the Department of Defense

John P. Nelson

INTRODUCTION

The mission of the Family Advocacy Program (FAP) in the Department of Defense (DoD) is to prevent, identify, intervene, and treat all aspects of child abuse and neglect and spouse abuse. Also, FAPs are designed to support family preservation without compromising the health, welfare, and safety of the victim; strengthen family functioning in a manner that increases the competency and self-sufficiency of military members; and collaborate with state and local civilian child protective services. To achieve these ends the Service FAPs provide a comprehensive range of programs and services in addition to intervention and treatment. These activities include training and education, primary and secondary prevention programs ranging from advocacy for nonviolent communities to programs targeted to at-risk populations, program evaluation to measure trends and outcomes of prevention and treatment, and, a central registry of all maltreatment reports. The Department of Defense, through the Office of Family Policy, in conjunction with headquarters-level organizations at each Service, funds, develops, and implements policy, manages, and evaluates child and spouse abuse prevention and intervention programs.

The issues and problems associated with family violence are a concern of the Department of Defense just as they are a societal

The opinions expressed in this chapter are the author's and should not be interpreted as the policy or opinions of the United States Air Force.

concern. As with other military family support programs, an additional rationale for military-sponsored family advocacy programs is the recognition that military members and their families face a number of unique demands and risks. These include separation from natural support networks; frequent separation due to temporary duty and deployments; increased stress due to drawdowns, funding reductions, and mission change; intensified operations tempo; and a high number of young families with young children. Paired with these factors is the recognition that a service member's family life can have a direct impact on performance, retention, and readiness. It is clear that family maltreatment among service members is incompatible with military service. Therefore, attending to the health, safety, and social development of military family members is a concern to commanders at all levels.

By 1998 the Department of Defense (DoD) Family Advocacy Programs were large, comprehensive, multidisciplinary operations funded at over $100 million per year and employing over 2,000 staff providing a wide range of intervention and prevention services. These programs had achieved demonstrated successes including: providing for safety of victims by reducing the DoD's rate of family violence and severity of reported cases; providing cost-effective services and significant savings to the DoD; developing a template for comprehensive community-based prevention services; improving morale and productivity; and having a positive impact on readiness. However, these programs were not always so robust. The first DoD Directive on Family Advocacy was not published until 1981. The foundation of the current program was formed at least a decade earlier in the grassroots efforts of individuals.

BACKGROUND AND HISTORY

A powerful convergence of events inside and outside the Department of Defense in the early 1970s focused attention and led to the development of early family violence prevention programs—with an initial focus exclusively on child abuse. Child advocacy programs began appearing at military treatment facilities (MTFs) all across the military in the late 1960s and early 1970s. As awareness of child maltreatment increased, individual clinicians, primarily social workers in the Army and Air Force, and pediatricians in the Navy, became involved in developing local, grassroots initiatives to identify and treat victims. Many programs initially focused on the medical aspects of child maltreatment. As these local programs developed, so did a recognition of the importance of prevention and education services and the acknowledgment that line support was required for such programs.

Events of the 1960s, such as rising national consciousness and heightened awareness of the impact of child abuse, began to affect the military more formally in the early 1970s. On the national scene there was lack of agreement about the extent of child maltreatment. However, speculation regarding the military services during the period suggested that child maltreatment was endemic, exceeding the incidence in the civilian world. It was argued that individuals within an organization such as the military would manifest greater degrees of family violence due to their training for "violent" missions. Although recently compiled statistics suggest that the DoD incidence of child abuse is approximately half of the U.S. estimate prepared by the National Center on Child Abuse and Neglect (NCCAN), no centralized data reporting mechanism was in place in the Services (Figure 4.1 indicates the DoD Family Advocacy Substantiated Maltreatment Fiscal Year [FY] 88-96; the FY96 incidence of child maltreatment in DoD was 6.2 per 1,000—less than half the national incidence reported by NCCAN). The DoD could not adequately address these concerns.

Dr. C. Henry Kempe addressed a meeting of the American Academy of Pediatrics (AAP) on "The Problems of Managing Child Abuse in the Armed Services" in March 1973. Subsequently, the AAP proposed recommendations to the Assistant Secretary of Defense for Health and Environment—ASD(H&E)—for the development of specific child abuse policies and programs as well as ongoing education for medical and ancillary personnel dealing with family violence problems.

In June 1974, an American Medical Association conference on child maltreatment in the military recommended that DoD develop specific guidelines for the management of child abuse. The ASD (H&E) responded to these recommendations by initiating planning for a Tri-Service Child Advocacy Working Group, representing command and medical proponents charged with monitoring existing Service child abuse programs.

FIGURE 4.1. DoD Family Advocacy Substantiated Maltreatment—FY88-96

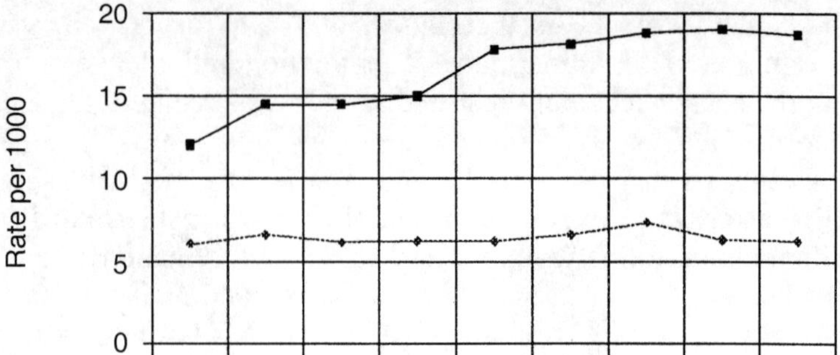

	FY88	FY89	FY90	FY91	FY92	FY93	FY94	FY95	FY96
Child Abuse	6	6.6	6.1	6.2	6.2	6.6	7.3	6.3	6.2
Spouse Abuse	12	14.5	14.5	15	17.8	18.1	18.8	19	18.7

PL 93-247

The passage of Public Law 93-247, "Child Abuse Prevention Treatment Act," in July 1974 provided additional focus and push for the development of military child abuse programs. This legislation authorized federal grants to states to develop and strengthen child abuse prevention and treatment programs, exclusively to states with an established system for reporting and investigation of incidents of suspected child abuse. The act also established the National Center on Child Abuse and Neglect (NCCAN), which was to become a strong advocate for programs in the DoD.

Following PL 93-247, pressure increased on the DoD to formalize programs directed at the identification and treatment of child abuse. DoD, however, was reluctant to take a direct management role. Rather, it defined its role as monitoring and encouraged the Services, through the Tri-Service Working Group established in January 1975, to continue work on developing Service child abuse programs and regulations.

The reluctance at the DoD level regarding how to manage the child abuse issue was reflected in each of the Services. In the Army, Navy, and Air Force extensive dialogue took place regarding where to place the program. Social workers carrying out child advocacy duties urged placement within the Surgeons General Staff while more senior medical officials saw the program as a broader social problem belonging to the line.

In 1975, the Air Force, with the publication of AFR 168-38, became the first service to establish a Child Advocacy Program. The Air Force program was managed in the Office of the Surgeon General. By 1976 each of the Services had adopted Child Advocacy Program regulations. The Navy had the early foresight to include spouse abuse in its program. Initially, the Navy program was established in the Bureau of Medicine and Surgery (BUMED). In the Army the debate swung the other way. Overall management of the Army program was given to the Deputy Chief of Staff for Personnel with the publication of Army Regulation 600-48.

During this period the Tri-Service working group served as the primary vehicle for interservice communication regarding child advocacy programs in the DoD (Myers, 1977). The General Accounting Office (GAO) (1979) reported that a good indicator of the low priority given to these programs was the fact that none were directly funded and all operated with staff assigned as additional or collateral duties. As such, the programs were little more than administrative mechanisms to formalize the existing structure. Additional resources to attack the problem and develop prevention programs were not available.

GAO Report

It was external impetus in the form of a 1979 GAO report, "Military Child Advocacy Programs: Victims of Neglect" that documented the need for overall DoD guidance in implementing military family violence programs. This report characterized Service programs as inconsistent and understaffed and labeled the DoD role as "limited." It identified the need for unified and consistent DoD policies, greater resource allocation, expanded education and training, and the creation of a small centralized group to serve as the focal point for all DoD child abuse programs. In response to the GAO report, a number of significant events were set into motion. Three key outcomes that emerged were the establishment of the Military Family Resource Center, the publication of the first DoD directive on family violence, and appropriated funding for the military family advocacy programs.

Military Family Resource Center

The first direct result of the GAO report, the Military Family Resource Center (MFRC), was established in October 1980 as a Health and Human Services-sponsored, three-year demonstration project. The grant called for gradual transfer of funding from DHHS to DoD. By FY83 DoD was entirely responsible for funding the MFRC. Grant funds were provided to the Armed Services YMCA on a contract basis to establish a Military Family Resource Center for the Department of Defense. This resource center was the sole mission of this branch of the ASYMCA.

As the focal point for military family violence programs, the MFRC was chartered to provide information and technical assistance to professionals serving military families, facilitate inter-Service and interdisciplinary cooperation, maintain liaison with other federal and civilian agencies serving families, and provide fiscal oversight to all of the military family violence programs. A small staff was hired to carry out the primary functions of clearinghouse, communications, resource, training, and research.

Following the success of the MFRC demonstration project, the DoD acted to institutionalize its operations. In October 1984, the MFRC was brought into DoD as a Defense Field Operation Agency of the Office of the Assistant Secretary of Defense for Health Affairs (OASD (HA)). The MFRC Director served as chair of a Joint-Service Family Advocacy Committee tasked to assist and advise in the identification of joint-service family violence issues.

When the MFRC was transferred to DoD(HA), the clearinghouse, resource, and training functions were maintained by the ASYMCA, under the name Military Family Support Center, through an ongoing contract with DoD. What began as a reference and resource library to provide information on child abuse had expanded its focus to include other military family issues. The ASYMCA functioned as consultant to the military services as they initiated new family programs. Initially conceptualized as a means to share information, the Military Family Support Center became a vehicle to manage activities such as program development and training and a catalyst for focus on prevention and family support programs. As expertise grew in the Services, the ASYMCA's activities once again returned to their primary clearinghouse function. By 1990 the ASYMCA had relinquished the contract for the clearinghouse. However, for the decade of the1980s, the role of the ASYMCA in the DoD evolution of family advocacy (if not the entire family) programs was as critical as the role of the AMA in the 1970s.

The second key outcome of the GAO report was the promulgation of DoD Directive 6400.1, "Family Advocacy Program," in May 1981. This directive expanded the scope of the program to include spouse abuse. It established the DoD Family Advocacy Program, the DoD Family Advocacy Committee, a set of common definitions, and required each of the services to establish a broad-based program providing for the prevention, identification, reporting, treatment, and follow-up of child and spouse abuse. The third key outcome of the GAO report was increased congressional interest and oversight. In response to the GAO report, the DoD commented that obtaining necessary personnel and financial support to improve the family advocacy programs could be difficult because of budget constraints and the concern that such programs do not directly contribute to the DoD's main mission of supporting active duty forces. In FY82, Congress appropriated $5 million to develop a DoD Family Advocacy Program. Senator Daniel Inouye (D, HI) is frequently recognized as an early and staunch supporter of military child advocacy programs. In FY83 the FAP funds were appropriated directly to DoD. This centralization of family maltreatment funding (often referred to as "fenced funding") was a key prerequisite in consolidating individual and uncoordinated service activities into a coherent DoD program such as recommended by the GAO in 1979.

The Military Family Act of 1985

The Military Family Act of 1985 directed the establishment of a new Office of Family Policy, under the Assistant Secretary of Defense for Force Management and Personnel. This office was charged with coordinating all programs and activities of the military departments regarding military families. This act also directed the transfer of the MFRC from Health Affairs to the Office of the Assistant Secretary of Force Management and Personnel. At that time, the FAP budget, DoD-wide, was $5 million. In July 1986, DoD Instruction 6400.1 was revised, and a year later DoD Instruction 6400.2, "Child and Spouse Abuse Report," created the first standardized central registry reporting requirements.

Office of Family Policy

In 1988, DoD realized the recommendations of the 1970s from the early Kempe-inspired Tri-Service Child Advocacy Committee and culminating with the 1979 GAO report. The Office of Family Policy became the centralized agency to serve as focal point for all DoD family programs. It assumed responsibility for programming, budgeting and allocating, funds for the FAP throughout DoD. Now all the pieces were in place and the guiding vision of the AMA and the GAO achieved—DoD had established the mechanism to provide for centralized oversight and management of the Family Advocacy Program. This Office of Family Policy provided the platform for a period of extraordinary growth in funding, which translated to growth in treatment and prevention programming. The FY88 FAP budget of $14.2 million grew fourfold by FY93 to $62.2 million and then doubled in two years to $124.8 million in FY95 (see Figure 4.2).

1988-1995

The period from 1988 to 1995 was one of extensive growth, both in policy and service standardization, quality assurance, and program services. The DoD developed policy for the Family Advocacy Command Assistant Team (FACAT), a joint-service multidisciplinary team trained to assist in cases of out-of-home child sexual abuse; moved aggressively to ensure standardization in reporting and in training; and developed a two-year contract with the Child Welfare League of America to develop and disseminate standards for practice. In particular, prevention services, long identified as crucial to reducing family violence and maltreatment, received strong support as report after report called for growth of outreach services (e.g., Caliber Associates, 1994). Not only were these programs identified

FIGURE 4.2. DoD Family Advocacy Budget—FY88-96 ($ Million)

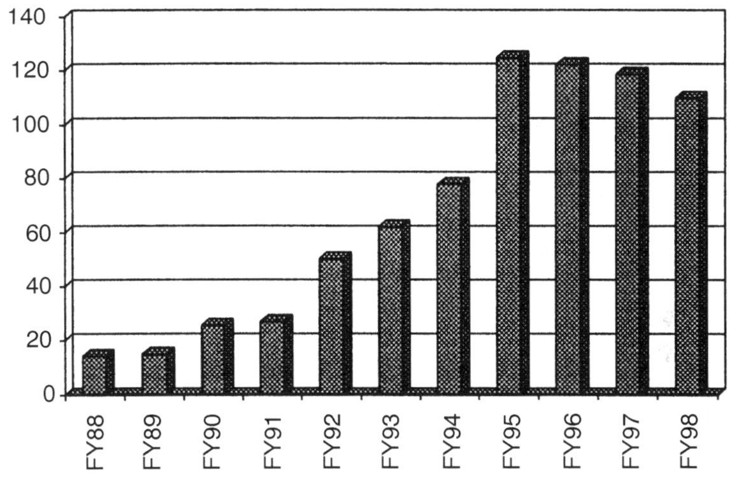

Note: FY95-97 includes $20 million for the New Parents Support Program. FY98 includes $10 million for the NPSP.

as critical, they were supported by funding. In addition to the growing prevention programs supported by the core FAP budget, in FY95 Congress appropriated an additional $20 million for the provision of New Parents Support Programs across the DoD.

1995-1998

The year 1995 represented the high-water mark in terms of funding growth (and the end of a period of extensive financial growth) for the DoD Family Advocacy Programs. Two key factors contributed to this state of affairs. The first was simply the impact of sweeping drawdown and changes in roles and missions occurring across the Department of Defense. By 1995 the DoD had approximately 1.5 million active duty members, approximately one-third less than even five years earlier. Numerous installations, particularly overseas, had been closed, initiating the movement toward homebasing. This drawdown, paired with an increase in complex and diverse missions around the globe, resulted in more frequent deployments, and increased OPTEMPO (operations tempo) and PERSTEMPO (personnel tempo). DoD budget reductions associated with the drawdown placed greater stress on the overall personnel and quality-of-life piece of the DoD budget pie. Ultimately, the cost associated with the critical need to modernize the force yielded an extremely tight fiscal environment. Quality of life issues that enjoyed high funding priority in the previous years were now viewed equally with other parts of the budget as a "bill payer" for force modernization. Ultimately, budget cuts and modernization requirements began to create pressures to eliminate or outsource nonwarfighting programs and services. In light of these pressures, it is extraordinary that the DoD FAP budget did not experience a serious reduction. In fact, it continued to grow on a proportional basis—declining less than the reduction in force structure. The other factor that was responsible for FAP budgets leveling off was a change in the mechanism DoD used to project requirements. In the mid-1980s an estimation framework was developed based on population. In 1996 DoD received its "workload" study (Caliber Associates, 1996), which provided a bottom-up or workload staffing model. While estimates from the old model suggested that FY95 funding met 77 percent of requirements, the workload model suggested that FY95 funding was adequate to provide for sufficient staff to accomplish the workload. With the publication of the workload study, it became hard, especially given the funding environment, for DoD to advocate for additional FAP funds.

Although funding growth began to level off in FY95, the period between then and FY98 was one of ongoing significant and positive developments in FAP standardization and programming. A number of important research initiatives were launched and completed. The Service FAPs began to work even more closely together in areas of domestic abuse, New Parents Support Programs, and additional improvements in central registry data collection and management.

SERVICE PROGRAM DEVELOPMENT

Army

The initial Army regulation establishing the Army Child Advocacy Program was issued by the Deputy Chief of Staff for Personnel (DCSPER). Over the years Army regulations have been modified and updated with expanded focus on prevention activities and programs to address spouse abuse. The Army program historically has been split. Treatment and case management activities are the responsibility of Surgeon General assets organized in the MTFs and overseen by Army Medical Command. Prevention activities are provided at the installation level by a Family Advocacy Manager working in the Army Community Services Center. The overall program receives oversight at Headquarters Army level from Army Community and Family Support Center (CFSC). The Army was the first Service to institutionalize required training with the Family Advocacy Staff Training course. In 1988 the Army FAP underwent a change in alignment that primarily changed the funding procedures. Essentially, Army Medical Command was removed from the funding process. Dollars flow from CFSC at the Department of the Army to Army MACOMS (major commands), then to installations. This change allows installation line commanders more direct control over their resources and their mission. Such a realignment has a rationale similar to the Navy Department program transfer that occurred in 1987. In the Navy's case, however, medical resources were realigned to the line.

Navy

The Navy Family Advocacy Program began in the Navy Medical Department in the late 1970s. The regulation establishing the program, BUMED Instruction 6320.53, was published in 1976. Hospital Family Advocacy representative positions, held by social workers, were created to manage the medical aspects of the program. In January 1984, the Navy Military Personnel Command was assigned overall responsibility for the Family Advocacy Program and, by way of the Family Service Centers, managed the nonmedical aspects of the program. The medical community continued to provide critical clinical services in support. The Navy Family Advocacy Program was realigned effective October 1997. At that time the program became a line responsibility completely under the auspices of Bureau of Naval Personnel. On Navy installations, the FAP is operated as part of the Family Service Center, with the exception of San Diego and Norfolk, where freestanding Family Advocacy Centers exist. Just under 200 Navy medical personnel resources were transferred to the line to work in the Family Advocacy Program.

Marine Corps

Prior to the publication of Marine Corps Order 1752.3, "Marine Corps Family Advocacy Program" in March 1983, the Marine Corps relied upon the Navy Medical Command for management of child and spouse abuse. The Marine Corps guidance supplements this assistance and adds the Marine Corps Family Service Centers (FSC) as having primary responsibility for identification, assessment, prevention, rehabilitation, and follow-up of family advocacy cases. Each FSC has full-time family advocacy staff including at least a Family Advocacy Program Officer.

Air Force

Because the author is more familiar with the Air Force, it will be used as the example to illustrate the growth, development, and evolution of the Family Advocacy Program in the services. The Air Force Child Advocacy Program (CAP) was established with the publication of AFR 168-38 on April 25, 1975, giving birth to the first servicewide child abuse and neglect program within DoD. The Air Force CAP was organized within the Office of the Surgeon General, reflecting the close ties to early grassroots efforts by social workers in establishing child abuse programs. In 1985, the Air Force began to expand family advocacy services, utilizing DoD funding provided by Congress to focus on preventing family maltreatment. With new approval to use Congressional funding to hire staff, the Air Force hired outreach workers to implement prevention services at selected Air Force bases. Ironically, in performing their jobs, outreach workers initially increased the rate and number of referrals for family maltreatment. Treatment staff, assigned only part-time to family advocacy duties, were overwhelmed with the scope and magnitude of the problems and the need for services.

The Air Force program was extensively revised and expanded in 1988-1989 with the publication of the standards that became the model for DoD standards published in 1991. In 1988 the Air Force was able to obtain additional funds to augment family advocacy staff trained in direct work with victims, offenders, and families (Mollerstrom, Patchner, and Milner, 1995). Also, comprehensive, multiyear treatment and program evaluation research was designed into the program.

In 1988, the Air Force FAP had approximately 150 staff. This number had grown to over 500 by 1998. Every Air Force installation had a core FAP team including a Family Advocacy Officer, Treatment Manager, Outreach Manager, Nurse Specialist, and Data Specialist. Most installations had additional personnel based on local population. The Air Force program, still organized under the Surgeon General, provided a complete range of treatment and prevention services and evolved into a comprehensive community-based program focused foremost on preventing family violence and building healthy communities by working in collaboration with other community agencies and programs.

Air Force-sponsored research clearly shows that interventions with abusive and nonabusive families reduce child abuse potential, reduce distress, and increase family cohesion and marital satisfaction. Child abuse rates in the Air Force (and DoD) are substantially below what is reported in the civilian sector. In FY97 the Air Force child abuse rate was 6.07 per 1,000. The Air Force spouse abuse rate in FY97 was 12.9 per 1,000 spouses. No comparable civilian rates are available for spouse abuse. Even more importantly, the severity of both child and spouse maltreatment cases has consistently declined since FY91.

ROLE OF SOCIAL WORKERS

Early child advocacy programs were managed by social workers, generally assigned as mental health officers. Social work training with its person-in-environment or ecological perspective and generalist orientation proved to be a strong fit with the demands and challenges of the job. The role of child advocacy officer was an additional duty. These workers were called upon to balance numerous competing demands including command-directed evaluations, counseling, and consulting, as well as the evaluation, treatment, and case management of child abuse cases—not infrequently, these cases were not the highest priority. From these early days, social workers have identified not only the need for more treatment resources, but for a focus on prevention. (Myers, 1977, 1979). This call for prevention has been a consistent theme as the programs grew. Certainly, those clinicians present during the 1973 DoD meetings with Dr. Kempe would be gratified to see the growth, development, and evolution that has taken place in twenty-five years.

Treatment

The Air Force FAP calls for mandatory reporting, offender accountability, and services to victim and offender. Therefore, historically the primary role of social workers in the child and family advocacy program has been clinical. Practitioners generally have been generalists, having the opportunity to utilize a wide range of modalities and approaches. Treatment includes identification, assessment, diagnosis, intervention including counseling, psychoeducational support, rehabilitation and referral services. Specific services include crisis intervention; case management; individual, group, and family counseling; support groups; respite and foster care; and shelter. The goals of direct services are first to protect the victim and then to provide alternatives to violent behavior to prevent abuse from recurring. Air Force and community goals include enhancing the health and well-being of military families and their communities so that military members can concentrate on their assigned duties and job performance.

Prevention

Prevention includes efforts to educate military communities regarding child abuse and neglect, spouse abuse, and activities that provide support to individuals and families vulnerable to the types of stress that may trigger abusive or neglectful behavior. The goal is to improve family functioning in order to reduce potentially abusive situations. Prevention services include community, command, and professional educational programs; parent education; safety education for children; family life education; and new parents support programs. They are provided by FAP staff—uniformed, civil service, and contract employees who are responsible for prevention services.

It has long been recognized that young military families are an at-risk population. These families are characterized by young age, strained finances, social isolation, and limited coping skills. Military demands and deployments increase spousal absence and financial concerns. Also, those with newborn children are considered at greatest risk. Finally, due to their isolation, transportation difficulties, and unfamiliarity with the system, they are difficult to reach. The DoD New Parents Support Program was specifically developed to target this population with the establishment of prenatal and postnatal home visiting programs. Such homevisiting programs were initiated in the Air Force in 1989. They were bolstered with the 1990 GAO report, "Home Visiting: A Promising Early Intervention Strategy for At-Risk Families," which showed that programs employing home visitors plus community services produce a range of positive outcomes for families and children. It appears that such outreach and early intervention programs are the single most effective strategy for preventing child abuse. In 1993 the Marine Corps established the second home visitation program in conjunction with Children's Hospital of San Diego. The Navy and Army followed suit. Beginning in FY95, congressional staff added an additional appropriation for these NPSP programs.

CONCLUSION

The issues surrounding the FAP are as complex as are the systems required to intervene. Command support is essential to program success. The program is truly interdisciplinary, depending upon an interface between social work, law enforcement, judicial and legal services, shelters, medical providers, clergy, educational programs, child care services, and others, both on and off the installation. From the early beginning in local MTFs in the 1960s, driven primarily by the activities of individual social workers and psychologists, the combined DoD FAP programs now employ over 2,000 personnel. Over half are devoted to providing primary and secondary prevention services. These services aimed at addressing the underlying causes (individual, family, and institutional) of family violence include: advocacy for nonviolent communitics; command and community education; training for medical, education, and child care staff; parenting education and couples communication classes; and targeted outreach programs focused on at-risk groups such as young, first-term families and families having children.

A review of the history suggests that resource and programmatic needs were consistently identified by staff working the program; but financial support typically was based on external forces, most typically congressional push. Indeed, a consistent theme across the evolution of the department's program has been congressional interest, attention, and support. The intersection of the grassroots efforts of clinicians at the local level, including social workers, psychologists, pediatricians, and others, working and advocating on behalf of military families and congressional interest, has yielded one of the most potent family advocacy programs in our nation—perhaps a benchmark in prevention and case management for all communities. DoD has come a long way in a short time and has become a national leader in developing and providing comprehensive services to deal with family abuse.

BIBLIOGRAPHY

Acord, L. D. (1977). Child abuse and neglect in the Navy. *Military Medicine*, 142(3), 862-864.

Caliber Associates (1994). *Abuse Victims Study—Disincentives. Disincentives to Report Abuse by Victims*. Alexandria, VA: Author.

Caliber Associates (1996). *Family Advocacy Program (FAP) Workload Study: Data Analysis and Development of FAP Personnel Staffing Model*. Alexandria, VA: Author.

General Accounting Office (1979). *Military Child Advocacy Programs—Victims of Neglect*. Washington, DC: Author.

General Accounting Office (1990). *Home Visiting: A Promising Early Intervention Strategy for At-Risk Families*. Washington DC: Author.

Military Family Resource Center (1987). *History of the Department of Defense Family Advocacy Program.* Alexandria, VA: Office of the Assistant Secretary of Defense (Force Management and Personnel).

Miller, J. K. (1977). Perspectives on child maltreatment in the military. In R. E. Helfer and C. H. Kempe (Eds.), *Child Abuse and Neglect: The Family and the Community* (pp. 267-291). Cambridge, MA: Ballinger Publishing Co.

Mollerstrom, W. W., Patchner, M. A., and Milner, J. S. (1995). Child maltreatment: The United States Air Force's response. *Child Abuse and Neglect*, 19(3), 325-334.

Myers, S. S. (1979). Child abuse and the military community. *Military Medicine*, 144(1), 22-23.

Myers, S. S. (1977). Child advocacy program: A brief history and status report. *Air Force Medical Service Digest*, 28(4), 3-7.

Chapter 5

TRICARE and Its Impact on Military Social Work Practice

Carla A. Monroe-Posey

TRICARE, the Department of Defense (DoD) managed care program initiated in 1993, is fundamentally changing the delivery of health care to beneficiaries of the Military Health System (MHS). This chapter includes a brief history of TRICARE, an overview of the uniform benefit established with TRICARE, and a summary of TRICARE structure and operations, successes and challenges. The initial effects of TRICARE implementation on the delivery of military social work services, which include medical social work, mental health, and family advocacy, are then addressed and conclusions drawn.

OVERVIEW OF TRICARE

CHAMPUS and the Development of TRICARE

The delivery of military medical services to family members of active duty personnel began with a congressional direction in 1884 that "medical officers of the Army and contract surgeons shall whenever possible attend the families of officers and soldiers free of charge" (TRICARE, 1997b). The Emergency Maternal and Infant Care Pro-

The opinions expressed in this chapter are the author's and should not be interpreted as the policy or opinions of the United States Air Force.

gram (EMIC) was established by Congress in 1943 to provide medical care to wives and infants of soldiers, sailors, and marines during World War II when the military medical system was unavailable to nonactive duty personnel. The Korean War again strained the capacity of the military system, so a more systematic approach to supplementing available military medical care began with the 1956 Dependents Medical Care Act. A 1966 amendment to this act established the Civilian Health and Medical Program of the Uniformed Services (CHAMPUS) to provide civilian medical care to active duty family members, retirees and their families, and survivors of deceased military sponsors (TRICARE, 1997b).

CHAMPUS expanded the medical benefit for military beneficiaries from traditional "space available" care at military medical treatment facilities (MTFs) to a comprehensive service available across the country. Benefits were more expansive, yet costs to beneficiaries were more moderate than those of traditional medical insurance. Although some restrictions applied, benefits continued to expand through the years, which resulted in significant increases in program costs. The fiscal year (FY) 1967 $106 million budget was by FY 1996 more than $3.5 billion (TRICARE, 1997b). CHAMPUS costs actually doubled between FY 1985 and FY 1993.

Although similar in some ways to an insurance system, CHAMPUS is a program through which the federal government pays certain authorized civilian health care providers to deliver medically and psychologically necessary care to eligible beneficiaries. The associated requirements for rendering care and for obtaining payment are detailed, and the resulting system is complex. CHAMPUS coverage includes most inpatient and outpatient services. Substantial portions of physician and hospital charges, medical equipment and supplies, and mental health care are also included. Beneficiaries pay no premiums, but they are responsible for a portion of the costs of care after their annual deductible is paid. The CHAMPUS Program for the Handicapped was designed to help families cope with the extraordinary costs associated with some physical disabilities (Boyer and Sobel, 1993). Under TRICARE the Program for the Handicapped has been reorganized as the Program for Persons with Disabilities.

Efforts to curtail CHAMPUS costs by making the system more efficient began in the 1980s with several demonstration projects, including:

- the CHAMPUS reform initiative (CRI) in California and Hawaii;
- the New Orleans managed care demonstration;
- several catchment area management (CAM) projects;
- the southeast region/preferred provider organization (SER/PPO) demonstration; and
- the contracted provider arrangement (CPA)-Norfolk.

The CRI and CAM projects illustrate the types of managed care systems that were demonstrated. CRI launched CHAMPUS into the managed care world in 1988 by competitively selecting an at-risk contractor to underwrite CHAMPUS services in California and Hawaii. Its goal was to increase the quality and decrease the costs of services. Approximately 800,000 beneficiaries in the demonstration area received three benefit options roughly similar to the TRICARE Prime, Extra, and Standard options described below. Later surveys indicated that the beneficiaries were pleased with their care and that network health care providers appreciated CRI's reduction in payment paperwork. Utilization management services, including utilization review, case management, and discharge planning, common to managed care programs, were initiated. Resource sharing agreements were used that allowed military medical facilities to work with the contractor to provide services using combined resources, so long as the project lowered costs. This demonstration continued until TRICARE was launched in 1993 (Boyer and Sobel, 1993).

By contrast, the catchment area management (CAM) projects initiated in 1989 expanded to five sites by 1993. They gave control of the budget for each military hospital and CHAMPUS services in an associated forty-mile area to the hospital commander. The commander had discretion in developing managed care practices and contracts so long as costs did not exceed the amount projected for the catchment area under traditional CHAMPUS requirements. All sites had a voluntary enrollment plan for families that featured benefit modifications to make enrollment more attractive. Utilization management practices, such as preadmission reviews of proposed inpatient care and retrospective case audits, were also used. Mechanisms for simplifying claims processing varied by site (Boyer and Sobel, 1993). The CAM demonstrations ended when their regions obtained TRICARE managed care support (MCS) contractors.

TRICARE had its beginnings in the CHAMPUS demonstration projects and in the creation in 1991 of the Office of the Assistant Secretary of Defense for Health Affairs (OASD(HA)) with centralized defense health program (DHP) funding. Traditionally, the Army, Navy, and Air Force have maintained their own health care systems, each functioning independently of the others. The peacetime use of the air evacuation system linked military medical facilities in each system to allow transfer of patients to other facilities. In most cases, patients remained within their own Service medical system.

Creation of the OASD(HA) and centralized funding facilitated the design of a single defense managed care system. The resources of the direct care system, namely, the military health care systems of each of the Uniformed Services, were supplemented with the services of a managed care support (MCS) contractor. The congressional goal was to reduce costs and to make systematic the managed care reforms of the CHAMPUS demonstration projects. This TRICARE system was announced in 1993. Twelve regions were designated in the United States, each of which would integrate its regional direct care system resources, supplementing them with the services provided by the MCS contractor. The commander of the largest medical center in the region was designated the lead agent. With a staff of approximately thirty-two, the lead agent was charged with integrating the regional direct care system and working with OASD(HA) and the Office of CHAMPUS (OCHAMPUS; now the TRICARE Management Activity [TMA]) to develop, award, and monitor the MCS contract for the region. The procurement process was combined for regions 9, 10, and 12; 7 and 8; 3 and 4; and 2 and 5. In all, seven contracts were awarded to cover the twelve regions, as noted in Table 5.1. Regions 7 and 8 were later combined under a single Army lead agent at Fort Carson, Colorado. Locations of military forces and their families in the Pacific Rim were later added to region 12, and those in Europe were designated region 13. Region 1 lead agent responsibilities are rotated annually among the commanders of the medical centers of each Service located in the National Capital area (i.e., Washington, DC, and surrounding area).

TABLE 5.1. TRICARE Regions, Contractors, and Health Care Start Dates

Region	Title/Area	MCS Contractor	Healthcare Start Date
1	Northeast (National Capital)	Sierra	May 1998
2	Mid-Atlantic	Anthem	May 1998
3	Southeast	Humana	July 1996
4	Gulfsouth	Humana	July 1996
5	Heartland	Anthem	May 1998
6	Southwest	Foundation Health Federal Service (FHFS)	November 1995
7 and 8	Central	Tri-West	April 1997
9	Southern California	FHFS	April 1996
10	Golden Gate	FFS	April 1996
11	Northwest	FHFS	March 1995
12	Hawaii, Alaska, and the Pacific	FHFS	March 1996-October 1997
13	Europe	Humana	October 1996
	Latin America	Humana	October 1996

Adapted from Department of Defense Health Services Regions Map (TRICARE, 1997c).

The TRICARE Uniform Benefit

Depending on geographic availability of TRICARE networks, military beneficiaries have three options in meeting their health care needs: TRICARE Prime, TRICARE Extra, or TRICARE Standard. TRICARE Prime is available in the forty-mile catchment areas of all military treatment facilities, at all Base Realignment and Closure (BRAC) sites, at locations where geographically separate military units (GSUs) are deployed and at other locations where there are sufficient military beneficiaries to make this option economically feasible for the government.

TRICARE Prime is a health maintenance organization-type (HMO) option in which beneficiaries enroll and are assigned a primary care manager (PCM) in the direct care system or the MCS contractor's network. The PCM provides routine care and also monitors and approves any referral for specialty care. With the exception of the first eight sessions of outpatient mental health care, the beneficiary agrees to work with the PCM for all health care needs while the PCM ensures quality, appropriateness, and continuity of care. Beneficiaries may enroll as individuals or families, with the same or different PCMs. PCMs may be family practice physicians, physician assistants, nurse practitioners, internists or, in special circumstances, other physician specialties.

TRICARE Prime enrollees receive enhanced benefits, which include preventive health care services such as physical screenings. They do not file claims and generally pay lower fees. However, they agree to use only network providers and hospitals for specialty care with the approval of their PCMs. Network providers must meet certain standards for proximity to the patient and waiting time for appointments. Active duty personnel are automatically enrolled and must use the direct care system. Their family members may enroll free of charge. Retirees and their family members may enroll for an annual fee of $230 for an individual or $460 for a family. Non-active duty enrollees may use their point-of-service (POS) option to obtain care outside the network without PCM approval, but they must pay an annual deductible of $300 for an individual or $600 for a family, plus 50 percent of the TRICARE allowable charge. These costs are considerably more than those of a nonenrolled individual using TRICARE Standard.

TRICARE Extra is a preferred provider organization (PPO) network of primary care and specialty individual and institutional providers. Beneficiaries use TRICARE Extra when they choose a network provider for care. Network providers agree to accept a discount on the TRICARE maximum charge for covered services. After satisfying their annual deductible amount, beneficiaries receive a discount of 5 percent on their cost share payment, and they generally do not have to file claim forms. Active duty members are not eligible for TRICARE Extra or TRICARE Standard.

TRICARE Standard, which is comparable to the traditional CHAMPUS system, provides payment for covered services with nonnetwork authorized providers. Generally, the patient files claim forms and pays the deductibles and cost shares listed in Tables 5.2 and 5.3 (TRICARE,

TABLE 5.2. TRICARE Costs for Active-Duty Family Members

	TRICARE Prime E-1—E-4	TRICARE Prime E-5 and up	TRICARE Extra	TRICARE Standard
Annual Deductible	None	None	$150/individual or $300/family for E-5 and above; $50/$100 for E-4 and below	$150/individual or $300/family for E-5 and above; $50/$100 for E-4 and below
Civilian Outpatient Visit	$6/visit	$12/visit	15% of negotiated fee	20% of allowable charge
Civilian Inpatient Admission	$11/day ($25 minimum)	$11/day ($25 minimum)	Greater of $25 or $9.90/day	Greater of $25 or $9.90/day
Civilian Inpatient Mental Health	$20/day	$20/day	$20/day	$20/day

TABLE 5.3. TRICARE Costs for Retirees, Their Families, and Others

	TRICARE Prime	TRICARE Extra	TRICARE Standard (CHAMPUS)
Annual Deductible	None	$150/individual or $300/family	$150/individual or $300/family
Annual Enrollment Fees	$230/individual $460/family	None	None
Civilian Provider Co-Pays:		20% of negotiated fees	25% of allowed charges
Outpatient Visit	$12		
Emergency Care	$30		
Mental Health Visit	$25		
Civilian Inpatient Cost Share	$11/day ($25 minimum)	Lesser of $250/day or 25% of billed charges plus 20% of allowed professional fees	Lesser of $360/day or 25% of billed charges plus 25% of allowed professional fees
Civilian Inpatient Mental Health	$40/day	20% of institutional and professional charges	Lesser of $137/day or 25% of institutional and professional charges

1997a). There are no charges for services when benefi-ciaries use the military direct care system. Priorities for care in the direct care system go to active duty military; to their family members who are Prime enrollees; to retirees, their family members, and surviving family members who are Prime enrollees; to active duty family members who are not Prime enrollees; and finally to all others (Office of Assistant Secretary of Defense, Health Affairs, 1997).

TRICARE Operations: Successes and Challenges

The Military Health System (MHS), which consists of the direct care system and the managed care support contracted systems, must be ready for and responsive to the health care needs of active duty members of all services who are deployed around the world. It must also be able competitively to provide peacetime health care to active duty members and military beneficiaries. (The recently revised mission and goals of the Military Health System are detailed in Table 5.4.)

The Congressional Budget Office (CBO) has contended that each of the two primary MHS goals dictates quite different medical systems, creating a conflict (Congressional Budgeting Office, 1995). Unless opportunities are specially created, military providers have few chances in peacetime to treat the types of conditions and injuries common in wartime and peacekeeping operations. To support the warfighting role, deployed military medical units and providers care for combatants and civilians with disease and nonbattle injuries (DNBI), and for individuals with combat-induced wounds as well as combatants wounded in action (WIA) in a variety of environments during conflicts. About 75 percent of peacetime diagnoses at military medical facilities match DNBI diagnoses, including inguinal hernia, uncomplicated births, pneumonia, coronary atherosclerosis, and chest pain. However, based on data reported for Marines in Vietnam, only about ten of the twenty-five DNBI primary diagnoses most common during conflicts and peacekeeping missions are among the top fifty peacetime diagnoses by volume in the direct care system. Only about 5 percent of the primary diagnoses treated at military facilities match the diagnosis of a battle-related injury, and none of the top fifty most frequent primary diagnoses at military facilities match a wounded in action condition. The CBO therefore recommended enhanced training opportunities, including peacetime practice in civilian trauma centers.

TABLE 5.4. MHS Mission and Goals

Mission:
The MHS supports the Department of Defense (DoD) and our nation's security by providing health support for the full range of military deployments and sustaining the health of members of the Armed Forces, their families, and others to advance our national security interests.
Goals:
1. **Joint Medical Readiness:** Ensure that military members of the Armed Forces attain an optimal level of fitness and health and are protected from the full spectrum of medical and environmental hazards. Our medical forces will meet the challenges of a rapidly changing continuum of Service-specific, joint, and combined military operations anywhere at any time. 2. **Benchmark Health System:** We will be the world's best integrated health system. Optimize use of the three Service medical departments to meet the MHS mission . . . (to) be health- and fitness-focused and responsive to customer needs where cost, quality, and access are paramount. 3. **Healthy Communities:** Forge partnerships to create a common culture that values health and fitness and empowers individuals and organizations to actualize those values. 4. **Resources and Structure:** Identify and prioritize resource requirements and establish effective and efficient organizations to support the readiness and benefit missions. 5. **Training and Skill Development:** Train and develop our people for their role in war and peace . . . developing plans to educate, train, and retain highly qualified and diverse personnel at all levels of the system. 6. **Technology Integration:** Integrate technologies into best practices designed to achieve high-quality clinical outcomes, decrease health care delivery costs, and improve management processes.

The CBO also advocated that the direct care system should be significantly scaled down to a deployable, medical readiness force dividing its time between mission training activities and practice in civilian settings giving the most opportunities to treat DNBI and WIA diagnoses. Active duty personnel would receive some of their peacetime health care in civilian facilities and other military beneficiaries would use civilian systems exclusively. The Federal Employees Health Benefits Program (FEHBP) was specifically recommended.

The DoD is adamant that its peacetime service delivery system is an integral part of its training and preparations for its wartime and peacekeeping missions. In addition, the direct care system is more cost effective than civilian alternatives in providing care to eligible beneficiaries. The DoD argument is that direct care should therefore be maintained in the TRICARE system with reductions in size geared to any further cuts in the active duty forces.

There have been numerous evaluations of the TRICARE system. In March 1995, the same month that the first region (Northwest) started health care delivery with their managed care support contractor, the General Accounting Office (GAO) published its Report to Congressional Requesters—*Defense Health Care: Issues and Challenges Confronting Military Medicine* (1995). Among its criticisms were:

- The regional structure established does not give sufficient authority to the lead agent commander to integrate the regional direct care system and facilitate work with the MCS contractor. Each Service retains command, control, and budget authority over its own medical facilities, making the lead agent dependent on the goodwill of the region's medical commanders in order to effect some degree of integration.
- TRICARE involves a cumbersome and contentious procurement system with a complex, detailed request for proposal. The procurement process is often delayed and unsuccessful bidders always contest awards.
- The direct care system has persistent problems with access to care, including delays and inconvenience in obtaining appointments.
- Lack of consistency in the uniform benefit across geographic areas maintains and strengthens inequities among categories of beneficiaries.
- TRICARE will not result in cost savings over the projected costs of the direct care system and traditional CHAMPUS. TRICARE's additional Prime prevention benefit and administrative costs could outweigh TRICARE's management and clinical efficiencies.

This report predicted that access to space-available care would be constrained for nonenrolled low-priority beneficiaries as military medical facilities attempted to enroll maximum numbers of beneficiaries, with first priority to active duty personnel and their families. Most beneficiaries over sixty-five would be unable to enroll and would likely have lowest priority for shrinking space-available care. An additional inequity cited was the predicted lack of availability of TRICARE Prime and Extra in areas outside military facility catchment areas that are sparsely populated with military beneficiaries. Availability of Prime enrollment with military primary care managers, the option with the lowest cost for care, might also be limited as the military continues to reduce the size of its forces, further restricting the number of enrollees who could obtain lowest cost care.

Finally, the GAO recommended that DoD and Congress agree on the actual size of the military medical force structure needed to meet wartime requirements. This determination would then drive the number and type of medical specialties required, their training needs, and the number of MTFs required. The scope and organization of the direct care system could then be accurately based on medical readiness requirements. The GAO seconded the CBO recommendation to make the Federal Employees Health Benefits Program (FEHBP) the primary mechanism for providing health care to military beneficiaries.

Since the Northwest Region (#11) first started health care delivery in March 1995, GAO officials have testified to Congress and prepared letter reports about numerous TRICARE issues. Early implementation in Region 11 was hampered by delays in approving the uniform benefit guidelines, which differed from draft versions that had been used to publicize TRICARE options with the region's beneficiaries. Larger than expected enrollments occurred, nevertheless, and lessons learned from this experience were shared with the other regions so that their implementation processes could be smoothed. A significant problem was the incompatibility between direct care system and MCS contractor computer systems, resulting in arduous double entry of data and later interoperability requirements. There were major concerns that projected cost savings would not be realized as few resource sharing agreements between military facility commanders and MCS contractors were executed. Thus, the associated cost savings could not be realized. Utilization management activities, another projected source of cost savings, were slow to be implemented in the direct care system and the contracted networks. Although annual surveys asked beneficiaries about delays in obtaining appointments, computer systems did not collect appointment availability data and so consistent, objective measurement of access performance was not possible (General Accounting Office, 1996).

TRICARE costs continue to be an issue. In a February 1997 briefing report, the GAO questioned DoD projected health care costs, citing two questionable assumptions. DoD had assumed *no* increase in health care costs would occur due to advances in medical technology and intensity of treatment while industry experts projected 1 to 2 percent growth for the same period. Using a rate of 1.5 percent growth, the GAO estimated that DoD costs could increase as much as $3.2 billion for fiscal years 1998 through 2003. The GAO also questioned DoD's assumption that 5 percent savings would occur due to utilization management activities. DoD officials had subjectively chosen this figure from a range of 2 to 14 percent savings in civilian systems (General Accounting Office, 1997a).

Small savings from resource sharing, initiatives in which military facility commanders and MCS contractors combine their resources to provide needed services at reduced cost, have persisted as a concern, with the GAO estimating that DoD would realize only 5 percent of its projected $700 million savings during a five-year period. Resource sharing contracts have been inhibited by lack of clear guidelines, the complexity of required cost analyses, lack of financial incentives for military facilities to participate, and changes in military direct care system capacity because of continued cost pressures and downsizing. The GAO also questioned DoD projected cost savings with TRICARE because they were based on estimates of traditional CHAMPUS costs for future years made with 1993 data. This report also described new DoD plans for revised financing in the requests for proposal for Regions 1, 2, and 5. Revised financing gives military facility commanders control of a variable budget capitated by the number of their Prime enrollees to cover enrollee costs of care in the direct care system as well as any services purchased for them from the MCS contractor. While acknowledging the desire to fix problems associated with resource sharing, the GAO criticized DoD's lack of "a simple, stable, long-term approach to TRICARE budgeting and contracting that provides clear managed care incentives and accountability and avoids the complexities and disincentives of resource sharing" (General Accounting Office, 1997a, p. 13).

Concerns about care access in the direct care system, beneficiary satisfaction with services, and equity among beneficiary categories have continued as well. In June 1997, the GAO reviewed options available to DoD for extending services to military beneficiaries over the age of sixty-five who are no longer covered by CHAMPUS, are not permitted to enroll in TRICARE Prime, and are not generally given other than lowest priority for shrinking space-available care in MTFs. A range of options was explored, including DoD providing a Medicare HMO option (called subvention), DoD funding various supplements of Medicare for these beneficiaries, or DoD expanding the mail-order pharmacy program to all Medicare-eligible military beneficiaries. Subvention would likely be limited to about 75,000 beneficiaries due to the lack of required military facility capacity. Other options ranged in estimated costs from $229 million for the pharmacy program to $2.2 billion for DoD-funded Medicare Part B and Medigap policies. Costs were deemed prohibitive, so only the pharmacy program was recommended (General Accounting Office, 1997b).

In a later report, the GAO critiqued DoD's mechanisms for obtaining beneficiary feedback, recommending regular surveys of beneficiaries receiving inpatient care, and systematic approaches to collecting and analyzing unsolicited beneficiary feedback regarding the direct care and the contractor's systems. These would supplement DoD's annual beneficiary surveys and monthly military facility surveys of beneficiaries receiving ambulatory services. This more comprehensive feedback system, which would be comparable to civilian systems, could then be used to monitor outcomes associated with beneficiary access to care and satisfaction with services (General Accounting Office, 1998).

With the start of health care delivery for Regions 1, 2, and 5 on May 1, 1998, TRICARE health care services have been implemented worldwide. While criticisms have been numerous, clear changes in the direct care system have been occurring. In most regions, medical facilities of all three Services cooperate to their mutual benefit in coordinating care for their patients. Case management and discharge planning activities have increased as military facilities struggled to meet utilization review criteria. Implementation of the primary care manager model of service delivery has created numerous challenges for most facilities. With fiscal year 1998, DoD began its use of enrollment-based capitation (EBC) budgeting for MTFs. While costs of medical readiness requirements and graduate medical education and training are separately funded, the military facility budget for peacetime medical care is now largely dependent on the number of its Prime enrollees. As a result, commanders have new pressures to increase their Prime enrollment and efficiency of service delivery. Many military facilities enroll virtually all the beneficiaries in their forty-mile catchment areas who select TRICARE Prime. Military facility leaders have been learning the intricacies of providing optimal access for the greatest number of enrollees to high-quality services delivered at low cost. Trying to recapture the business of beneficiaries previously sent to the civilian community for care has taught many commanders the importance of direct and indirect marketing. Only teaching hospitals and medical centers, which must meet the requirements of their sponsored educational programs, consistently maintain services available to nonenrollees, particularly Medicare-eligible patients who are not able to enroll. It is in this environment, with knowledge of the competing pressures on commander and staff, that the effects of TRICARE on military social work practice must be studied.

MILITARY SOCIAL WORK PRACTICE IN A TRICARE ENVIRONMENT

To gauge the impact of TRICARE on military social work practice, sixteen social workers at seven military facilities were interviewed using two single-facility focus group meetings and seven individual telephone sessions. The military facilities included medical centers, medium and small hospitals, and small outpatient clinics from Regions 3, 6, 8, 9, and 11. These regions were among the first to start health care delivery with their TRICARE managed care support contractors. Army, Navy, and Air Force facilities were included, most of which were urban or near an urban area. One small facility in an isolated area was also included.

Medical Social Work Services

With TRICARE, the direct care system of military medical facilities adopted managed care principles. The requirement for utilization management (UM) services began with the September 1994 publication of the DoD Utilization Management Plan. Use of Inter-Qual criteria for physical illness and Health Management Strategies (HMS) international mental health criteria were mandated, as were more extensive, cost-sensitive case management and discharge planning services. Use of provider profiling, care paths, and practice guidelines were encouraged. Some regions chose to have their managed care support contractors provide all or most military facility utilization management services. Other locations provided all their UM services internally.

Hampered by information systems that were not supportive of the types of data collection and analyses required, most facilities were slow to implement all UM practices. Computer interoperability problems made it difficult to identify a military facility Prime enrollee's primary care manager (PCM). Even with these problems, many providers found their practice patterns questioned for the first time as the traditional belief that an unoccupied bed can be filled without substantive additional cost was challenged. The so-called "churn and earn" strategy associated with workload-based dissemination of resources was seriously questioned for the first time at many facilities.

There is a wide variety in the staff size and hierarchical placement of the social work departments surveyed for this chapter. Social work services were a separate unit in larger facilities, but were most often a part of the mental health service in smaller facilities. Generally, the Army has more extensive social work departments, while the Air Force and Navy tend to have fewer services per capita (see Chapters 1, 2, and 3). In smaller facilities, provision of social work services is an additional duty for mental health social workers. Most social workers contacted for this study reported that their social work departments were not encountering significant size reduction pressures because there is clear recognition of the departments' importance in a managed care environment. One social worker at a medium-sized facility reported pressures to reduce the number of staff and voiced her belief that medical social work services in military facilities would eventually all be contracted. Some of the social workers interviewed were aware of military facilities whose social work services and staff were integrated with those of the UM department, but this integration had not occurred at any of their facilities. However, one social worker was assigned to the UM service at a few of the facilities whose personnel were contacted. Most social workers reported close working relationships with UM services intended to facilitate more efficient care with effective referrals.

The PCM model of service delivery had been deployed with varying levels of success at the military facilities surveyed. Some of the regions had been more active than others in assisting their facilities to make the system changes necessary to facilitate the oversight and approval of specialty care by PCMs. At one medium and one large facility the transitions were smooth as primary care providers already had a tradition of following their patients through episodes of care. The staff was accustomed to consulting a patient's primary care practitioner when specialty services were needed. One of these facilities had devised special discharge planning forms to ensure that the PCM was notified of plans made for patients in his or her care.

Other facilities, large and small, have had great difficulty with implementing the PCM model. At one small facility, social workers failed to recognize the implications of the PCM model in making referrals for care in the contractor's network. Their approach was to send the patient to the TRICARE Service Center to obtain a network referral without coordinating their plans with the patient's PCM or informing the patient that such coordination was necessary.

At one large facility, Prime enrollees were generally unfamiliar with Prime services and requirements. They could not state whether they had a PCM or who that individual or team might be. Assignment to a team or clinic instead of an individual provider was for others so impersonal that they failed to understand or to use the unique features of the Prime option. PCMs were not familiar with the patients assigned to their teams, nor did they want to be consulted about these patients. Some specialists functioned as PCMs for their chronically ill patients without sanction, leaving the actual PCMs uninformed about their patients' care. The number enrolled exceeded this facility's capacity to provide care efficiently without redesigning the service delivery system. Although active duty and Prime enrollees had priority for treatment, services were difficult for these patients to obtain. The beneficiaries frequently had to advocate for their own care. Parents often functioned as the care managers for their chronically ill children.

Medical social workers at this large facility did not routinely consult Prime enrollees' primary care managers to arrange care. These social workers did coordinate plans with the primary care or specialty provider when one was clearly taking the PCM role. By using the informal network of relationships they had built throughout the facility, these social workers could promptly obtain the specialty care needed for some of their patients. The specialty care system was so overloaded that social workers used their informal networks only in the most precarious cases. When no PCM was taking the PCM role for an enrollee, the patient was sent to the contractor's TRICARE Service Center (TSC) to obtain referrals. One social worker stated she had a policy of returning with the patient to the center when there were difficulties in obtaining a referral.

Medical social workers at all facilities surveyed reported few substantive changes in the nature of referrals to their services. At military facilities where the MCS contractor was providing some or all of the UM services, the social workers interviewed believed that the contractor referred to them the patients with the most complex medical and psychosocial needs. A social worker at one of the smaller facilities reported an increase in the number of referrals of Medicare-eligible patients for whom TRICARE services were not available.

The extent of discharge planning services at a military facility depended on its size and the nature of services provided as well as the type of patients served. Older retired patients and their families generally required more frequent and complex medical care and more extensive discharge planning than younger beneficiaries did. Increasing pressures to effect a discharge plan without incurring "avoidable days" (i.e., days for which inpatient care was not medically necessary) had resulted in preadmission discharge planning for many patients, and there was generally less time to work with all patients on their discharge plans. The MCS contractor provided discharge planning services at some military facilities, while at others the ward nursing staff provided the bulk of discharge planning services using guidelines provided by medical social workers. In the latter case, social work referrals were limited to those of inpatients with complex psychosocial issues and needs.

At some military facilities, case management was limited to Prime enrollees, while at others, only the services of specialty case managers were available. According to the medical social workers interviewed, discharge planning and case management services provided to their facilities by MCS contractors were most often delivered by telephone. The TRICARE Service Center, where contract staff are generally located, is not always in the military medical facility or even on the base or post, thus making in-person services more difficult and costly to provide. In addition, the contractor's discharge planners and case managers reportedly did not always consult with military PCMs on plans for their patients' care.

Many military facility medical social workers stated that the roles and functions they shared with contractor personnel could be difficult. These social workers felt that the contractor's staff had a high turnover rate because the contractor offered fewer benefits and less time for interacting with patients, which is often more rewarding for social workers than the details of coordinating services. Generally, these military facility social workers believed that they received the referrals of patients with more complex psychosocial situations and needs, while the contractor's personnel faced even greater pressures than they to move patients to lower levels of care swiftly.

TRICARE has heightened attention and sometimes brought more complex referrals to military medical social work departments because of pressures to increase the efficiency of service delivery and ensure care is medically necessary. The majority of social workers interviewed believed that TRICARE had enhanced the credibility of and demand for military medical social work services in the direct care system.

Mental Health Services Provided by Clinical Social Workers

Clinical social workers have traditionally had significant roles in the provision of military mental health and substance abuse rehabilitation services, with some social workers specializing in these services (see Chapter 9). At many facilities, mental health care had been largely limited to active duty personnel with few space-available services. Some mental health services have been cut as the number of mental health providers is reduced due to cost-cutting initiatives. One social worker expressed concern that the coming absence of psychiatrists in his facility might result in some quality of care problems as PCMs tried to respond to some challenging mental health care needs without readily available psychiatric consultation.

Although historically patients air-evacuated for inpatient care in the military direct care system have most frequently had mental health and substance abuse diagnoses, there has been a systemwide reduction in the number of inpatient beds available for mental health and substance abuse rehabilitation services in recent years. The additional pressure on military facility commanders to increase the cost efficiency and effectiveness of their service delivery systems has resulted in the closure of inpatient mental health and substance abuse rehabilitation services or in their conversion to partial hospitalization and/or day treatment programs. Frequently these units served few patients, so they had high per patient-day costs.

The onset of TRICARE and enrollment-based capitation budgets for military facilities has heightened commanders' attention to their costs for Prime enrollees referred to the contractor's mental health network for care. All facilities must provide all the mental health and substance abuse rehabilitative care required by their active duty populations, or they must pay for the care when an enrollee is referred to the contractor's mental health network. Military facility mental health case managers are active in working with providers and PCMs to arrange quality, cost-effective treatment at the medically necessary level of care.

Of the facilities surveyed, most provided mental health care solely to active duty personnel and military facility Prime enrollees unless there was a teaching mission requiring a wider range of patients. Although DoD mandates their use, not all facilities were aware of nor were they using Health Management Strategies (HMS) International criteria for utilization review of mental health services. A few larger facilities had dedicated mental health case managers, either social workers or mental health nurses, who applied the mental health and substance abuse rehabilitation criteria for inpatients while on the wards. Consistent use of the criteria to review outpatient mental health care was rare.

Whether the criteria were used or not, all facilities felt pressure to increase the efficiency and capacity of their outpatient services. One social worker at a smaller, isolated facility reported a significant deterioration in the availability of care when the new MCS contractor was unable to provide replacements for civilian mental health providers who had been working under a demonstration resource sharing agreement in the military facility.

Larger facilities were more likely to provide the care of the chronically mentally ill and to refer patients needing short-term services to the network. Some large facilities used screening questionnaires as tools to determine which patients to see in-house and which to refer to the contractor's providers. Smaller facilities were more likely to accept clients needing short-term services for discreet problems and to refer those with chronic mental illness or complex life circumstance issues whose care needs might overwhelm their in-house capacities.

One social worker noted with pleasure the ability of Prime enrollees to seek up to eight sessions of mental health care in the network without PCM awareness or approval. Many active duty personnel and their families prefer to seek mental health care outside the direct care system because of the greater degree of privacy afforded with civilian services. At the same time, a dilemma for many social workers was the likelihood that patients referred to the network would not act on their referrals.

Some of the social workers interviewed reported a paucity of network providers available to provide specialized care. Child and adolescent inpatient and outpatient services were particularly lacking in the local networks of most of the military facilities whose social workers were interviewed. Specialty providers in the network may be inconveniently located, especially when the MTF is in a medically underserved area. Furthermore, these providers are reportedly more likely to leave the network if problems develop in claims processing or payment. As noted in Tables 5.2 and 5.3, co-payments for inpatient and outpatient mental health services are higher than for other types of care. When these factors compound with the reluctance that many people feel to seek mental health or substance abuse rehabilitative care, the number of failed referrals for these treatments is understandable and concerning.

It is clear that TRICARE has had significant impact on the delivery of mental health care in the military direct care system. While the resulting increase in the efficiency of mental health service delivery in military facilities is noteworthy, concern remains for the:

- relative paucity of specialized mental health services in some areas of the contractors' networks;
- increased financial burden to patients no longer able to obtain care in the military facility; and
- resulting number of eligible individuals and families who will decide not to obtain care.

Family Advocacy Program Services

Although implemented somewhat differently by each of the Uniformed Services, the Family Advocacy Program (FAP) is the DoD-mandated program intended to prevent and treat child and spouse abuse (see Chapter 4). Social workers from all seven MTFs reported that referrals to the FAP have been largely unaffected by the advent of TRICARE. Network providers do not refer suspected maltreatment to the FAP any more frequently than CHAMPUS providers did. FAP social workers at two installations having agreements with state child protective services (CPS) to cover reporting of cases by CPS to the FAP confirmed that they have not received cases from CPS that originated with TRICARE providers.

The only substantive change in patterns of incoming referrals has occurred at medium and smaller military facilities where closure of the emergency service has ended ER referrals to the FAP. In these locations, active duty personnel and other beneficiaries must now use emergency services at civilian facilities. These facilities must report suspected child abuse to the local CPS agency, which may result in a referral to the FAP depending on state law and local agreements. A problem arises with suspected spouse abuse because so few states have mandatory reporting laws. Civilian facilities may or may not be aware of FAP services available on the post or base. One FAP director stated that she was actively seeking to execute agreements with local civilian emergency services to cover referrals of families in suspected spouse abuse situations.

Most FAPs offer the bulk of the maltreatment intervention services provided to their clients. FAP clients with substantiated cases of maltreatment and with active intervention plans receive priority for mental health services at some military facilities. When clients voice their preference to seek mental health services with civilian TRICARE providers, FAP providers are generally receptive, so long as a release of information can be executed. This allows the social workers to learn about client treatment attendance and about the effectiveness of the treatment in reducing the risk of further maltreatment. Thus, FAP providers must be familiar with the methods for making referrals under TRICARE. Determining clearance for overseas travel of FAP families is generally not a problem because the majority of services to such families are provided and documented by the FAP staff. The Service central registry of substantiated cases can be consulted for any incidents occurring at prior bases. Thus, the FAP is the area of military social work practice least affected by TRICARE.

Other Effects of TRICARE

As the military direct care system has adopted managed care principles, many military facility social workers have worried about the financial costs to patients when they are moved from military facility inpatient care to their homes when they have some continuing medical needs that may not be covered by TRICARE benefits. These patients are more reliant on any available informal support systems to obtain the assistance they need. Some military medical social workers have become adept at assisting patients in obtaining Medicaid, Medicare, or other state benefits for home care.

A significant issue for Prime patients at most facilities was the limited range of some specialty services in the Prime network, especially child and adolescent mental health services. Providers in high-demand specialties are frequently reluctant to accept the reduced fees generally associated with joining the contractor's network. The Prime patient is restricted to the available network providers, so they can seek the often more experienced nonnetwork specialty providers only by incurring prohibitive point-of-service costs.

Concern was also expressed for patients' confusion about TRICARE options and requirements as they made their health care choices.

These decisions can be difficult when family members have complex medical needs and incorrect choices can be costly, either in financial terms or in terms of freedom of choice of favored providers or types of care. Although most families with members having exceptional medical needs were initially urged to enroll these members in the lower-cost TRICARE Prime, some learned that they could not obtain their preferred providers or forms of treatment except under the point-of-service option. One social worker reported on the difficulties some patients have had in getting the MCS contractor to reimburse emergency care obtained while traveling.

Another issue mentioned by the social workers interviewed is the accurate clearance of active-duty family members accompanying their military sponsor to overseas assignments. Reductions in military forces have greatly reduced the availability of military medical services overseas. The implementation of TRICARE overseas is greatly hampered by local differences in language, culture, and medical care standards. To the extent that TRICARE places active duty family members in the contractor's network for care, these families will have incomplete military medical records. Accordingly, there will be increased risk that family members could be cleared for overseas travel in error. Some of these family members would suffer from the paucity or absence of needed services, and as a result the military might incur the additional costs of returning the family to an area where needed care is available. Unfortunately, some active duty members and their families may minimize their special needs to avoid losing a desired assignment.

Some social workers expressed anxiety for social work department staff as they experienced increased pressures for efficiency in delivering services, which frequently resulted in less time to work with patients. They voiced their ethical dilemmas in making care arrangements when the focus on reducing costs competes with patient and family benefits. Some felt that the staff at their agencies was increasingly stressed since the advent of TRICARE while others reported that they had learned to cope with the different and sometimes more extensive demands after an initial period of confusion and stress. Many of the examples given seemed to reflect the traditional conflict for military and other social workers between functioning as client advocates and as agents of social control. Some expressed their excitement because of TRICARE's recognition of the value of social work services, and because of the opportunities for personal and professional development as they faced new TRICARE challenges.

REFERENCES

Boyer, J. and Sobel, L. (1993). CHAMPUS and the Department of Defense managed care program. In Kongstvedt, P. (Ed.), *The Managed Health Care Handbook* (Second Edition). Gaithersburg, MD: Aspen, pp. 382-391.

Congressional Budget Office (1995). *Restructuring Military Medical Care.* Washington, DC: CBO Papers.

General Accounting Office (1995). *Defense Health Care: Issues and Challenges Confronting Military Medicine: Report to Congressional Requesters*. Washington, DC: GAO/HEHS-95-104.

General Accounting Office (1996). *Defense Health Care: New Managed Care Plan Progressing, But Cost and Performance Issues Remain.* Letter Report. Washington, DC: GAO/HEHS-96-128.

General Accounting Office (1997a). *Defense Health Program: Future Costs Are Likely to Be Greater Than Estimated.* Briefing Report. Washington, DC: GAO/NSAID-97-83BR.

General Accounting Office (1997b). *Military Retiree Health Care: Costs and Other Implications of Options to Enhance Older Retirees Benefits.* Letter Report. Washington, DC: GAO/HEHS-97-134.

General Accounting Office (1998). *Defense Health Care: DoD Could Improve Its Beneficiary Feedback Approaches.* Letter Report. Washington, DC: GAO/HEHS-98-51.

Office of Assistant Secretary of Defense, Health Affairs (1997). *Policy 97-41: Use of Medical Treatment Facilities by TRICARE Prime Enrollees.* Washington, DC: Office of Assistant Secretary of Defense, Health Affairs.

TRICARE (1997a). *TRICARE Standard Handbook.* Denver, CO: TRICARE Support Office.

TRICARE (1997b, August). TRICARE Support Office Fact Sheet 1. Denver, CO: TRICARE Support Office.

TRICARE (1997c). *DoD Health Services Region Map.* Denver CO: TRICARE Support Office.

Chapter 6

Military Social Work Practice in Substance Abuse Programs

Richard Newsome

Structured provision of substance abuse treatment in the military dates back to 1971 federal legislation sponsored by Senator Harold Hughes of Iowa. Through Senator Hughes' efforts, Public Law 92-129 was enacted, mandating a program for the identification and treatment of drug and alcohol dependent individuals in the armed forces. Senator Hughes' focus on the establishment of substance abuse treatment services at the federal level was at least partially related to his own publicly revealed recovery status.

CONCEPTUAL MODEL FOR SUBSTANCE ABUSE PREVENTION AND TREATMENT SERVICES IN THE MILITARY

Substance abuse prevention and treatment in the military is primarily a readiness activity. It parallels the Employee Assistance Program (EAP) activities in civilian institutions. It is unlike civilian EAPs, which are primarily driven by the economic benefits derived from a stable and healthy workforce (Claunch, 1996). Military substance abuse prevention and treatment programs are primarily targeted at assuring force readiness.

"Constructive confrontation" has been the basic approach for dealing with substance abuse prevention and treatment in the occupational

---

The opinions expressed in this chapter are the author's and do not represent United States Air Force policy or opinion.

setting (Strauss and Sayles, 1980). Constructive confrontation calls for supervisors to confront unacceptable performance solely on the basis of deficiencies in performance. In a constructive manner, the confronted individual is told about the consequences of continued unacceptable performance and offered nonpunitive, nonjudgmental rehabilitative help (Trice and Beyer, 1982). As much as possible, the constructive confrontation avoids using diagnostic labels in the referral process (Trice and Roman, 1972).

Fundamentally, all military substance abuse prevention and treatment programs have operated on the basis of constructive confrontation concepts. Effective constructive confrontation has strongly depended on coordinated efforts between the military member's commander addressing the individual's behavior and substance abuse treatment personnel offering hope through behavior change avenues. This combination of confrontation and resources for help provides the type of motivation for change that Perlman (1957) referred to in her definition of motivation as the combination of discomfort plus hope.

DEVELOPMENT OF SUBSTANCE ABUSE TREATMENT PROGRAMS IN THE ARMED FORCES

With the enactment of PL 92-129, each branch of the armed forces established its own substance abuse treatment program. Early in the military's provision of substance abuse treatment services, the primary treatment model was the twelve-step model of Alcoholics Anonymous. The status of "being in recovery" was often the primary criterion for being a provider of substance abuse recovery services. Both inpatient and outpatient programs relied heavily on a twelve-step treatment model.

A paraprofessional approach to substance abuse service delivery continued through the early 1980s. In the Army and the Navy, there was a strong reliance on using individuals recovering from their own alcohol use disorders. The Army established the counselor role as a specific duty position. In the Navy, the counselor role functioned as an additional duty, with the counselor maintaining a Navy operations role as his or her primary duty designation. In the Air Force, the provision of substance abuse services was assigned to the Department of Personnel. Rehabilitative services were provided by paraprofessional counselors assigned to a multiservice agency called Social Actions. Along with addressing substance abuse issues, this agency was also responsible for addressing employee relations, racial relations, and equal opportunity issues.

The Air Force substance abuse evaluation process combined an initial assessment by the Social Actions counselor and a subsequent assessment by the medical consultant. The medical consultant roles were primarily filled by active-duty social workers assigned to the base mental health clinic. Only the medical consultant was authorized to render an alcohol use disorder diagnosis.

The treatment regimen for individuals given an alcohol dependence or alcohol abuse diagnosis was generally a referral to one of the regionalized inpatient treatment centers operating a fixed-interval twenty-eight-day inpatient treatment program. Following discharge from the inpatient program, the individual participated in outpatient counseling at Social Actions. Mental health providers assigned to the base medical facility generally had minimal direct involvement in the delivery of follow-up (aftercare) substance abuse treatment services.

A major change in the identification and treatment of substance abusers in the Air Force occurred in the early 1980s when a new policy mandated referral for evaluation following any incident in which substance abuse was suspected. Prior to 1980, referral for an incident was at the discretion of the individual's commander.

Discretionary referral had the potential to set the "bar" quite high to determine how bad is bad enough. Referrals tended to be delayed in identification of substance abuse problems. Individuals in their first term of enlistment (generally the first four years of active duty) and, interestingly enough, individuals nearing retirement were the primary referral groups. Referring those nearing retirement appeared to reflect the extent the individual's alcohol use disorder was known by the commander but had not been addressed earlier. Referrals of mid-career individuals were rare.

With the change in policy, commanders were required to refer any individual in his or her unit involved in an incident in which substance abuse was suspected. Although the mandated referral requirement may have appeared to be a loss in a commander's authority, it functioned to benefit commanders by being no longer required to prediagnose. During the era of discretionary referrals following incidents, referred individuals had a tendency to question whether the commander had decided that the individual was an "alcoholic." With mandatory referral, commanders were no longer in a position of having to prediagnose and provide supporting evidence to justify the referral. Instead of providing an extensive explanation to support a discretionary referral, the commander, by citing the mandatory referral policy, could state he or she did not know whether or not the individual had a substance abuse problem. The commander could state that the point of the referral was to assess the presence of a substance abuse problem.

Establishment of the mandatory policy quickly led to an increase in the number and types of referrals. A broader spectrum of individuals was seen. Those who were seen tended to be referred at earlier phases of substance abuse problems. The transition to mandatory referral functioned to enhance the prevention potential of more extensively developed substance abuse problems. This change was a benefit to the individual and his or her family, as well as the military.

CERTIFICATION/PROFESSIONALIZATION

During the era of fixed-interval treatment, the Air Force operated twelve regionalized treatment programs. The program director was almost always a clinical social worker with a physician supervising medical management of the inpatients. Prior to 1986, the program directors were not required to have any specialized training in substance abuse. In 1986, the Air Force directed that all inpatient treatment staff should be certified as substance abuse counselors. The Air Force established reciprocal certification privileges with the International Certification and Reciprocity Consortium (ICRC). Once Air Force certification had been obtained, it could be used to obtain state certification. The Air Force was the first armed forces service to establish reciprocal certification relationships with state certification authorities.

With the advent of certification status for addiction counselors, each service took steps toward a more professional level of service delivery. Each service made a commitment to service providers achieving certification status. The Army at Fort Sam Houston, San

Antonio, Texas, and the Air Force at Sheppard Air Force Base, Wichita Falls, Texas, established training programs specifically for substance abuse counselors. The Navy established an extensive structured internship program (United States Navy, 1991a, b) for the training of substance abuse counselors.

CHANGES IN TREATMENT MODALITY

Addictions treatment historian Ernest Kurtz has suggested that all substance abuse treatment primarily involves two steps (Kurtz, 1979). Step One occurs when the individual comes to the belief that he or she cannot use that drug safely. Step Two focuses on the individual recognizing that he or she has the personal power to choose not to drink. In other words, Step One focuses on the person recognizing that there is no way he or she can drink safely. But Step Two focuses on the person's recognition that he or she has the choice of not drinking. In other words, "I *can* not drink" is the belief indicating self-control over the choice of drinking. The person is choosing abstinence. Achievement of Kurtz's Step Two requires the development of skills associated with having the ability to make the choice to not engage in the addictive behavior.

From the perspective of Kurtz's typology, armed forces substance abuse programs through most of the 1970s and 1980s were primarily Step One programs with Step Two a function of the outpatient program mainly through focus on active participation in AA. By the mid-1980s, there were initiatives developing skill-based treatment approaches requiring more than acknowledgment of addiction as the goal of initial treatment.

The development of skill-based approaches was enhanced in the late 1980s with an individualized treatment focus heralded by the Joint Commission on the Accreditation of Healthcare Organizations (JCAHO). Providing individualized treatment flew in the face of what had been for many treatment programs a "cookie cutter" approach to treatment, with all individuals going through the same treatment program for the same length of time.

Moving into the 1990s, military treatment programs, paralleling practices in the civilian sector, were placing an increasing emphasis on outpatient treatment following relatively brief inpatient stays when required. As the shift to outpatient service delivery occurred, accomplishing both of Kurtz's steps became more a function for provision by outpatient service providers.

Paralleling the moves in the civilian community to individualize treatment plans and lengths, a reduction was made in the early 1990s in the number of Department of Defense (DoD) inpatient treatment facilities. Using the American Society of Addiction Medicine (ASAM) criteria for determining level of care, the trend for treatment of alcohol use disorders diagnosed under DSM-IV criteria moved toward outpatient rather than inpatient treatment. This trend also paralleled practice pattern changes in the civilian community.

With the use of ASAM criteria for determining level of care, most active duty members with diagnosed alcohol use disorders do not meet the criteria for extended inpatient treatment. This is primarily due to the relatively early identification of alcohol use disorders that can be accomplished in the military with the must-refer criteria following an incident. The level of substance abuse severity for active duty members is often well short of the extensive biological/medical consequences that might be seen in a civilian population of individuals with alcohol use disorders.

With the intent to meet JCAHO standards for certification, military treatment programs by the early 1990's were developing individualized treatment programs identifying a broad spectrum of issues specific to the individual. These treatment plans addressed areas such as nuclear family issues, family of origin issues, physical, and emotional well being, spiritual issues, and job skill issues.

The potential for losing focus on the individual's addiction/alcohol use disorder was an undesired outcome from individualized treatment plans addressing a broad spectrum of issues. Patients would often be quite willing to address marital problems or communication problems but maintained a high level of avoidance in addressing changes directly associated with substance use. Counselors, perceiving the need to address all problems identified in the individualized treatment plan, were vulnerable to losing perspective on the priority of addressing the addiction/alcohol use disorder.

One technique developed for addressing loss of focus by the patient, as well as the counselor, was utilizing repeated measuring techniques that gauged the individual's progress in moving from denial to acceptance of his or her alcohol use disorder (Newsome and Ditzler, 1993). Repeated assessment of the individual's progress was included in reports to supervisory staff as well as to the patient. All parties involved had a more structured process for ensuring maintained focus on the addiction while efforts were made to address the additional identified individual problems.

SOCIAL WORKER SKILLS FOR PROVIDING SUBSTANCE ABUSE SERVICES IN THE MILITARY

Substance-abusing individuals in the military tend to be identified at earlier levels of abuse due to the mandatory referral requirements. Early identification presents challenges to service providers in conducting substance abuse prevention and treatment. The individual undergoing assessment will be better armed to minimize his or her alcohol use disorder by asserting the ability to maintain employment and overall physical well being. The treatment staff has to develop skills in detecting relatively early levels of alcohol use disorder. Assessment needs to be multimodal in methodology to ensure a comprehensive assessment. Collateral information from supervisors and family, if available, are important to supplement the individual's self-reports. The use of screening instruments with well-established sensitivity and specificity such as the World Health Organization's Alcohol Use Disorders Identification Test (AUDIT) (Saunders et al., 1993) is critical to enhance the accuracy of assessments.

Due to the frequency of relatively early identification of an alcohol use disorder, successful practice with a population of military members having alcohol use disorders often requires well-developed skills in constructive confrontation. The practitioner may need to focus extensively on the risks of continued alcohol use to enhance the individual's investment in behavioral changes. This utilization of "leverage" to remain in the military may initially be the only investment the individual has in considering the impact of the alcohol abuse. The individual developing awareness of additional reasons for changing in drinking behavior and developing skills enhancing sobriety may also require much collateral input and involvement from supervisors, peers, and family.

ADDRESSING ILLEGAL DRUG USE IN THE ARMED FORCES

During the early 1980s, there was a period in which individuals with a substance abuse problem involving illegal drugs could be treated under the Limited Privilege Communication Program (LPCP). Numerous program restrictions ensured that an individual did not use the program to avoid prosecution for behavior that was under investigation. The LPCP program was replaced in the mid-1980s by the "zero tolerance" concept. Under zero tolerance, any report by self or others regarding illegal drug use could result at a minimum in administrative discharge if not criminal prosecution.

Recognizing the potential for experimental use by younger people, the Army encourages commanders to utilize administrative and disciplinary actions short of discharge for junior enlisted individuals identified for marijuana use (Army Regulation 600-85, 1996). If marijuana or any other illegal drug is used by a noncommissioned officer (enlisted grade of E-5 or higher) or by a commissioned officer, all of the armed forces branches pursue separating the member from the military.

In the Air Force, self-reporting of personal illegal drug use remained at the individual's peril until the establishment of the Alcohol and Drug Abuse Prevention and Control (ADAPT) program in January 1998. Under the ADAPT program (Air Force Instruction 44-121, 1998), self-identification of personal illegal drug use was given limited protection from criminal prosecution as long as the self-report was not made to avoid prosecution in an ongoing investigation. The new limited privilege program carries the protection from criminal prosecution of the old LPCP program, but does not include treatment by the Air Force for illegal drug use. Treatment is available from the Veteran's Administration in association with an administrative discharge from the military.

Congressionally mandated guidance requires the expenditure of funds to address the prevention of illegal drug use by military members. The prevention efforts are referred to as "demand reduction." Each service has a program designed to conduct drug demand reduction activities. Military social workers, whether or not they are directly involved in conducting the prevention-oriented drug demand reduction activities, often are involved in supervising the deliverers of drug demand reduction activities.

The demand reduction programs often function as a cooperative effort between the active duty armed forces units and the state National Guard units. During the 1990s, National Guard units, with their local community basing, have taken active roles in conducting drug demand reduction activities.

The National Interagency Counterdrug Institute (NICI) is a specific drug demand reduction resource funded by DoD through the National Guard Bureau. NICI, located in San Luis Obispo, California, conducts training for both military and civilian individuals in conducting drug demand reduction activities.

Drug Testing Program

During the 1996 presidential campaign, both major candidates addressed the reports of increasing drug use among high school seniors. While each candidate attempted to put the responsibility for the increase on the other candidate's political party, neither denied that during the 1990s there has been an increase in drug use by high school students. One study of reported marijuana use in the previous thirty days by high school seniors found a reversal in the steady trend of decreased use during the 1980s to a steady trend of increased use since the early 1990s. Although the reported rate in 1996 of approximately 25 percent of high school seniors using marijuana in the previous thirty days was below the peak reported rates of the 1970s, which neared 40 percent, the steady upward trend in the 1990s suggests a change in attitude toward increased acceptance of drug use (Manning, 1997).

Increased use as well as acceptance of illegal drug use by the nation's youth is especially of concern to the armed forces since new military members come primarily from the nation's population of young people. The average new recruit is in his or her late teens or early twenties. Individuals coming into the armed forces in the later 1990s have lived their most recent six or seven years in environments of increasing drug use as well as increasing acceptance of drug use. Historically, drug use levels for new recruits have mirrored the rate reported for American high school seniors (Romberg et al., 1993).

Considering the armed forces' zero tolerance policy toward illegal drug use, education about the policy and monitoring compliance is especially important with a contrast between norms in the civilian and military sectors. Military substance abuse prevention and treatment program managers, often social workers, have the additional responsibility of ensuring the lowest possible illegal drug use in the armed forces to maximize the military's operational readiness.

Unlike the national trend of increased drug use during the 1990s, in DoD there has been no upward trend in the 1990s (Bray, 1996). The Worldwide Survey of Alcohol and Nonmedical Drug Use Among Military Personnel has revealed a relatively stable level of drug use in the military over the past ten years (Bray, 1996). The self-reported rates by active duty military members of any illegal drug use in the past thirty days declined from 6 percent to 3 percent during the first half of the 1990s.

The Worldwide Survey is an externally contracted study conducted primarily in five-year intervals since 1980. It includes an anonymous sample of approximately 20,000 active duty members with extensive matching for accurate proportions by service, gender, and rank.

As with any self-report instrument, there can be concerns regarding accuracy. One measure that provides additional reliability for the self-reports of the Worldwide Survey is the drug testing program's detection rate for illegal drug use. In 1995, the self-report rate by Air Force members for any illegal drug use in the past thirty days was 1 percent (Bray, 1996). The rate of positive drug tests in the Air Force for 1995 was .7 percent. This close agreement between reported and detected levels of use serves to enhance confidence in the accuracy of the Worldwide Surveys' self-reports.

The relative stability over the past ten years in the rate of reported illegal drug use has the potential for creating a picture that distorts historical appreciation of changes that have occurred over the past twenty years. The Worldwide Survey results in 1980 indicated that the rate of illegal drug use during the previous thirty days was 28 percent. More than one out of four active members reported engaging in illegal drug use during the previous thirty days.

Prior to 1980, DoD did not conduct routine testing for tetrahydrocannabinol (THC), an active ingredient of cannabis/marijuana. Drug testing for THC prior to 1980 was by specific request. Early in the

Reagan Administration, the decision was made to routinely test for marijuana (THC).

Initiation of routine testing for marijuana use did not immediately achieve the more recently experienced relatively low reported levels of drug use (Allen and Mazzuchi, 1985). Close examination of the 1982 Worldwide Survey results revealed a low confidence level in the armed forces of the drug testing program results. Only 36 percent of the survey respondents believed the drug tests were reliable (Bray, 1983).

The confidence issues were at least partially related to startup problems in quality control that the drug testing laboratories experienced. Other confidence problems were related to the difficulty commanders had in believing that an identified individual was actually a user. This difficulty in trusting the accuracy of the results was at least partially associated with an institutional belief that drug users would be obviously incapacitated individuals and could easily be identified. When someone in more senior enlisted or officer ranks was identified as testing positive for illegal drug use, the individual's overall performance of meeting or exceeding standards was often used as evidence that he or she could not possibly be engaging in illegal drug use.

Belief that obvious deterioration in work performance must accompany illegal drug use reflected stereotypical characterizations of drug culture youth from the 1960s and 1970s. Experience in providing rehabilitation services in the occupational setting often suggests just the opposite picture. A substance-abusing employee's performance may belie the actual extent of the substance abuse. This is not a new observation. The AA book written in the late 1930s, *Alcoholics Anonymous*, often referred to as "The Big Book," in its chapter "To Employers" speaks of substance-abusing employees in the following terms:

> A look at the alcoholic in your organization is many times illuminating. Is he [she] not unusually brilliant, fast thinking, imaginative and likable? When sober, does he [she] not work hard and have a knack of getting things done? If he [she] had these qualities and did not drink, would he [she] be worth retaining? (Alcoholics Anonymous, 1939, p. 139)

It is not atypical for an individual engaged in illegal drug use to be perceived as a superior performer. Investment in performance often functions for the individual as a means for self-denial of addiction as well as a means to defend self from external confrontations—"If I was a user, how could I possibly be performing so well?"

The employed drug-using individual is often quite economically motivated to maintain job performance standards to ensure the income needed to purchase drugs. The effort to maintain job performance standards can often result in overcompensation, with focus on maintaining employment functioning at the expense of all other relationships. A vicious cycle functions between the focus on job performance and maintaining a financial resource for drug use. Stress mounts as the individual dually tries to perform at a level high enough to hide problems and seeks relief through drug use. This cycle is set up for an eventual collapse, with either the loss of the ability to physically maintain the desired performance level or the increasing drug use reaching a point that causes incapacitation.

Not surprisingly, early in the period of implementing routine testing for marijuana use, commanders were able to discount initial results detecting illegal drug use if subsequent repeated tests were negative for illegal drug use. Although the subsequent negative findings may have served the function of disavowing the initial result, it could not be determined that the negative findings were not the result of the individual discontinuing use after initial detection.

By 1985, the Worldwide Survey was finding that confidence in the testing results had markedly improved. Over 80 percent of the survey respondents believed the results of the drug tests were reliable (Bray, 1986). The increased confidence related to improved quality control at the testing laboratories and to commanders more consistently taking action on initial results. As military members more frequently experienced peers being separated from the military for drug use, the perceived risk of illegal drug use being detected by the drug testing program increased.

The relatively low, stable rate of drug use in DoD over the past ten years appears to show that a drug testing program can be highly effective if it:

1. tests for the actual drugs being abused;
2. is perceived as reliable and professionally managed; and
3. applies undesired consequences to those the program detects.

In addition to testing active-duty members for illegal drug use, the armed forces also tests selected civilian DoD members. President Reagan issued Executive Order 12564 in 1986, establishing the goal of a drug-free federal workplace. Department of Defense Directive (DoDD) 1010.9 was published in 1988. It established authority for a civilian drug testing program, defined policy, described procedures, and assigned responsibilities.

With the establishment of DoDD 1010.9, each service developed its own specific drug testing program for civilians. Testing focused on individuals whose drug use might most affect mission accomplishment or pose a high risk for injury to personnel or property. These positions were labeled Testing Designated Positions. Unlike the military program, the civilian program does not randomly test all civilian DoD employees.

Outcome Assessment

Assessment of outcome by armed forces substance abuse treatment programs has historically been a piecemeal process, with various local programs conducting outcome studies. These studies have primarily looked at outcome intervals of twelve months or less.

Systematic assessment of outcome—especially beyond twelve months—has been lacking in armed forces programs. Due to the relatively transient nature of the military lifestyle, it is difficult for local treatment providers to conduct long-term studies. Many of the individuals who received services from a local program will not be in the local area two years later.

Although it might appear that armed forces centralized computer databases could support longer-term outcome studies on individuals receiving substance abuse treatment services, systematic assessment has not been accomplished. The primary barrier has been concern that longer-term follow-up may reidentify an individual as a one-time substance abuser. In the context of the armed forces, a premium is placed on an individual's record being "clean." Long-term codings that reflect a history of substance abuse treatment could easily be perceived as a potential factor that might restrict an opportunity for promotion or a desired assignment.

The establishment in January 1998 of the Air Force's Alcohol and Drug Abuse Prevention and Treatment Program (ADAPT) included for the first time in the Air Force, a requirement that all treatment programs —inpatient and outpatient—conduct follow-up at the three-, six-, and twelve-month posttreatment intervals on the drinking behavior and duty performance of all individuals who received substance abuse treatment. This initiative provides the first opportunity for a force-wide effort to assess outcome.

Ethical Aspects

Unlike civilian EAP programs, which generally subcontract/outsource the actual provision of services, the military uses its own force members to provide services. Substance abuse prevention and treatment service provision by military members to military members creates a primary ethical dilemma for military social workers. In the delivery of services to the individual, the social worker is responsible for assuring the armed forces that the individual is capable of performing his or her national defense duties. Fundamentally, the military social worker must develop skills to maintain a delicate balance based on a relationship of trust with the individual receiving services and a trust with the armed forces that necessary information will be provided for preventing incidents negatively affecting the mission.

These necessary trust relationships result from actively working with both client groups—the individual, including his or her family, and the service provider's armed forces branch. The substance abuse prevention and treatment social worker in the military must directly communicate to service recipients these dual roles. He or she must communicate competency in effectively discriminating between information that remains in the treatment relationship and information that is shared with the individual's commander. The social worker's effective balancing of roles ultimately depends on the level of trust both direct and indirect service recipients develop in the social worker's judgment.

Establishment of trust relationships with commanders requires being known by commanders. The social worker must make time to get out to the commander's unit to develop the type of relationship that will enhance the commander's trust in the social worker's communication and noncommunication of information on individuals receiving substance abuse prevention and treatment services. Many of the problems that can arise in providing substance abuse prevention and treatment services in the military can be prevented and alleviated through the nurturing of trust relationships with both the individual receiving services and his or her commander.

REFERENCES

Air Force Instruction 44-121 (1998). *Alcohol and Drug Abuse Prevention and Treatment (ADAPT) Program.* United States Air Force.

Alcoholics Anonymous (1939). *Alcoholics Anonymous.* New York: Alcoholics Anonymous World Services, Inc.

Allen, J. and Mazzuchi, J. (1985). Alcohol and drug abuse among American military personnel: Prevalence and policy implications. *Alcohol and Research World, 150*(5), 250-255.

Army Regulation 600-85 (1996). *Alcohol and Drug Abuse Prevention and Control Program.* United States Army.

Bray, R.M. (1983). *1982 Worldwide Survey of Alcohol and Nonmedical Drug Use Among Military Personnel.* Research Triangle Park, NC: Research Triangle Institute.

Bray, R.M. (1986). *1985 Worldwide Survey of Alcohol and Nonmedical Drug Use Among Military Personnel.* Research Triangle Park, NC: Research Triangle Institute.

Bray, R.M. (1996). *1995 Worldwide Survey of Alcohol and Nonmedical Drug Use Among Military Personnel.* Research Triangle Park, NC: Research Triangle Institute.

Claunch, T. (1996, March). An EAP—An American Historical Perspective. Paper presented at the Third National Conference on Alcohol and Other Drugs in the Workplace, Sydney, Australia.

Kurtz, E. (1979). *Not God: A History of Alcoholics Anonymous.* Minneapolis, MN: Hazelden Educational Services.

Manning, A. (1997, August 7). Teen drug abuse decline yields hope. *USA Today,* p. 3D.

Newsome, R.D. and Ditzler, T. (1993). Assessing alcoholic denial: Further examination of the denial rating scale. *Journal of Nervous and Mental Disease, 181*(11), 689-694.

Perlman, H.H. (1957). *Social Casework: A Problem-Solving Process.* Chicago: University of Chicago Press.

Romberg, R.W., Needleman, S.B., Porvaznik, M., Past, M., and Beasley, W. (1993). Effect of pre-enlistment testing on the confirmed drug-positive rate for Navy recruits. *Military Medicine, 158*(1):14-19.

Saunders, J.B., Aasland, O.G., Babor, T.F., de la Fuente, J.R., and Grant, M. (1993). Development of the alcohol use disorders identification test (AUDIT): WHO collaborative project on early detection of persons with harmful alcohol consumption—II. *Addiction, 88*(6), 791-804.

Strauss, G. and Sayles, L.R. (1980). *Personnel: The Human Problems of Management.* Englewood Cliffs, NJ: Prentice Hall, Inc.

Trice, H.M. and Beyer, J.M. (1982). Social control in worksettings: Using the constructive confrontation strategy with problem-drinking employees. *Journal of Drug Issues, 12*(1), 21-49.

Trice, H.M. and Roman, P.M. (1972). *Spirits and Demons at Work: Alcohol and Other Drugs on the Job.* Ithaca, NY: Cornell University, New York School of Industrial and Labor Relations.

United States Navy (1991a). *Structured Internship: Counselor/Intern Workbook.* Windsor, CT: ETP, Inc.

United States Navy (1991b). *Structured Internship: Clinical Supervision Guidelines.* Windsor, CT: ETP, Inc.

Chapter 7

Medical Social Work in the U.S. Armed Forces

Nancy K. Raiha

Soldiers, sailors, airmen, retirees, and family members face illness, injury, dismemberment, and death in times of both war and peace. Medical social workers assist these patients and their families in coping with medical conditions, resolving psychosocial issues, and implementing plans for further care and adaptation.

HISTORICAL BACKGROUND

The beginnings of medical social work practice in the U.S. military can be traced back to the Civil War, when volunteers visited hospitalized Union soldiers. Subsequently, the American Red Cross was the primary source of social services for soldiers. World War I saw the emergence of a social work staff for military hospitals. The American Red Cross assigned a psychiatric worker to the military hospital at Plattsburgh, New York in September 1918. This worker was assigned five enlisted men to assist in the social work mission. The Red Cross continued to staff seventeen military hospitals with social work personnel between World Wars I and II. Additionally, visiting nurses from the Navy Relief Society provided counseling and social service referral to sailors and their families.

The opinions expressed in this chapter are the author's and should not be interpreted as the policy or opinions of the United States Army. The author gratefully acknowledges the assistance of USA Colonel Elwood Hamlin; USAF Major Sarah Moore; Ken Lee, DA Civilian Social Worker; and many medical social workers throughout the Department of Defense.

Much of the massive need for social services for medical patients in World War II was met by American Red Cross and Navy Relief Society volunteers and staff, along with physicians, nurses, psychologists, and patient affairs officers. Social workers joining the armed forces often worked as enlisted men in psychiatric settings. In 1945 the Army designated its first commissioned social work officer (Garber and McNelis, 1995). At the end of World War II, the Navy Relief Society employed its first professional social worker (Medical Service Corps, 1997).

The years following World War II were marked by a decrease in medical social work services provided by the American Red Cross and a buildup of Army social work programs. In 1951 the Red Cross withdrew support of medical and surgical social work activities. The medical social work orientation within the Army was accelerated. Most Army hospitals contained an independent Social Work Service that included medical-surgical and maternal/child sections. The Navy, lacking a military social work program, and the Air Force, emphasizing psychiatric social work services, continued to rely on the diminishing medical social services provided by the American Red Cross and Navy Relief Society.

The disparity between the services' medical social work programs reached a critical level in the 1970s. The American Red Cross further withdrew from the provision of psychosocial services. The Joint Commission on the Accreditation of Hospitals required all hospitals to have a social work program. In 1979, only twenty-nine civilian social workers were employed in naval hospitals. The Air Force's social work program was more robust, but primarily focused on psychiatric services. Neither service could meet the standards for hospital social work set by accrediting agencies and civilian practice. By the early 1980s both the Navy and Air Force were establishing medical social work sections in accordance with Joint Commission on Hospital standards. The first uniformed Navy social worker was commissioned. By 1985, the largest Air Force hospital employed social workers in nephrology, hematology/oncology, neonatal and pediatric intensive care, rehabilitation medicine, and adult medical and surgical intensive care units.

For all three services, the 1980s were marked by a stabilization of the medical social work role. Before the large-scale implementation of managed care, most patients remained in the hospital until they were able to return home. Medical social workers concerned themselves primarily with permanent nursing home placements, home health needs, financial assistance, psychosocial issues, crisis intervention, grief, and problem or unwanted pregnancies. The relatively lengthy hospitalizations allowed for the establishment of therapeutic relationships over time. The amount of time available for clinical services varied according to patient ratio and workload. Special funding for the treatment of patients with HIV enriched many hospitals with the addition of social workers with expertise in catastrophic illness.

TODAY'S MEDICAL SOCIAL WORKER

The 1990s have ushered in an era of change and variation. Military health care reflects the changing face of U.S. health care. The advent of managed care and resultant dramatic changes in the delivery of health care have led to definitive changes in medical social work. The structure and roles in today's medical social worker's world vary throughout the military and through each of the services. The following paragraphs summarize current trends.

Multidisciplinary Structure

Social workers continue to provide medical social work in most military hospitals, but the structure in which they work varies widely. Reengineering initiatives, the move away from a standardized hospital structure prescribed by the medical higher headquarters (Cameron, 1993), and the Joint Commission's emphasis on interdisciplinary cooperation have resulted in a variety of structural models for medical social work, discharge planning, and case management. Some hospitals maintain a separate social work service or department of social work that includes a medical social work section. In other medical treatment facilities, medical social work is decentralized or enfolded into another department. A 1996 survey of thirty-nine Army medical treatment facilities (Hamlin, Pehrson, and Gemmill, 1996) found that 43 percent had experienced or expected a structural reorganization of social work services. Whatever the structural model, medical social workers function in close partnership with nurses, utilization management staff, and specific medical functional areas or "product lines." The roles of each discipline in providing care for a specific medical problem is often standardized as a "clinical pathway." In a number of military hospitals, the traditional organization by department and medical specialty is supplemented by interdisciplinary groups working on related functions and processes. Because of social work's systems orientation and integration with services throughout the hospital, social workers find themselves included in almost every facet of hospital functions, including inpatient services, primary care, family practice, specialty care, intensive care, emergency care, mental health, and health promotion. In fact, military social workers routinely are assigned on faculty teaching positions in family practice residency programs.

Varied Roles and Functions

The roles and functions assumed by medical social workers also vary among medical facilities. In most cases, psychosocial assessment and support, and assistance with complex family issues and adjustment to illness are provided by professional social workers. In a few smaller facilities social workers are removed from the medical arena, confining their activities to mental health, community, and family violence issues. The multidisciplinary process of discharge planning almost always includes social workers, but the extent of their involvement varies. In large medical centers with many complex cases, social workers generally continue to play a focal role in orchestrating safe and effective discharge plans. At Walter Reed, Tripler, and Madigan Army Medical Centers, and Balboa and Bethesda Naval Medical Centers, medical social workers are the primary coordinators of discharge plans. Social work discharge planners are experts in resource finding and medical benefits, as well as in identifying and addressing the concerns of patients and families. Social workers' unique strengths in providing discharge planning stems from the ability to simultaneously provide psychosocial and "concrete" services (Humphreys and Falck, 1990).

Case management is another role that may involve teamwork with a number of specialties. In the managed care environment, the case manager plays a vital role in keeping selected patients healthy, reducing reliance on physicians, and lowering costs. Social workers often play a leadership role in the management of cases involving psychosocial or community resource issues. Cases that involve medical monitoring are more often managed primarily by nurse case managers, and those which involve limiting costly expenditures are often managed by TRICARE case managers.

The initial screening for factors that may require medical social work assistance may be accomplished by nurses, physicians, social workers, or some combination of health care providers. Social workers may also be involved in mental health treatment, staff consultation, support for caregivers, and utilization review. They often play a major role in physician training programs and provide expertise to hospital human use and ethics committees. Most medical social workers find that an important part of their job involves providing support to health care providers facing the stress of a fast-paced, life-and-death environment. For example, military social workers on faculty in family practice residency programs offer all-day retreats for medical residents (e.g., family practice, obstetrics, pediatrics) that help normalize the medical care and training process. Many social workers have specialized in specific areas such as hemodialysis, neonatal intensive care, oncology, burns, emergency medicine, rehabilitation medicine, maternal/child issues, and developmental pediatrics.

TRICARE Contractor Role

As the delivery of military medical care converted to a managed care model, each Department of Defense health care region contracted with a civilian contractor to provide managed care services. (Also see Chapter 5 for an expanded discussion of TRICARE.) Each beneficiary has the choice of participating in a health maintenance organization (TRICARE Prime), preferred provider network (TRICARE Extra), or fee-for-service (TRICARE Standard) plan. Those who elect the more managed options have a more limited choice of providers, but pay a lower contribution to cost of care. The TRICARE contractor manages the HMO and preferred provider networks, and contracts for services the military medical treatment facilities in the region cannot provide. The extent to which the TRICARE contractor's employees are involved in case management and discharge planning varies between facilities and regions. Contractor employees are often involved in case management, especially in the fiscal management of high-cost cases. In some facilities they are also involved in discharge planning. Contractor services are often restricted to those groups eligible for TRICARE plans (usually active duty family members, retirees, and retiree family members under sixty-five), but in some cases the contractor may be involved in case management and discharge planning for active duty and Medicare-eligible patients. Even in locations such as Wilford Hall Air Force Medical Center and Brooke Army Medical Center in San Antonio, Texas, where most of the routine work of finding resources has been assumed by the TRICARE contractor, medical social workers assist with psychosocial problems, adjustment to illness, family issues, and crisis intervention.

Six military medical sites are presently participating in "Medicare subvention" demonstrations. Hospitals and their associated TRICARE contractors enroll a limited number of Medicare-age military retirees and their spouses in TRICARE Senior Prime, which will provide all TRICARE Prime benefits plus Medicare-unique benefits such as skilled nursing facility, home health, and durable medical equipment benefits. If hospitals provide more care to Medicare-eligible beneficiaries than in previous years, these hospitals receive additional funding from the Medicare budget.

Rapid Pace

The transition to managed care and to capitated budgeting has also brought many changes to military medical social work. When hospital budgets were based on the number of patient bed days, there was little pressure for swift discharges. In the new era of capitated budgets, a hospital's funding is based on the number of beneficiaries served. It is now in the hospital's best interest to minimize inpatient stays. The emphasis has shifted from an illness-based model to a wellness focused model. The push for rapid discharges that ensure patient well-being requires instant availability of social work staff and careful balancing of competing demands for rapid service. There is limited time to form therapeutic relationships. Discharge planning must often be initiated before a patient is hospitalized. Many patients who need assistance are never formally hospitalized; they receive ambulatory surgery or are housed for less than twenty-four hours in an observation unit. Social workers find the work of discharge planning places them under close scrutiny. For example, a multidisciplinary team at Madigan Army Medical Center is conducting a study of "avoidable days" (cases in which the patient remains in the hospital beyond the time he or she is medically ready for release). Any cases in which the social worker did not respond to consultation or coordinate a discharge plan in a timely manner are reported to hospital-wide oversight committees. Also, a daily discharge planning status report on all cases with extended stays is presented to the hospital commander.

Increased Complexity

The process of planning for a patient's continuing care needs has become increasingly complex in recent years. Advances in medicine have increased the survival rate for life-threatening conditions, but the surviving patients often require long-term intensive services (Stamper, 1998). The dramatic decrease in acute facility length of stay means that many patients are discharged with significant care needs. The process of arranging needed care has also become more complicated as each source of medical benefits develops its own managed care plan with individualized restrictions. Many patients have more than one source of health care benefits. The social worker must sort through multiple entitlements to determine which is primary, secondary, and tertiary. The discharge plan often depends on the entitlements of the patient's insurance plans and upon which community agencies have contracts with the insurers. Each potential payer has a voice in the post-hospitalization plan and the social worker must obtain an authorization for the planned care from each payer.

Focus on Outpatient and Primary Care

The managed care model focuses on keeping patients well in order to avoid costly episodes of illness. The primary care manager is the focal point of medical care. Social workers play an important role in keeping patients out of the hospital and preventing unnecessary outpatient visits and procedures. Social work functions include linking patients with community resources, overcoming barriers to compliance with medical recommendations, and providing psychosocial support and short-term mental health interventions. Numerous studies have shown that psychosocial interventions can significantly reduce the cost of medical care (Berkman, 1996; Cancer and the Mind, 1998; Cummins, 1994; Hearts and Minds, 1997). Many social workers are involved in the case management of "frequent flyer" patients (Rengo and Kune, 1995). Balboa Navy Medical Center has initiated a pilot case management program including home visits by social workers and nurses.

A number of military medical treatment facilities have instituted programs addressing critical health-related areas such as smoking, stress management, alcohol and drug abuse prevention, and early identification of hypertension. Social workers are involved in these programs at various levels from identification of patient needs to implementation and clinical interventions. The Wellness Program at Madigan Army Medical Center has found that patients who complete a four-session psychoeducational program emphasizing stress management and biofeedback have significantly fewer medical appointments than a control group. Another social worker at Madigan has reduced the need for gynecological surgery by using biofeedback to teach patients to strengthen pelvic floor muscles. Outpatient social workers are often physically located in the medical treatment facility's primary care clinics. Three large Army medical centers, Walter Reed, Tripler, and Madigan, have initiated aggressive and well-publicized outpatient medical social work programs. Bridges are being built between medical and community agencies to better serve soldiers and their family members. Examples include the WIC nutrition program, which is sponsored by Social Work Service at Tripler Army Medical Center, drop-in centers sponsored by military social workers and community agencies, and the planning of and participation in health fairs.

Emphasis on Measures

In the present era, health care delivery involves intensive resource management and frequent reengineering and downsizing (Berger et al., 1996). Each health care functional area must not only deliver a quality service, but also document the efficacy and cost effectiveness of that service (Scesny, 1997). Many military social work sections participate in local outcome studies designed to measure the efficiency and effectiveness of their services. The local hospital often reviews such studies regularly and compares performance with other civilian and military benchmarks. Also, the Department of Defense (Health Affairs) publishes standardized "report cards" summarizing local, regional, and national data on such issues as length of inpatient stays, utilization rates for selected diagnoses, health promotion activities, and inpatient treatment utilization rates. The future role of medical social workers in military facilities depends on the ability of social workers to show that their interventions are effective and contribute to a lower overall cost of medical care.

Change in Social Work Identity and Culture

In successfully coping with the demands for change presented above, military social workers have had to redefine many aspects of their own professional identities and traditional culture. Rather than limiting clients to patients and families, an expanded vision now includes the providers, clinics, and health service organizations served.

Social workers no longer view themselves as being respondent providers, passively waiting for requests for services. Managed care demands have empowered them to actively engage in case finding, and to use their professional expertise to identify and recommend program changes and interventions to further the goals of managed care. Because of their pivotal role in utilization management, social workers often find themselves becoming recognized as experts in managed care and training other health care providers. Social Work Service at Madigan Army Medical Center has published both a pocket-sized manual, "The Kwik-Key Guide to Discharge Planning" and electronically published "Discharge Planning Diamonds." These documents are also available on the Social Work Service Web page. Medical social work staff also help teach managed care concepts to new interns, new nursing staff, new case managers, and "Health Care 101," a class for all health care providers. At times the goals of managed care and patient care appear to conflict, causing ethical dilemmas and questions as to which "client" should be served (Poole, 1996). While these and other questions are not easily answered, they have caused many social workers to reevaluate their own professional identities and reexamine their perceptions of the value of the profession itself.

UNIQUE ASPECTS OF MILITARY SOCIAL WORK

Although changes in military medical social work mirror many of the trends found throughout the health care arena, some aspects of medical social work remain unique to the military environment.

Patients

The majority of patients in military medical facilities are active duty service members, their family members, retirees and family members, and family members of deceased service members and retirees. Civilian employees of the Department of Defense are eligible for care in overseas commands. Less frequent users of the military medical system include civilian emergency cases, ROTC cadets and Reserve and National Guard members injured on active duty, Alaskan natives, and government officials. When military medical units are tasked with humanitarian missions, social workers may also find themselves in other countries assisting local patients with complex social, political, and physical concerns. On occasion, local nationals are brought to military facilities within the United States for care, and medical social workers may collaborate with the local United States Immigration and Naturalization Service. Social workers will also assist these foreign nationals with financial assistance, translation, and discharge planning services.

Military patients present a somewhat different picture than the typical civilian patient population. Military patients are often stationed and hospitalized far from extended family and support systems. The active duty service member is subject to frequent deployments. Thus, when the service member's spouse becomes ill or gives birth there is often no family member to provide care for children or to assist with convalescence. Social workers often depend on the unit's family support group to assist a needy family until the deployed spouse returns. Also, the military aeromedical evacuation system provides worldwide transport of patients, usually from smaller facilities and field deployments to larger facilities where more comprehensive services are available. Patients and families who arrive via the aeromedical evacuation system are faced with both serious medical problems and displacement from their home environment. The Fisher Houses at twenty-five military medical treatment facilities provide housing for the families of such patients in a supportive, homelike environment. Medical social workers work closely with the Fisher Houses in recommending and screening families for admission. Several Army Fisher Houses are operated by Social Work Service.

Military patients also have a different attitude toward their medical care than civilian patients. There is both a sense of entitlement and a sense of family. The familiarity of the military setting is reassuring and comfortable to many patients. Most retirees have sacrificed much in the course of a military career and believe they have "earned" lifetime medical care. Many report being promised lifetime care. Under the TRICARE system, retirees who are not enrolled in TRICARE Prime or TRICARE Senior are seen on a space available basis. Most beneficiaries over the age of sixty-five are not eligible for either TRICARE program, and many under sixty-five refuse to pay to join TRICARE Prime. Situations where retirees can only be seen on a space available basis invoke much anger. Patients also often resist being moved from the comfort of the medical treatment facility to an unknown (and more expensive) skilled nursing or rehabilitation facility. Some patients even resist being sent home with home health care. The social worker must often deal with a patient and family who feel betrayed and rejected. Military patients sometimes must stay in the medical facility beyond the time when a civilian patient would be discharged. Service members who live in group housing (barracks, dorms, billets) often must stay in the medical facility with medical conditions that would normally require home care. A young soldier, sailor, or airman cannot expect monitoring or assistance in the barracks. Contagious diseases, however minor, cannot be introduced into crowded group housing. Other active duty patients remain in the medical facility awaiting air transport back to their home station.

While military patients can have special needs, this population also excludes some factors that are common in the civilian world. Military beneficiaries are seldom indigent or homeless. Almost all beneficiary families include at least one member who receives either a regular pay check or pension. Likewise, military hospitals seldom treat patients lacking medical insurance. Military beneficiaries are generally entitled to the TRICARE programs, Medicare, or the coverage for active duty service members. Civilians involved in a traumatic accident near a military hospital may be brought to that facility for emergency care.

These patients may be indigent or uninsured, but are usually transferred to a civilian facility when stable.

The last characteristic that differentiates the military patient population is the nature of injuries. Military service is, in the final analysis, a deadly profession. In peacetime many of the injuries are related to training for war. Training accidents are inevitable when a young, active population simulates the activities of war. Such accidents can involve parachutes, artillery shells, helicopters, tanks, snakes, hand grenades, and many other war-related items. Illness, too, can follow training in less-developed countries with different standards of hygiene. War accelerates injuries and illness and adds patients injured by enemy weapons. In war and peace, social workers must assist patients and families in dealing with the tragedy of young service members killed or disabled in the prime of life. More assistance may be required after an armed conflict. A number of facilities have created support groups for Persian Gulf operations veterans reporting health issues. Post-traumatic stress disorder is also common in the aftermath of military operations.

Relationship with the Military Community

The line between the military hospital and community is less definitive than that between a typical civilian hospital and the community it serves. All of the employees on a military installation, including medical staff, answer to the same organization and are expected to support the overall mission. Thus, the hospital's goal is not only to serve patients in an efficient and cost-effective manner, but to ensure that soldiers, sailors, and airmen are able to do their jobs. The Army Medical Department's motto is "preserve the fighting strength." The shared mission colors medical units' priorities and leads to joint ventures with community agencies. Hospital staff will suspend routine activities to assist with support to deploying units and unit family members and to intervene in community emergencies. In addition to participating in the hospital's Emergency Preparedness Plan, medical social work staff will often participate in planning for and operating the installation's Family Assistance Center. Family Assistance Centers are typically opened during deployments and at other times when there is a mass casualty situation. The shared mission also leads medical social workers to work closely with installation units. It would be unusual to look to a civilian patient's employer as a source of social support. In a military hospital, however, when an active duty patient or family member needs assistance, the unit and unit family support group is one of the most common sources of assistance. The welfare of the entire family is seen as part of the unit's mission. Unit and support group members provide transportation, child care, food, supervision, companionship, monitoring, shopping, and so on.

Medical social workers also have close relationships with community agencies. They will often sit on the governing councils for agencies such as the New Parent Support Program and the Exceptional Family Member Program. They depend on community agencies to provide financial assistance to patients. They often work closely with or lead the installation Rape Crisis Team.

Staffing Patterns

Military medical social work staffing is often less stable than that of its civilian counterparts. Uniformed military social workers rotate to a new station every few years. Because active duty social workers should be exposed to as many facets of social work as possible, they may work in medical social work for only part of their tour at an installation. Even when uniformed social workers are assigned to a medical social work position, many contingencies can remove them from the work area. They may be deployed around the world on a few hours' notice. Many uniformed hospital social workers are assigned to "professional filler" positions in deployable units or psychiatric rapid reaction teams. Others are selected for special missions. At the installation, service members must often complete military training and extra duties ranging from weapons firing to court-martial officer and drug destruction officer. In time of war many active duty social workers from a medical treatment facility will join field medical or mental health units. These workers will be replaced by reservists. Reservists often train each year in social work service in preparation for their wartime missions. Civilian social workers often provide stability and historical perspective in hospital social work sections.

CONCLUSION

According to a 1995 study (Applewhite et al., 1995), 25 percent of Army active duty and civilian social workers participated in medical social work. Social workers selected medical social work as their primary field of practice more often than any other field. Medical social work is also an important field of practice in the Navy and Air Force. Medical social work is practiced in settings ranging from the large flagship medical centers such as the Army's Walter Reed, the Air Force's Wilford Hall, and the Navy's Bethesda to field hospitals and small installation hospitals and clinics and field hospitals. The delivery of medicine is changing in all these settings, but medical social workers adapt to and even embrace change. The Department of Defense medical social workers continue to assist military members, retirees, and families in dealing with the psychological, social, and physical consequences of illness and injury.

REFERENCES

Applewhite, L., Brintzenhofe-Szoc, K., Hamlin, E., and Timberlake, E. (1995). Clinical social work practice in the U.S. Army: An update. *Military Medicine*, 160, (January), pp. 283-288.

Berger, C.S., Cayner, J., Jensen, G., Mizrahi, T., Scesny, A., and Trachtenberg, T. (1996). The changing scene of social work in hospitals: A report of a national study by the Society for Social Work Administrators in Health Care and NASW. *Health and Social Work,* 21(3), 167-177.

Berkman, B. (1996). The emerging health care world: Implications for social work practice and education. *Social Work,* 41(5), 541-551.

Cameron, R.D. (1993). Cameron lists do's and don'ts of budget cuts. *Health Services Command,* 20(1), 7.

Cancer and the mind. (1998, March). *The Harvard Mental Health Letter,* 14(9), 1-5.

Cummins, N.A. (1994). The successful application of medical offset in program planning and in clinical delivery. *Managed Care Quarterly,* 2(2), 1-6.

Garber, D.L. and McNelis, P.J. (1995). Military social work. In R.L. Edwards (Ed-in-chief), *Encyclopedia of Social Work,* Nineteenth Edition, Volume II (pp. 1726-1735). Washington, DC: NASW Press.

Hamlin, E.R., Pehrson, K.L., and Gemmill, R. (1996). Social work services in Army medical treatment facilities: Are they reorganizing? *Military Medicine,* 161(1), 33-36.

Hearts and minds—Part II. (1997, August). *The Harvard Mental Health Letter,* 14(2), 1-4.

Humphreys, M. and Falck, H.S. (1990). Point/counterpoint: Maintaining social work standards in for-profit hospitals. *Health and Social Work,* 15(1), 75-77.

Medical Service Corps (1997). The clinicians. In *Many Specialties, One Corps: A Pictorial History of the U.S. Navy Medical Service Corps* (pp. 151-153). Washington, DC: Department of the Navy.

Poole, D.L. (1996). Keeping managed care in balance. *Health and Social Work,* 21(3), 163-166.

Rengo, R. and Kunes, C. (1995). Outpatient case management: A role for social work. *Social Work Administration,* 21(1), Winter, 1-6.

Scesny, A.M. (1997). Measuring the effectiveness of social interventions on health outcomes. *Social Work Administration,* 23(5), 1-10.

Stamper, J. (1998, April 12). The dark side of longer life: Evidence mounts that medical gains make the end harder for many. *The Tacoma News Tribune,* A-5.

Chapter 8

Military Social Work Practice in Mental Health Programs

James G. Daley

This chapter outlines the varied and significant roles military social workers have served within the mental health service component of military medicine. After a brief overview of military mental health programs, the chapter discusses the clinical services and unique military requirements provided within the mental health programs. The chapter then contrasts mental health and other social welfare programs within the military. The chapter concludes with a reassertion that military social workers need to continue this vital role.

OVERVIEW OF MENTAL HEALTH SERVICES WITHIN THE MILITARY

Staffing

Regardless of service branch, mental health services have always been a subcomponent of and accountable to the military medicine chain of command. Further, mental health services have always consisted of five disciplines: psychiatry, psychology (typically clinical PhD), social work (always MSW), psychiatric nursing (typically inpatient settings), and enlisted mental health technicians (wide range of professional preparation and experience from PhD to high school graduate). Though other social service programs (e.g., family support centers) have allowed great variance in professional degrees (e.g.,

PhD in guidance and counseling, MA in marriage and family therapy, MBA), the mental health programs have rigorously maintained a profession-defined cadre of providers. Mental health services increase the quantity and breadth of providers as the program increases in size. For example, a small mental health clinic on a small base or post might be staffed with a social worker and two technicians whereas a major medical center would have a psychiatric ward (or two) and the full range of mental health staff. Personnel requirements are built upon an expectation of triage. The small clinics handle most outpatient needs, and the medical centers receive the patients triaged as needing inpatient or more complex (e.g., neuropsychological testing) services (Jones, 1980).

Paying Homage to the Medical Model

The above-described service delivery system most commonly functions within a medical model format (e.g., diagnosis, treatment, resolution). Leadership has traditionally always been physician-dominated, with military social workers accountable to psychiatrists (or other physicians in smaller locations) as the boss. Nonmedically based programs (e.g., family advocacy, combat stress teams, outreach programs) have functioned within the mental health program authority with some periodic tension or conflict over priority of funding, documentation (e.g., "patient count"), program goals, and accountability. A common result has been a reduction of nonmedical programs or even elimination of some programs as not mission essential or less significant than in-clinic therapy. For example, military social workers, in the early days of family advocacy program (FAP) development, were expected to do FAP requirements as an additional duty after completing all of the primary mental health services (Myers, 1977; see Chapter 4 for more description). Another example is the human development centers (HDC), prevention-oriented programs centered on facilitating the successful completion of technical training by airmen. I was director of an HDC when the command surgeon general (SG) relocated and the new SG eliminated all HDCs as "not necessary" and redirected the funding to other medical priorities. In sum, mental health programs have kept as highest priority the patient-centered clinical treatment format and expanded to a greater prevention orientation only "when staffing allowed." Prevention-focused programs have only blossomed when carved out and funded, staffed, and implemented separate from the MHC (see FAP and divisional mental health examples in following paragraphs).

This clinic-centered focus was often based on inadequate staffing, provision of tertiary care as a top priority, and a massive caseload always bursting at the seams. The consumer was (and is) the military hierarchy, and getting rapid treatment for the mentally distressed soldier, sailor, or airman was the top priority (Diebold, 1997; Kutz, 1996). Delivery of service was (and is) prioritized as military, then military dependents, and finally (if you had time left over) retirees and their dependents. Often the delivery of service was capped due to staffing shortages at military only, and dependents and retirees were referred out to CHAMPUS providers. (See Chapter 5 for a more extensive discussion of the transition from CHAMPUS to TRICARE and efforts to improve the service to family members and retirees.)

Blending EAP and Clinical Services

The services within the mental health clinic (MHC) are best conceptualized as a blend of an employee assistance program (EAP) and a full range of clinical services (outpatient and inpatient therapy, substance abuse screening and treatment, consultation service, etc.). The EAP services include mental health evaluations, screening interviews for specialty jobs (e.g., recruiter, drill sergeant), and recommendations for retention in the military. The MHC is seen as a consultant for the commander, providing what service is necessary for the soldier, sailor, or airman to become worldwide qualified or expediting the patient's departure from the military. This service has a long tradition in all military branches and is institutionalized as an expectation (Will, 1946; Maas, 1951; Bailey, 1980; Jeffer, 1979; Hibler, 1985; Norwood, 1997). An uneasy balance occurs between mission requirements and the individual needs of the patient (see ethics scenarios in Chapter 11; Johnson, 1995; Page, 1996). A lament from a provider more than eighteen years ago that the MHC is "seen as a 'body and fender shop' where they are supposed to make soldiers over to return to duty or send them out" (Mitchell and Orlin, 1980, p. 56) is often still true in today's downsizing environment.

Ironically, the cutting edge efforts in EAP services are actually occurring within outreach programs functioning outside the MHC. The FAP has a very progressive, nonpathologizing blend of clinical and primary prevention services focused on family violence (see Chapter 4 for more discussion). FAP has taken a dominant role as the image of the military social worker and has moved much of the duties of the military social worker away from being a clinician within the MHC (much to the chagrin of some chiefs of MHC). Some FAPs have bypassed the MHC reporting official and report directly to the chief of hospital services. Within the Air Force, regulations require FAP to be located outside of the MHC and an oversight committee for FAP to be chaired by the hospital commander. Congressionally fenced funding and top-down social work leadership have produced a high visibility, rapidly expanding social welfare program. Within the Navy, FAP is now designated a line (rather than a medical) position (see Chapter 20) and the Army has line positions within FAP (prevention portion is line, clinical services are medical). Further discussion of FAP is beyond this chapter's focus and is covered in Chapter 4. The point is that FAP originated in the MHC and has bypassed the MHC goals and leadership to produce a template of a successful EAP format.

In addition to family advocacy, the divisional mental health teams (DMHT) within the Army have excelled as an EAP function. The Navy has SPRINT teams and the Air Force is just institutionalizing their combat stress teams, but the Army's DMHT are most effectively integrated at this time. A much more comprehensive discussion of the tri-service efforts at combat stress teams is provided in Chapter 9. However, the DMHT concept is worth highlighting in the EAP discussion. The DMHT is composed of a combination of the five mental health professions depending on size of team and deployment. The DMHT is assigned to the division commander, not the hospital. Extensive outreach, preventive education, and formal and informal consultation with the line leadership are primary job functions of the DMHT members. When the division deploys, the DMHT deploys with it. When the division trains, the DMHT trains with it. Military social workers join the DMHT as an assignment, not an additional duty. In sum, the DMHT is a fully deployed mental health function embedded within the daily life of the soldier. The implications are clear: better access, higher credibility, better understanding of the daily issues facing the division, and direct presence in combat scenarios. The value of the DMHT in assessment and rapid intervention has been discussed widely in literature (e.g., Martin, Sparacino, and Belenky, 1996; Hall, Cipriano, and Bicknell, 1997).

Besides an EAP function, the MHC provides a wide range of clinical services. Individual, group, and family therapy are provided. Specialized credentials are required for provision of sex therapy (AASECT certification), biofeedback (proof of adequate training), or hypnosis (proof of adequate training). The documentation requirements and service parameters mimic most civilian MHCs and meet Joint Commission on Accreditation of Hospital Organizations (JCAHO) standards. Some MHCs have training programs (psychiatry residency, psychology residency, MSW field placements) linked to their program. Clinical services tend to be short-term, problem-focused, and most often centered on "problems of living" (marital strain, adjustment to military, parent-child conflict, phase of life issues) (McKain, 1973; Lagrone, 1978; Baresch, 1979; Bailey, 1980; Rodriguez, 1980; Creel, 1981; Ursano et al., 1989; Figley, 1993; Nice, 1993; Kelleher et al., 1996). Substance abuse treatment services have been provided through a combination of MHC and a paraprofessional program called Social Actions (Myers, 1978) but have now become an exclusive MHC function except in the Navy, which still uses paraprofessionals for triage and outpatient services (see Chapter 6 for extensive discussion of history and current status of substance abuse treatment). Significant efforts are made to focus on assessment of and intervention in military deployment stressors within the military person and family members (McCubbin, Dahl, and Hunter, 1976; Kaslow and Ridenour, 1984; Kaslow, 1993; Martin, Sparacino, and Belenky, 1996; Ursano and Norwood, 1996; Litz et al., 1997). The managed care revolution has had some impact on prevention orientation (see Chapter 5) and there have been exceptional location-unique demonstration projects (e.g., Saxe and Cross, 1997). But the primary day-to-day operations continue as a tertiary therapy service providing recovery efforts for dysfunctional patients brought for or seeking resolution of the impairment.

The Erosion of Military Social Work Within the MHC

Military social workers have been an integral part of the MHC since before the first uniformed military social worker was sworn in. They have provided the full array of services (excluding prescribing medication or psychological testing) and, as the cadre of military social workers have advanced in rank, they have provided leadership as chiefs of mental health clinics throughout the world. Substance abuse services have been predominantly staffed by military social workers, with almost every inpatient alcoholism treatment program having a military social worker as program chief (Myers, 1984). Military social workers have developed highly innovative programs, provided successful management, and contributed to the professional literature on relevant topics. In sum, they have been very successful wherever they have worked.

Unfortunately, the MHC function of military social work is eroding. Because military social workers have been so successful, they have expanded into many career paths and reduced their presence within the MHC. Military social workers are teaching at the military academies and professional military education schools, involved with psychological operations, serving as squadron commanders, running medical social work programs, heading up family support centers, and overseeing family advocacy programs. In fact, the wide array of jobs within which military social workers function is only limited by the tenacity of the worker to achieve that position. Military social workers have pushed the parameters of the military social work mission and succeeded repeatedly in expanding an added job responsibility into a regulation-supported permanent requirement. As military social workers increased in rank, they became more sophisticated in how to create and solidify programs, gained access to higher level military leadership positions, and learned how to win within the military bureaucracy.

With this programmatic success, military social workers shifted from being primarily clinicians to being primarily program managers. FAP changed from an additional duty to a full-time, very intensively demanding job. The identity of the military social worker evolved from MHC clinician to a highly diversified entity. In other words, our success eroded our past clear identity as MHC clinicians. Military social workers spent less time honing MHC skills and more time rotating among other positions (FSC director, alcoholism treatment program director, recruiter, FAP manager).

This transformation of military social work from MHC clinician to social service entrepreneur produced a subtle tension in job demands. A military social worker is deployed as part of a mental health team. Therefore the military social worker's MHC skills must be fine-tuned. The less involved in MHC services the military social worker becomes, the less practice and refinement occurs. Granted, the deployed social worker does much more than just diagnose mental illness (see Chapter 9 for an in-depth discussion on the deployed social worker), but the MHC skills are still a necessary component. In addition to deployability, the tension in job demands affects MHC mission progression. Military social workers have put their primary energy and focus on non-MHC issues and yet the non-social work leadership in MHC has still been evolving (Kelleher et al., 1996; Page, 1996; Diebold, 1997; Norwood, 1997).

Some of the efforts by non-social work leadership have directly damaged the ability of military social workers to function within a MHC. Sadly, the evaluation of "fitness for duty," which has been successfully done for many years by military social workers (Thom, 1942; Will, 1946; Maas, 1951), has recently been eliminated as an independent decision and must now be completed or co-signed by a psychologist or psychiatrist unless the social worker has a PhD (see discussion in chapters 19, 20, and 21 on DoD Instruction 6490.4, Requirements for Mental Health Evaluations of Members of the Armed Forces, and the DoD Directive Number 6490.1, Mental Health Evaluations of Members of the Armed Forces). Further, the 1982 DoD Directive 1332.14, Enlisted Administrative Separations, and the subsequent October 1982 Air Force Regulations 39-10 specifically stated that only a psychologist or a psychiatrist could make a personality disorder diagnosis for administrative separation purposes. These regulation changes have each occurred without prior consultation with senior social work leadership and erode credibility of social work within the line leadership. In short, we were broadsided by changes within MHC and have not remedied the situation. If military social work is not carefully attuned to advances in MHCs, it will have eroded our current primary readiness mission. And without a readiness mission, the civilianization of military social work positions becomes inevitable. It is possible that the combat stress teams will reassert the readiness role of military social workers. But the place of military social workers within the MHC must be watched carefully.

CONTRAST OF MENTAL HEALTH AND OTHER SOCIAL WELFARE PROGRAMS WITHIN THE MILITARY

The military provides a wide array of social support systems (see Chapters 12-15). Finance and personnel offices provide advice and monitoring of benefits. Housing offices help place military families in housing on base or post. Informal support organizations such as the officers' or enlisted spouses' clubs reach out to newcomers and serve as a conduit for a myriad of personal or family needs. The military aid society expedites emergency financial assistance. And the list goes on. But two key programs warrant more extensive discussion: the chaplains and the family support centers. These two programs provide a profound additive social welfare resource for military families beyond what the mental health programs offer. Further, the two programs commonly work in conjunction with the MHC. And yet they have very different lines of authority and missions than the MHC.

The Chaplains

Chaplains within the military are significant personal resources for the military member and family. Chaplains are ordained ministers of a purposefully wide range of religious orders from Southern Baptist to Catholic to Buddhist. Chaplains, regardless of background, have a direct chain of command through chaplains all the way up to a general officer chief of chaplains. Besides providing religious services within their general religious discipline (e.g., Protestant, Catholic, Jewish), the chaplains serve as roaming consultants for the commander. Like flight surgeons, they make "rounds" within the units to which they are deemed responsible. They provide counseling with complete confidentiality, a feat not permitted to MHC staff. When the unit deploys, they deploy with them (somewhat like the division mental health teams), and are often in the most high-risk combat situations sharing the experience with the troops. Becoming a military chaplain is a highly competitive task for a civilian minister and nearly all military chaplains arrive in the service with extensive ministerial experience. The chaplain focuses this expertise on facilitating personal, family, and organizational well being. Chaplains frequently serve on most social welfare committees on base or post and usually have a solid grasp of the pulsebeat of the unit. Multidisciplinary efforts to work with multiproblem families often include chaplains in the team planning and intervention. In short, chaplains are solid allies for the MHC staff member smart enough to utilize their expertise while respecting their mission.

The Family Support Center/Family Service Center

The family support center (FSC) (or family service centers within the Navy) offers extensive social welfare programs including financial counseling, relocation assistance, job training and placement assistance, brief crisis counseling, a myriad of preventive education on topics such as parenting, personal happiness, and coping with a military deployment. The FSC director can be trained in any of a wide range of human resource disciplines (at least master's level and often PhD level) and reports directly to the base or post commander or designee. FSCs were developed to facilitate families getting preventive and "problems of living" assistance without the assumed (and sometimes real) stigma of going to the MHC. FSCs' primary mission is to enhance family wellness and thereby improve military readiness. Many FSCs were created as a result of studies showing the negative impact of family distress on career retention and deployment capability of military members. Effective care of the family produces soldiers and sailors who can deploy more effectively. FSCs also have a direct mission of handling family evacuations during high-risk overseas scenarios (e.g., the volcano eruption in the Philippines, invasion of South Korea by North Korea). FSC directors are usually civilian professional, though they are not credentialled within the hospital and the FSC is not inspected as part of the JCAHO guidelines. FSC staff include a senior enlisted person (usually designated as assistant director) and a range of paraprofessional and professional staff members. FSCs are housed completely outside the hospital, usually in a nicely renovated building (though a few are in buildings that should be and sometimes are condemned). FSCs are high-visibility programs to the line command and directly reflect the base commander's (and operational commander's) ability to "take care of my people." The FSC director reports directly to the base commander, but is part of the personnel chain of command. All FSCs also are linked and accountable to command and Pentagon-level family matters offices.

Some very effective partnerships have emerged between MHCs and FSCs. MHC staff have provided educational topics (e.g., depression prevention, improving parent-child communication), with the FSC doing all the marketing and setup of workshops. FSC staff often work closely with family advocacy staff and serve as members of the family advocacy treatment team and family advocacy committee. FSC works closely with division mental health teams and sets up support groups for spouses of deployed personnel (e.g., Black, 1993).

However, there are concerns about some of the FSC services and professional services offered without adequate malpractice protection. By regulation, FSCs cannot provide therapy and only offer short-term crisis counseling. Record keeping is not consistent with typical mental health records and they are not accessible to MHC staff when needed. Clinical supervision is sometimes problematic due to a lack of depth of expertise (e.g., an MSW as FSC director and no other clinically trained FSC staff to provide consultation or supervision). Informal supervision arrangements can sometimes be developed between MHC and FSC, but liability is a major concern as the FSC has no formal chain of authority within the medical arena and the existing chain of command is line officers with little clinical preparation and very different missions than the MHC.

Regardless of the concerns, the FSC is an excellent resource and very inventive when developing new programs for military families. The FSC is akin to a civilian family counseling agency but ingrained in the military institution. FSCs often have budget and line authority to develop programs that MHCs do not have the resources to create. The best scenario is an effective partnership between the MHC, FAP, and FSC.

THE FUTURE OF MILITARY SOCIAL WORKERS WITHIN THE MENTAL HEALTH CLINIC

The proud heritage of military social workers within the MHC is in jeopardy of becoming a historical footnote. The proven clinical capability of military social workers has been subtly challenged by regulation changes and our own aggressive expansion beyond the MHC. The diverse new "career broadening" opportunities have led to highly successful new definitions of what military social work is. In our zeal to prove additional capability, we must ensure that we retain old territory. Military social workers must have a vital role within the MHC. Positions must be maintained and not converted to psychologist slots (which has occurred) or simply deleted in the next round of downsizing efforts (which has occurred). We must be careful that we do not weaken our clout simply by benign disinterest.

There has been talk throughout the history of military social work about "breaking away" from psychiatry and creating a purely social work function. FAP has achieved some of that goal. However, we should progress with great caution and awareness that our professional growth is not occurring within a vacuum. There are other professions with their own agendas and growth. The smartest strategy is to embrace advances while maintaining established roles. In other words, we should strongly reassert our MHC skills, highlighting our proud history of service, and ensure that every military social worker obtains and retains basic MHC skills. All military social workers should rotate through a MHC as part of their skill building. The trends and advocacy by non-social work leadership should be attended to carefully and, where appropriate, social work's role inserted. Too often I have seen a deaf ear turned toward base or post-level MHC chiefs who are trying to embrace military social workers within the MHC. We have the skills but must flex them periodically to maintain credibility.

REFERENCES

Bailey, L.W. (1980). Outpatient mental health services in the Navy: Referral patterns, demographics, and clinical implications. *Military Medicine*, (February), 106-110.

Baresch, R. (1979). A joint treatment "package" of the Army and a child welfare agency. *Child Welfare*, 58(5), 333-338.

Black, W.G. (1993). Military-induced family separation: A stress reduction intervention. *Social Work*, 38(3), 273-280.

Creel, S.M. (1981). Patient appraisal of current life and social stressors in a military community. *Military Medicine*, 146(11), 797-801.

Diebold, C.J. (1997). Military administrative psychiatry. In R.G. Lande and D.T. Armitage (Eds.), *Principles and practice of military forensic psychiatry.* Springfield, IL: Charles C Thomas Publisher (pp. 269-304).

Figley, C.R. (1993). Coping with stressors on the home front. *Journal of Social Issues*, 49(4), 51-71.

Hall, D.P., Cipriano, E.D., and Bicknell, G. (1997). Preventive mental health interventions in peacekeeping missions to Somalia and Haiti. *Military Medicine,* 162(1), 41-43.

Hibler, R.J. (1985, October). *Behavioral security evaluations.* Unpublished manuscript. Fort Meade, MD: National Security Agency.

Jeffer, E.K. (1979). Psychiatric evaluations for administrative purposes. *Military Medicine*, (August), 526-528.

Johnson, W.B. (1995). Perennial ethical quandaries in military psychology: Toward American Psychological Association and Department of Defense collaboration. *Professional Psychology: Research and Practice,* 26(3), 281-287.

Jones, D.R. (1980). Aeromedical transportation of psychiatric patients: Historical review and present management. *Aviation, Space, and Environmental Medicine*, 51(7), 709-716.

Kaslow, F.W. (Ed.) (1993). *The military family in peace and war.* New York: Springer.

Kaslow, F.W. and Ridenour, R.I. (Eds.)(1984). *The military family: Dynamics and treatment.* New York: Guilford Press.

Kelleher, W.J., Talcott, G.W., Haddock, C.K., and Freeman, R.K. (1996). Military psychology in the age of managed care: The Wilford Hall model. *Applied and Preventive Psychology,* 5(2), 101-110.

Kutz, D.L. (1996). Military psychiatry: A cross-cultural perspective. *Military Medicine*, 161(2), 78-83.

Lagrone, D.M. (1978). The military family syndrome. *American Journal of Psychiatry,* 135(9), 1040-1043.

Litz, B.T., Orsillo, S.M., Friedman, M., and Ehlich, P. (1997). Post-traumatic stress disorder associated with peacekeeping duty in Somalia for U.S. military personnel. *American Journal of Psychiatry,* 154(2), 178-184.

Maas, H.S. (1951). *Adventure in mental health: Psychiatric social work with the armed forces in World War II.* New York: Columbia University Press.

Martin, J.A., Sparacino, L.R., and Belenky, G. (Eds.) (1996). *The Gulf War and mental health.* Westport, CT: Praeger.

McCubbin, H.I., Dahl, B.B., and Hunter, E.J. (1976). *Families in the military system.* Beverly Hills, CA: Sage.

McKain, J.L. (1973). Relocation in the military: Alienation and family problems. *Journal of Marriage and the Family,* (May), 205-209.

Mitchell, G.W. and Orlin, M.B. (1980). Service delivery in the military: Training issues. *Social Casework*, (January), 54-57.

Myers, S.S. (1977). A brief history and status report: Child advocacy program. *USAF Medical Service Digest*, (Winter), 21-25.

Myers, S.S. (1978). Alcoholism treatment: Where are we today? *USAF Medical Service Digest*, (May-June), 5-9.

Myers, S.S. (1984). Reflections. *Jetlag*, (Winter 1983-1984), 21-23.

Nice, D.S. (1993). The military family and the health care system. In F.W. Kaslow (Ed.), *The military family in peace and war.* New York: Springer Publishing Company (pp. 191-213).

Norwood, A.E. (1997). William C Porter lecture award: Joining forces: Psychiatry and readiness. *Military Medicine*, 162(4), 225-228.

Page, G.D. (1996). Clinical psychology in the military: Developments and issues. *Clinical Psychology Review*, 16(5), 383-396.

Rodriguez, A.R. (1980). The family in the military community: Issues for the military psychiatrist. *Military Medicine,* (May), 316-319.

Saxe, L. and Cross, T.P. (1997). Interpreting the Fort Bragg children's mental health demonstration project: The cup is half full. *American Psychologist,* 52(5), 553-556.

Thom, D.A. (1942). The war and its effect upon the mental health of the armed forces. *Virginia Medical Monthly*, 69, 672-678.

Ursano, R.J., Holloway, H.C., Jones, D.R., Rodriguez, A.R., and Belenky, G.L. (1989). Psychiatric care in the military community: Family and military stressors. *Hospital and Community Psychiatry*, 40(12), 1284-1289.

Ursano, R.J. and Norwood, A.E. (1996). *Emotional aftermath of the Persian Gulf War: Veterans, families, communities, and nations.* Washington, DC: American Psychiatric Press.

Will, O.A. (1946). The value of the social service history in the detection of those psychiatrically unsuited for military service. *Naval Medical Bulletin*, 46, 1403-1407.

Chapter 9

The Role of the Social Work Officer in Support of Combat and Noncombat Operations

James A. Martin
Spencer J. Campbell

INTRODUCTION

Professional social workers serve as commissioned officers within the Army, Navy, and Air Force medical departments. Social work officers are assigned to a variety of health, mental health, and human service roles. These assignments include program management, policymaking, and research assignments. Military social workers are a select group of men and women who have obtained a master's degree in social work from a graduate school accredited by the Council on Social Work Education. Most are competitively selected for a direct commission. Some have previous military experience, usually as enlisted service members. Others received their commission after completing a Reserve Officers Training Corps (ROTC) program in college and subsequently enter one of the services' medical departments after completing their master's-level social work education.

Military social work officers are typically assigned to deployable mental health teams or units only after completing at least one tour of duty in a military hospital or mental health clinic. Individuals assigned to deployable mental health units are expected to be experienced mental health clinicians and capable of independent clinical practice.

The opinions expressed in this chapter are the authors' and should not be interpreted as the policy or opinions of the United States Army.

Social work officers who are involved in providing clinical services are typically required to maintain a social work state license. Many military social workers obtain an advanced practice license and/or advanced practice credentials from one of the national social work credentialing organizations.

Military social workers play an important role in support of the medical mission of "sustaining the fighting force." As members of military mental health units and teams, they provide services directed at the prevention of combat stress casualties, the sustainment of military members exposed to combat stress (and other traumatic stress events), and when necessary, the provision of supportive interventions designed to restore combat stress casualties to duty. They provide training in combat stress management and consultation to commanders on individual clinical matters, as well as on issues related to unit morale and cohesion. Military social work officers provide clinical mental health assessments, individual and group mental health interventions, supervision of enlisted mental health providers, and case management services. These individuals bring a unique biopsychosocial perspective to the role of military mental health officer.

A BRIEF HISTORICAL OVERVIEW OF SOCIAL WORK ROLES WITHIN THE CONTEXT OF MILITARY MENTAL HEALTH SUPPORT IN COMBAT OPERATIONS

Social work officers can trace their lineage back to the service of civilian Red Cross social workers in World War I Army hospitals. These professional social workers provided both medical and psychiatric services to returning combat casualties.

In World War II, enlisted social workers served in hospital units and newly constituted combat mental health teams. Professional social workers were first commissioned in the Army in 1947 (Ginn, 1997, p. 217) as a result of an initiative begun by Brigadier General William C. Menninger and subsequently by Colonel John Caldwell, Jr., both Army Medical Corps leaders who helped champion the concept of a combat mental health team. Social work officers served as key members of combat stress control units during the Korean War, the war in

Vietnam, the entire period of the Cold War, and during the Persian Gulf War. Today, social work officers are important members of military medical units and mental health teams. The roles these military social work officers perform in support of combat and other military operations have evolved from a long history of combat and other operational stress interventions.

The history of combat stress is as old as armed conflict (Holmes, 1985, p. 32). In modern history, the American Civil War provides numerous examples of what we now refer to as combat stress reaction; then it was referred to as "soldier's heart" (Marmar and Horowitz, 1988, p. 83).

American military mental health care (psychiatric units in military hospitals) dates back to World War I, and the initiatives led by Dr. (Major) Thomas Salmon (Copp and McAndrew, 1990, p. 13), who was the Director of Psychiatry in the American Expeditionary Forces and responsible for the development of a multiechelon and multidisciplinary (physician, nurse, and enlisted medical corpsmen) approach to the treatment of combat stress, which still forms the basis of our modern combat stress control approach (Jones, F. D., 1995a, p. 26). In this same era, civilian Red Cross social workers provided medical and mental health support to soldiers who had returned from Europe to military hospitals in the United States (Rock et al., 1995, p. 155).

At the outbreak of World War II, the mental health lessons learned from World War I had been all but forgotten. While psychiatrists were initially assigned to Army hospitals in 1941 (see Glass, 1966, 1973), an actual military mental health unit (which later became the basis for the Army's Mental Hygiene Consultation Services) was first established in 1942 as part of the training command at Fort Monmouth, New Jersey (Rock et al., 1995, pp. 155-156). This unit included a psychiatrist, an enlisted social worker, and a psychologist. By 1943, hastily formed mental health teams were established in the European Theater (Rock et al., 1995, p. 156). By the war's end, an extensive array of divisional, corps, and theater mental health teams and hospital-based mental health units had been developed, along with a mental health doctrine that still exists today (refer to Glass, 1966, 1973 for a complete description of these World War II teams and units).

Shortly after the end of World War II (1947), the specialty social work officer was established within the Army's Medical Service Corps (Rock et al., 1995, p. 157). Their assignments included membership on division mental health teams. Some of these first social work officers were recruited from officers who had line combat experience in World War II. It was believed that their military training and experience would help bring credibility to this new military specialty. Based on their previous military experience, these officers were believed to have a strong identification with Army life that would facilitate handling the problems of soldiers and their families (Ginn, 1997, p. 218). Major Elwood Camp, MSC, the second chief of Army social work (1948), sought to expand the number of social workers from the four serving on active duty in 1948. By 1951 there were 129 active duty and 89 reserve social work officers in the U.S. Army, including seven women who had received commissions under the provisions of the Women's Armed Forces Integration Act (Women's Army Corps Officers) (Ginn, 1997, p. 218).

By the late 1940s, the Army (and other services) had been substantially downsized and was generally unprepared for combat. The start of the Korean War, the losses sustained by Task Force Smith, and the American retreat to the Pusan perimeter resulted in numerous casualties, which included large numbers of combat stress casualties (Rock et al., 1995, pp. 157-158). Lieutenant Colonel Albert (Al) Glass (a psychiatrist) was assigned to Korea as the Neuropsychiatric Consultant. He reestablished an effective division mental health capability, backed by the creation of a small mobile psychiatric detachment (KO Team). He established a third-echelon psychiatric holding company in Korea. Army social work officers were assigned at each of these echelons of care (Rock et al., 1995, pp. 157-159).

This same model was employed during the Vietnam War (the late 1960s and early 1970s). Social work officers were deployed as members of the division mental health teams. The first KO Team deployed to Vietnam from Valley Forge General Hospital in 1965 included two Army social work officers. A second KO Team was added later in the war, which contained social work officers. Unlike World War I, World War II, and Korea, where combat stress reactions were manifested by physical and overt psychological reactions, these division and theater mental health units were confronted by a form of combat stress reaction that often exhibited itself in drug and alcohol abuse, disruptive behaviors, indiscipline, various criminal behaviors, and somatic complaints (Jones, F. D., 1995a, pp. 17-20).

The divisional mental health team concept, built around a psychiatrist, psychologist, and social work officer, continued throughout the Cold War among Army divisions in the United States, Europe, and Korea. The Gulf War deployment provided what may be the last twentieth century combat deployment of division mental health teams. Each Army division in the Gulf theater operated under this traditional multidisciplinary (psychiatry, psychology, and social work) team model. While a number of social work officers distinguished themselves in mental health assignments during the Gulf War, few teams were trained and ready. The majority of mental health units deployed to the Persian Gulf theater of operations initially lacked critical personnel and equipment. No unit had received adequate prior team training. Most reached an acceptable level of functioning, but only after a prolonged period in the combat theater (Martin and Fagan, 1996, pp. 19-32).

The Korean War and Vietnam War KO Teams that provided second echelon-level mental health care had been redesignated (and restructured) as OM Teams in 1973. The "K" designated a "hospital" augmentation unit. The "O" was a designation for an "area support unit" and OM Teams assumed responsibility for augmenting combat zone deployable hospitals. Each OM Team consisted of a small headquarters detachment and three mobile consultation teams. Each had a psychiatrist, social worker, and six enlisted behavioral science specialists. Unfortunately, only six of these teams were established during the Cold War period, and all were in the Army Reserve component. No doctrine was written for their deployment, and they were never deployed until the Gulf War. There were no active component OM teams when the Gulf War began. The consequences of this neglect have been documented in accounts of the activation and deployment of one of the OM Teams during the Gulf War (Holsenbeck, 1996, pp. 39-58; Martin and

Cline, 1996, pp. 161-178). While many members of this and other teams distinguished themselves as individual soldiers and mental health clinicians, none of the OM teams was able to perform their roles as intended. They were ill staffed, lacked unit-level operational training, were initially missing necessary equipment, and in general took months in theater before they became capable of performing basic operational requirements.

As part of the Army's 1980s "Air-Land Battle" plan designed to meet the perceived Soviet threat, the Medical Force 2000 component envisioned the establishment of new corps and theater-level mental health units called combat stress control (CSC) companies (containing eighty-five members) and detachments (containing twenty-three members). These modular units included both mental health prevention and treatment teams (Stokes and Jones, 1995, pp. 251-252). Social work officers were designated members of each prevention team. Unfortunately these units were not established until after the Gulf War. The Army's first Active Component CSC detachment was activated in 1991 and, since that time, CSC units have been involved in a number of peacemaking and peacekeeping activities including deployments to Somalia in 1993 and 1994, Haiti in 1994, Saudi Arabia in 1994, Guantanamo, Cuba, in 1994 and 1995, and most recently to Bosnia (Jones, F. D., 1995a, p. 28). Today there are six active CSC detachments. A social work officer is assigned to each of the three prevention teams in each detachment. While these units have been deployed in various peacemaking/peacekeeping roles, it remains unlikely that they would be deployed in support of brief combat operations such as the invasion of Panama. Typically in this type of rapid and brief operation, these units would not make it onto the constrained list of units to be airlifted into action.

What may be the future of the forward mental health care in combat operations was seen in the 1989 invasion of Panama where "combat heavy" (but lightly supported) divisional units conducted a rapid, very brief, and highly successful military operation. In the invasion of Panama, very few medical assets made the limited airlift roster. Neither the 82nd Airborne Division nor the 7th Light Infantry Division deployed their mental health teams. While this was a successful military operation, there were a number of psychologically traumatic incidents and soldiers might have benefited from the presence of mental health support (Jones, F. D., 1995a, p. 25). Unfortunately, in this operation, the concept of "return to duty" for any medical (or mental health) casualty meant rapid triage and a trip home. No efforts were made to restore soldiers to their units in the field; rather the operational doctrine called for immediate evacuation out of the theater for even the slightest physical and/or emotional injury. Anyone who needed to be held as a patient for even a few hours was air evacuated to his or her home base in the United States. It remains unclear if the "broken bonds" caused by this medical evacuation policy were restored when these units returned home or whether these soldiers remained to some degree detached from the group and/or were seen by group members as a potential liability or "weak link" in the unit. It is not clear if and/or how division (or other) mental health personnel were able to offer support to these service members.

This brief historical review of social work roles in combat and other military operations has focused on the U.S. Army and the Army medical units designated with a combat stress control function. Social work has a later history and somewhat different role in the Air Force and in the Navy. Today, in addition to various hospital-based medical and mental health assignments, Navy and Air Force social work officers are heavily engaged in an array of community-based service programs, for example, family advocacy positions.[1,2] In some cases, such as the loss of social work positions on Navy hospital ships, military social work has lost ground in its effort to provide combat mental health care. It is clear that in today's situation of constrained personnel resources, there will be additional threats to social work positions in all the services.

It is important to point out that military social workers (representing all the services) have performed important operational activities during many stressful noncombat events (Jones, F. D., 1995a, p. 28). These include mental health interventions after major training accidents, as well as other national and international disasters involving civilian populations (Stokes and Jones, 1995, pp. 263-264). Army social work officers have been involved in hostage retrieval and in support of refugee assistance. It is likely that these various noncombat stress-intervention roles will continue to be critical aspects of readiness for all military social work officers.

COMBAT AND OTHER OPERATIONAL MENTAL HEALTH PRINCIPLES AND THE ROLE OF THE SOCIAL WORK OFFICER

The modern history of recognition and forward care for combat stress casualties began with the efforts of Russian physicians in 1904 during the Russo-Japanese War (Jones, F. D., 1995a, p. 8). World War I established the importance of "proximity" or forward treatment as one of the core principles in the treatment of combat stress. Both British and French armies experienced large numbers of "shell-shocked" soldiers, many of whom became permanently disabled. An American psychiatrist, Thomas Salmon, studied the British and French experience with "war neurosis" and devised a program of intervention that placed psychiatrists with forward medical units. This system of providing "forward echelon care," combined with what Artis (1963) later described as the principles of "immediacy" and "expectancy" remain even today part of the core of combat stress care. These principles are summarized by F. D. Jones (1995a, p. 9) as:

> Proximity—treat the casualty in a safe place as close as possible to the battle scene.
>
> Immediacy—treat the casualty as soon as possible after the stressful event.
>
> Expectancy—provide a clear, explicitly stated expectation that the individual is not ill and will soon be rejoining his or her unit.

In addition, forward care is focused on providing very simple interventions highlighted by the additional principle of:

> Simplicity—provide rest, warm food, and fluids, perhaps even a warm shower and shave.

While the lessons of World War I were not rediscovered until well into World War II, Captain Fredrick Hanson, an American psychiatrist who had first entered World War II as a volunteer in the Canadian Army, applied these principles while serving as a consultant to General Omar Bradley's forces in the North Africa theater.

The rediscovery of these principles (highlighted by Copp and McAndrew, 1990) resulted in dramatic return-to-duty figures (in one case more than 70 percent of casualties were returned to their units within 48 hours) and the subsequent adoption of these combat stress principles in the entire European theater (Jones, F. D., 1995a, p. 12). World War II mental health efforts produced evidence for the importance of unit cohesion both in preventing breakdown and in enhancing combat effectiveness (Jones, F. D., 1995a, p. 12). World War II combat stress studies demonstrated the cumulative effects of wartime stress exposure, expressed by the concept "everyone has his breaking point" (Jones, F. D., 1995a, p. 14). This principle was later a factor in the establishment of the concept of rest and recreation periods and the concept of a rotation policy based on time in theater. Both of these principles were subsequently employed during the Vietnam War. Unfortunately, the rotation policy used in the Vietnam War was based on the individual's time in the combat theater. This policy of individual rotation (rather than unit rotation) actually diminished small unit cohesion, increasing rather than decreasing the risk for stress-related mental health problems among those serving in Vietnam—something that S.L.A. Marshall had warned about in his World War II writings (Marshall, 1956 and Marshall, 1947).

The Vietnam War demonstrated the limits of traditional combat stress treatment approaches (Jones, F. D., 1995a, p. 20). This prolonged, unpopular, low-intensity conflict resulted in many psychological casualties (Shay, 1994). The most important principle it added to our understanding of combat stress is the value of mental health prevention efforts focused on the critical importance of building well-equipped, well-trained, well-led, cohesive units, with clear and achievable missions, and the necessary means to carry out the associated mission tasks. From a mental health prevention perspective, competent training includes combat stress prevention measures practiced at every level from the unit leader to the individual soldier. These measures include actions focused on the well-being of the soldier's family. Unit leaders must establish and maintain unit-family bonds designed to diminish the potential that family factors will become an added psychological burden for the deployed soldier. These biopsychosocial readiness factors, with their focus on primary prevention, can be added to our list of core combat stress treatment principles:

> Primary (mental health) prevention is a critical aspect of building, sustaining, and employing combat forces.

Across the history of warfare, literature suggests that combatants benefit from the opportunity to "tell their story." S. L. A. Marshall (1956) provided evidence of the importance of debriefing as a means of restoring psychological equilibrium after exposure to extremely traumatic events. The chance to share one's story (and experiences) with members of one's group can have a powerful therapeutic effect (Belenky, Martin, and Marcey, 1996). Various forms of debriefing, after what have been labeled critical incidents (Mitchell, 1991, pp. 8-9), are now standard aspects of civilian emergency and disaster mental health interventions. The military equivalent of these exposures has involved events such as the Marine Corps barracks bombing in Beirut or the civilian equivalent bombing in Oklahoma City. The critical incident stress literature (reviewed in the context of combat by Koshes, Young, and Stokes, 1995, pp. 271-290) that has emerged in the 1980s and 1990s provides a final principle for combat stress interventions:

> Group psychological interventions (critical incident debriefings) need to be the standard response to traumatic stress exposure.

Every effort needs to be made to keep individuals with their peers (those also exposed) until group members have the opportunity to process their experiences within a supportive group environment. Such debriefings need to be directed by individuals who have been trained in the principles of psychological debriefing. Gulf War experiences (Martin and Cline, 1996) suggest that this intervention will only be successfully implemented when military leaders understand the importance of these interventions and are committed to their implementation. Military mental health professionals must address these leadership issues before, not after, the occurrence of a traumatic event. A comprehensive, ongoing command consultation and training program must focus on leadership training. Among others, social workers serving in a variety of military medical and community roles can be critical in sensitizing military leaders to these issues.

SOME EXAMPLES OF SOCIAL WORK OFFICER INVOLVEMENT IN COMBAT AND NONCOMBAT STRESS INTERVENTIONS

Prior to a deployment or a military operation, a social work officer can help soldiers prepare for the stress that they will encounter. The following is an example of a stress inoculation training session conducted during the Gulf War.

Prior to the ground war phase of the Gulf War many expected a high American casualty rate. Soldiers trained as combat medics were concerned about their ability to provide effective care in a mass casualty situation. Aware of these concerns, a social work officer conducted a stress inoculation training session with the enlisted medics in the Armor Taskforce he was supporting.

Based on his knowledge of research from World War II and his prior experience as a "grunt" in Vietnam, the social work officer knew the general level of anxiety in combat could be reduced if the medics could use their high level of training as a realistic basis for believing in themselves and their ability to perform their military medical skills. All of the medics in the forward support battalion (FSB) assigned to the mechanized armor task force had completed the combat medical training course. They had earned the Expert Field Medical Badge (EFMB). They had received the best available training to that point.

The session started with the social worker asking each medic to describe his or her training and experience in some detail. These medics had emergency room training and experience. Without exception they stated that if they received two or three wounded soldiers they were confident they could handle the situation. They were concerned about receiving five or ten casualties at once. They thought that this load would exceed their capabilities to save lives. The social work officer asked them what they thought of the Army's Combat Lifesaver Program. This program is designed to train "grunts" to provide immediate first aid to their fellow soldiers. These medics all agreed that this was a great training program and would be a combat multiplier. Several of the medics had actually served as Combat Lifesaver instructors.

The social worker pointed out that the combat medics would not be the only soldiers with medical training. He reminded them that every soldier had basic CPR and first aid training. He added that the Combat Lifesavers in most cases would be the medical person closest to the wounded soldier, and they were capable of providing immediate lifesaving treatment to stabilize wounded soldiers. After these points were made, the medics started to recognize that this combination of trained soldiers, their own presence, and the backup of a doctor or highly trained physician assistant at the battalion aid stations would allow them to handle almost any contingency. They realized that they were not the sole medical support for the task force and this alone was a source of support.

The social worker discussed the medics' fears about combat and pointed out that these were normal reactions. He talked about the lessons from military history that demonstrated that troops who expressed a high degree of self-confidence prior to combat were more likely to perform well and with relatively less fear during battle. In this discussion the medics started to share with each other how they saw the stabilization and evacuation process of wounded soldiers operating during the battle. They subsequently had a meeting with the battalion surgeon, who outlined the triage and evacuation plan. They also touched base with the Combat Lifesavers at the unit level and made sure that they had the supplies they needed.

A positive atmosphere developed during this session. It was similar to the atmosphere in a locker room prior to an important athletic event. These medics had experienced tough, realistic medical training. They had prior experience treating physical trauma in a community hospital emergency room. They were focused. They had a plan. The medics supported each other. They understood their responsibilities. They were ready.

When combat came, two soldiers in the task force were immediately killed by direct fire. Four soldiers were wounded. The combination of Combat Lifesavers, combat medics, and battalion aid station doctors worked in synchronization to stabilize and evacuate the wounded soldiers. These medics had received their "baptism by fire" and they rose to the occasion. Today, they proudly wear the Combat Medic Badge (CMB) of distinction for their service during the Gulf War.

A Social Work Officer's Experience While Assigned to a Combat Stress Team During the Gulf War

A brigade contact team supported several reconnaissance, or "berm buster," missions in the days just prior to the start of ground combat during the Gulf War. These missions involved movement of armored battalions beyond the massive sand berm that Iraq had placed along its southern border. During these operations, the division suffered the loss of four soldiers, with twelve soldiers wounded in action. What follows is an account of two separate mental health debriefings following combat engagements.

The enlisted mental health corpsman and I approached the M113 Air Defense Track that had taken a direct hit and lost two crew members. We found the crew inventorying their equipment and we were both immediately overwhelmed by these soldiers' heightened emotions. I spoke to a soldier standing on top of the track and saw that he was close to tears. I asked him if he had heard any news of his sergeant, who had been evacuated with second- and third-degree burns. When he said no, we told him the story of how we were with the medical unit that had treated his sergeant shortly after he was wounded. We told him that his sergeant was conscious and had spoken with us prior to being evacuated. We said that the sergeant had been in a lot of pain, and that he was not likely to return to the unit soon, but was sure to recover. This news appeared to make this soldier feel better. We asked if we could help him and the crew with their inventory, and he invited us to climb on board their vehicle.

Once on the track, we could see that its top part had been blown off in the battle. The soldier described to us how their sergeant had taken a direct hit from an artillery mortar round and was decapitated. Another sergeant, the one we helped, had been burned by the explosion because he was standing below where the first soldier was killed. He vividly described how the decapitated sergeant's lower body had fallen into the track and settled to the floor for the rest of the crew to see. The other crew members also began to talk to us about the experience while they continued to remove ammunition and equipment from the track. One soldier got angry and started to cry. He held out his hand and showed us pieces of skin and bone. "This is all that's left of my sergeant," he said.

We remained with these soldiers until they completed their inventory. We talked with the crew about returning to combat. All three of those remaining had less than three years in the Army. Two said it was important for them to go into Iraq. One said he wanted to be placed in a support position but remain with his unit even if it returned to combat. Eventually the first two soldiers stayed in their jobs and the third drove a fuel truck for his unit. All performed well during the subsequent ground campaign. All three received awards for outstanding combat service.

The second debriefing involved a Bradley scout crew that had also been hit in the same battle as the Air Defense Track. We met with the survivors and walked with them to the motor pool where their Bradley (an armored personnel carrier) had been towed. I asked the crew to describe what had occurred. A staff sergeant immediately crouched to the ground and used a stick in the sand to diagram the battle. His speech was rapid as he related how a track commander of another Bradley had been hit and killed with a round. "I remember it like slow motion. It's just so unreal," he said. He told of watching the same Bradley take three more direct hits. Almost without thinking, he and his crew had then left their Bradley while under fire, moved to the hit Bradley, and started performing first aid. One member of the sergeant's crew ran to a wounded soldier and initiated medical aid. As the rounds came closer, the crewman covered the wounded soldier with his body, taking a fatal head wound as a result. The staff sergeant became visibly angry as he told of going to his Bradley, positioning it behind the disabled Bradley, loading a round, locating the Iraqi position, and "terminating" it. Ground ambulance crews then arrived and stabilized and evacuated the wounded. Iraqi fire then started to focus on other locations.

We shifted the focus of the conversation to other crew members and sought their comments. The staff sergeant continued his pressured speech and started to go through the battle again. My behavioral science specialist took the sergeant aside, and the debriefing continued with the remaining crew members. These soldiers concurred with the sergeant's account of the battle. Some crew members said that they had blocked out many of the details, and the sergeant's description had brought them back. We opened the Bradley and saw its partially charred interior. The mood in the group was like a wake.

These soldiers knew that we had assisted their wounded and handled their dead. They asked about the "L Tee" (their lieutenant and platoon leader), who had been burned about the face, taken some shrapnel, and injured his back in the battle. I told them what I knew—that he was awake, talking, and in a lot of pain when he was loaded on the evacuation helicopter. He seemed OK, but probably would not return to the unit soon if at all.

These crew members were later assigned to other crews. We visited them prior to their next battle, and they had spray painted "We're Back" on the outside of their new Bradley. They all served well in the ground war, and three Silver Stars were awarded to the involved soldiers, one posthumously.

These powerful vignettes offer striking testimony to several principles. An outstanding feature of both debriefings is the quick rapport achieved by the mental health team with these crew members. In general, combat veterans' level of suspicion toward the "strangers" was in direct proportion to the person's distance from combat. The mental health team had positioned itself centrally so they could be aware of the status of casualties and even participate in their medical care. Consequently, an implicit bond existed that was based on a mutual combat experience. Thus, the mental health team was trusted by both track crews.

This mental health team was active both prior to and during the ground attack. The social work officer was aggressively involved in reaching out to medical and line unit leaders throughout the immediate operational area. All members of the combat stress team had assumed a very high profile within the maneuver elements in their brigade through the use of stress prevention briefings and regular attendance at command and staff meetings. Their perceived availability and their level of credibility were essential factors in their success. These "berm buster" operations were highly sensitive and dangerous. If the mental health team members were not viewed as combat ready, their presence on the forward-deployed medical team would never have been allowed.

A Combat Stress Debriefing Conducted with a Group of Soldiers Who Attempted to Render Medical Aid to a Soldier Who Committed Suicide

The debriefing started when the social work officer asked the participants to describe the events. One medic started by saying, "Sir, you know how it is on the range. The command, 'all ready on the left, all ready on the right,' had been given. I was looking down range and waiting for the command to 'commence firing.' When the command was given and my target appeared, I started firing, and I immediately heard screams coming from the left. I stopped firing and I looked to my left and saw one of the instructors, a sergeant, jump down into the firing position. At that time, I placed my weapon on safe, removed my magazine, and moved over to the firing position to assist the sergeant. Upon jumping down into the firing position with the sergeant, I identified myself as a medic. My first observation was that the soldier had placed the barrel of his M-16 into his mouth and pulled the trigger. His kevlar helmet was still on and the round had not exited the helmet. By this time, the others had arrived to assist me. The only other soldiers permitted to see the soldier who had killed himself were the range ambulance crew. The medic went on to describe how he removed the soldier's helmet and saw the broken skull and brains inside. The group confirmed the medic's factual account of the critical event by their verbal and nonverbal responses.

It was clear that everyone was in agreement with the factual account of the critical event that the medic had provided. At this point, I asked the medic how he felt about it. He stated, "I did not see anything like this in the war and did not expect to see anything like this at Fort Hood." I asked each group member to discuss his thoughts and feelings about the event he had experienced. The soldier who was not a medic and had not been in combat expressed surprise at how the event had been stressful for the medics. He stated that he was also surprised about the medics' willingness to discuss their thoughts and emotions. He went on to state that he was as shocked about the event as the medics were and felt his thoughts and feelings were "normal."

After the participants discussed the facts of the event and their thoughts, I asked the question, "What bothered you about this event?" The medics' responses were very similar. They stated they were bothered by the fact that the victim took the option away from them to save his life. They expressed some anger toward the victim. They all expressed the shock of knowing the soldier was dead when they saw his brains. One medic remarked, "He didn't even think of his parents or friends, because he can't have an open casket funeral." The group then talked about what emotional state an individual gets in, to see suicide as the only way out. The nonmedic described seeing the victim's brains and realizing he was dead as the most significant for him. He stated, "When they were putting him in the ambulance, I threw up.

That's the first dead body I ever saw." In this phase, the group provided mutual support for each other. I observed emotions of disbelief, shock, and anger. Each participant stated that life had a new meaning for him and that he didn't think he would ever forget this event.

The medics focused on feelings of unreality by making statements such as, "I can't believe this guy killed himself. In my mind I can still see the look on his face. I don't think I'll ever forget the sight of his brains in his helmet." The nonmedic also confirmed that he had a vivid memory of the look on the soldier's face and how limp his body was. The nonmedic was very emotional and went on to say he did not know if he could ever eat spaghetti again. This statement broke the tension of the group, but all participants were well aware of the impact of the critical event on themselves and each other. This was supported by their verbal and nonverbal reassurances for each other.

As the session moved into the teaching stage of the debriefing process, I focused on some symptoms that participants often experience three to five days later. I told them that some participants may dream about their experience and that it is OK to dream. I also shared with them that at the one-year anniversary, they could find themselves thinking about the event. I discussed the predictable phases of the vulnerable state an individual usually goes through. I also discussed the possibility that at some point in the future, they may experience feelings of depression, helplessness, and hopelessness. I advised them that these feelings could surface at any time, particularly around the anniversary date of the critical event. I made it clear that if these symptoms occurred and persisted, they should seek mental health intervention. I remembered to myself that during the teaching phase of a debriefing, the debriefer must not set the survivors up for follow-up treatment, but they must not be led to believe they might never require it either. The teaching stage must reinforce the debriefer's goals of: (1) relieving the symptoms; (2) restoring participants to a pre-event level of functioning; (3) connecting the current stress with past life experiences that take them back to feelings of a vulnerable state; and (4) discussion of new ways of perceiving, thinking, feeling, and developing new coping responses that can be used beyond the immediate crisis situation.

After the participants asked all their questions, I provided them with information on when and where they could obtain additional treatment if they felt the need. I then concluded the session. The session lasted one hour and twenty minutes. During the session, the verbal and nonverbal behavior displayed by the nonmedic indicated that this experience was having a severe impact on him. My observations were confirmed when one of the medics pulled me aside and recommended I spend a few minutes talking with the nonmedic. In the process of talking with the nonmedic, I was able to get his permission to refer him for follow-up treatment. The nonmedic participated in follow-up treatment for three months and returned to the rifle range and qualified with his weapon.

The medics returned to the rifle range the following week and qualified with their weapons. A follow-up with their company commander disclosed that they were taking medical training more seriously. One of the medics volunteered and returned to Kuwait. The sergeant, who was first to jump into the firing position, never participated in any type of treatment.

These accounts of stress interventions during combat operations and in training environments provide an example of how social work officers function within the broadly defined military operational environment. It is obvious that these roles demand advanced clinical skills as well as appropriate military training. The opportunity to function in these roles requires that the social worker (or other mental health professional) be present in the environment where these events occur and where these potential clients are located. Access is critical. Typically, such access only happens when the social worker has previously established credibility with unit leaders and has taken the organizational steps necessary to ensure that they will learn about and be able to respond to trauma in a timely manner. These considerations led us to some thoughts about the future roles and opportunities for military social workers in support of military operations.

THE FUTURE

Each of the military services will enter the twenty-first century having developed well-thought-out visions of future threats and the nature of future armed conflicts. In general, these visions are focused on a vast array of threats ranging from a major war with Russia or China, a more likely regional conflict with a nation such as North Korea or Iran, to a high-technology threat from a vast array of ideological and/or religious terrorists willing to use biological, chemical, nuclear, and information technology weapons. Most military leaders believe that there are no real threats to American military dominance until at least 2010 if not beyond—no one nation possesses America's superpower military capabilities so as to pose a direct threat. As Colonel Mike Starry has noted, "so we have a benign period where we can take some risks and do some different things" (Naylor, 1996, p. 18). For many this means the opportunity for sacrifices in current personnel areas (quality, quantity, and compensation of personnel), in order to build structure—defined as "modernization"—the development of new high-technology weapons and weapon systems.

The absence of a major threat does not mean that there will not be conflict and/or dangerous military missions during the rest of this century and into the next. Clearly, the world remains a dangerous place and the U.S. military will continue to be involved in peacemaking and peacekeeping operations that will create risks for military personnel. These roles involve danger while training for these missions, while executing missions, and as seen in the air crash at Gander, Newfoundland, that killed members of the 101st Airmobile Division, danger just coming and going to and from training and operational activities locally and around the globe.

The U.S. military provides a unique capability for humanitarian functions at home and abroad. While they are considered low-frequency events, major manmade and natural disasters will continue to demand the use of military resources. Finally, as seen in the Oklahoma federal building bombing or the World Trade Center explosion, domestic terrorism is an ever-present and growing threat. As demonstrated by current efforts to develop National Guard resources in preparation for biological and chemical terrorist attacks, the U.S. military must remain "always ready."

Military social workers are among those uniquely trained to help in the response to many of these operational activities. In addition to their core clinical skills, the social work professions' historical focus on the "person in the environment" equips military social workers with a broad range of nonclinical skills that are invaluable in establishing prevention interventions, as well as dealing with what can be defined as the requirement to create, to manage, to coordinate, and to utilize formal and informal human service networks in support of overwhelming stress events. Unfortunately, current efforts to downsize the Department of Defense may lead to a loss of military social work positions. Currently, military social workers assigned to hospital and various community functions such as family advocacy have to defend their positions from those who see these roles as ripe for conversion to civilian positions and subsequent privatization. At the same time, the Army and the other services are looking to establish smaller operational units. The Army wants smaller divisions, the Navy wants fewer people onboard ship, and the Air Force envisions pilotless combat aircraft. As all the services seek to downsize, regardless of the motivation, military medical structure will be among the first to feel the effects. There will be a smaller medical component in each of the services. What the services cannot do without in preparation for medical support of combat operations will be moved into the reserve component—this is likely to include Army combat stress control units.

Military social workers, as well as other military mental health professionals, need to continue to advocate for the capability to support the mental health needs of our soldiers, sailors, marines, and airmen and women. This includes their well-being within the context of their daily service, and personal and family lives. In the context of this chapter, it means meeting the mental health needs of combat and other operational duties.

At the individual level, military social workers, regardless of the nature of their assignments, need to be versed in the clinical skills needed to respond to traumatic stress events. They should be ready and able to "deploy" whether it is in support of combat or a disaster. Universally, military social workers need to be willing and able to engage those who seek their care, in the field, on board ship, or in a hospital setting, with skills that will "conserve the fighting strength" and promote the recovery of those who have volunteered to sacrifice their lives and well-being for our nation.

A GUIDE FOR SOCIAL WORK OFFICERS ASSIGNED TO DIVISION MENTAL HEALTH TEAMS OR OTHER COMBAT STRESS CONTROL SETTINGS

Social work officers have historically worked with psychologists and psychiatrists in a variety of settings to provide assessment and treatment to the individual soldiers and their families. Military social workers need to be able to conduct mental health diagnostic assessments, make provisional (DSM-IV) diagnosis, and develop a comprehensive treatment plan.

Social work officers are trained to assist soldiers in the management of anxiety, suicide prevention, assessment and treatment of combat stress and battle fatigue, and substance abuse and critical event stress debriefings. Social work officers must understand the concepts of battlefield management of combat stress and battle fatigue. In many cases social work officers are the first mental health practitioners available to evaluate combat stress and battle fatigue.

In combat divisions (and similar operational assignments in the Navy or Air Force) it is part of the social work officer's responsibility to work in a high-stress environment, whether it is in a training exercise, a peacekeeping role, or actual combat. In these situations social work officers are deployed as far forward as possible based on the combat psychiatry principles discussed earlier in this chapter. The social work officer's goal in combat or peacekeeping operations is to provide rest to the soldiers exhibiting signs of stress, with return to the unit as soon as possible.

Many aspects of providing division (and other operationally based) mental health services are unusual. Some of the critical functions required in this role include the following.

Knowledge of the Organization

The division social worker must know the units in the division, understand their unique missions, follow their command climates, and track their mental health utilization rates. It is essential to know the role of each member of the division's command and staff. This enhances the division social worker's ability to understand implicit factors contributing to organization conflict and devise efficacious solutions.

Maintain Proximity and Build Mission Credibility

Soldiers, perhaps even more than the civilian community, view the mental health mission with a mixture of suspicion, stigma, and fear of career damage. Also, soldiers generally regard physicians with a mixture of respect for their education and disdain for their apparent disregard for military mores. The division mental health team must nurture proximity to the division and its soldiers to reduce soldier concerns based upon negative stereotypes and, as previously mentioned, become credible players on the division team to have full division command.

Maintain Unit Integrity to Nurture Cohesion

The division mental health team must develop cohesion with the division and within itself to increase combat readiness. The generally unspoken reality for every mental health team is the possibility of imminent combat. Mental health team members are often only dimly aware that their fate may depend on the decisions of the division social worker and section noncommissioned officer in charge. Therefore, these leaders must know their soldiers and nurture their trust and allegiance. Mental health team members must have a sense of belonging to the section and division.

Operational Cohesion Is Essential

During the Gulf War, many division mental health teams developed "fast-teams," subelements designed to move immediately on initiation of ground combat. Prior to combat, fast-teams were often located 100 or 200 meters from the main element, allowing them to develop a sense of its equipment, transportation, personnel, supply, and other needs. In doing so, the likelihood of last-minute surprises was reduced. We view division mental health teams in garrison as a "mental health fast-team." It is the possibility of impending deployment and subsequent combat that truly separates the division mental health team concept from their installation community mental health activity.

Advocate for Division Mental Health Interests

The division social worker is a staff officer to division command regarding matters of division morale and mental welfare. To perform this function effectively, the social worker's allegiance to the division must remain relatively untarnished by nondivision interests. If division mental health team positions remain unfilled in favor of placing personnel in the garrison hospital (or community mental health activity), mental health advocacy for the division will be lost. This loss potentially compromises the division's ability to respond efficiently during times of maximum stress.

"Train As You Fight"

Individual soldier and unit training is essential for each to achieve maximum performance under duress. Division mental health team members must become experienced at providing care to their division. Such experience better equips them to understand the unique customs of particular units, build credibility and rapport with commanders, fully appreciate organizational problems, and institute essential preventive mental health programs. We have heard it said among combat arms professionals, "We will fight as we have trained, therefore we must train as we expect to fight." For medical and mental health care professionals, perhaps we might say, "We will support the fight as we have trained, hence we must train as we expect to support the fight."

SOME IMPORTANT CONSIDERATIONS FOR SOCIAL WORK OFFICERS ASSIGNED TO A DEPLOYABLE STATUS

It is important to achieve your own "readiness status." In addition to achieving competency in military mental health skills, you must be a competent soldier. This means being physically fit and technically competent in basic soldier skills. Achieving the Expert Field Medical Badge (EFMB), the mark of a soldier who is proficient in basic field medicine, should be a goal. While your skills as a mental health officer are critical, your skills as a soldier-medic will often be the most important factor in gaining initial acceptance among both the line and your field medical peers. In addition, being perceived as "one dimensional" (behavioral science-focused only) will not help you get to the critical locations when there are "limited seats available on the bus." If you can't get there, you can't help, and you will always be competing to get to the battle with others who feel that their role is just as important as yours.

You must have the capacity of grasping the reality of the physical, mental, and emotional stressors of combat (or peacekeeping operations), and the impact of the leadership challenges faced by combat arms officers, NCOs, and soldiers. You must be willing to face the hardships and be able to provide a stabilizing and calming force. When the social work officer is seen as a force for helping soldiers facing traumatic events, as well as loneliness, boredom, and homefront worries, he or she will be viewed as a valued combat multiplier rather than an unwanted straphanger.

Pay attention to your own personal preparation. This includes taking time to prepare your own family prior to deployment. If you don't develop and maintain your own personal support system, you are doomed to failure and a lot of pain.

CORE READINGS FOR A LIBRARY ON COMBAT AND OPERATIONAL MENTAL HEALTH

Belenky, G. (Ed.) (1987). *Contemporary Studies in Combat Psychiatry.* Westport, CT: Greenwood.

Bourne, P.G. (1970). *Man, Stress, and Vietnam.* Boston: Little, Brown.

Camp, N.M. (1993). "The Vietnam War and the ethics of combat psychiatry." *American Journal of Psychiatry,* 150(7):1000-1010.

Copp, T. and McAndrew, B. (1990). *Battle Exhaustion: Soldiers and Psychiatrists in the Canadian Army, 1939-1945*. Montreal: McGill Queen's University Press.

Field Manual 22-51 (1994). U.S. Department of the Army: *Leaders' Manual for Combat Stress Control*, Washington, DC: Department of the Army.

Figley, C.R. (Ed.) (1985). *Trauma and Its Wake: Study and Treatment of Post-Traumatic Stress Disorder.* New York: Brunner/Mazel.

Gal, R. and Mangelsdorff, A.D. (Eds.) (1991). *Handbook of Military Psychology.* West Sussex, England: John Wiley and Sons.

Glass, A.J. (1953). "Preventive psychiatry in the combat zone." *U.S. Armed Forces Medical Journal,* 4:683-692.

Grinker, R.R. and Spiegel, J.P. (1963). *Men Under Stress*. New York: McGraw-Hill.

Hendin, H. and Haas, A.P. (1984). *Wounds of War: The Psychological Aftermath of Combat in Vietnam*. New York: Basic Books.

Holmes, R. (1985). *Acts of War: The Behavior of Men in Battle*. New York: The Free Press.

Jones, F. D., Sparacino, L.R., Wilcox, V.L., and Rothberg, J.M. (Eds.) (1994). "Military psychiatry: Preparing in peace for war." In *Textbook of Military Medicine.* Washington, DC: Office of the Surgeon General of the Army and The Borden Institute.

Jones, F. D., Sparacino, L. R., Wilcox, V. L., Rothberg, J. M., and Stokes, J. W. (Eds.) (1995). "War psychiatry." In *Textbook of Military Medicine*. Washington, DC: Office of the Surgeon General of the Army and The Borden Institute.

Keegen, J. (1978). *The Face of Battle*. New York: Penguin Books.

Kellett, A. (1982). *Combat Motivation: The Behavior of Soldiers in Battle*. Boston: Kluwer Nijhoff.

Levav, I., Greenfield, H., and Baruch, E. (1979). "Psychiatric combat reactions during the Yom Kippur War." *American Journal of Psychiatry*, 136(5):637-641.

Manning, F.J. (1991). "Morale, cohesion, and esprit de corps." In A.D. Mangelsdorff and R. Gals (Eds.), *Handbook of Military Psychology*. New York: John Wiley and Sons, pp. 531-558.

Martin, J.A. (1989). "Future combat: Critical aspects of medical readiness." *Army Magazine*, September, pp. 42-48.

Martin, J.A., Sparacino, L.R., and Belenky, G. (Eds.) (1996). *The Gulf War and Mental Health*. Westport, CT: Praeger.

Rahe, R. H. (1988). "Acute versus chronic psychological reactions to combat." *Military Medicine*, 153(7):365-372.

Shalit, B. (1988). *The Psychology of Conflict and Combat*. New York: Praeger.

Shay, J. (1994). *Achilles in Vietnam: Combat Trauma and the Undoing of Character*. New York: Atheneum.

Soloman, Z. (1993). *Combat Stress Reaction: The Enduring Tool of War*. New York: Plenum Press.

Stouffer, S.A., Lumsdaine, M.H., Williams, R.M., Smith, M.B., Janis, I.L., Star, S.A., and Cottrell, L.S. (1949). *Studies in Social Psychology in World War II. Vol. 2. The American Soldier: Combat and Its Aftermath*. Princeton, NJ.: Princeton University Press.

Talbott, J.E. (1997). "Soldiers, psychiatrists, and combat trauma." *Journal of Interdisciplinary History*, 27:3 (Winter), 437-454.

Wilson, J.P., Harel, Z., and Kahana, B. (Eds.) (1988). *Human Adaptation to Extreme Stress*. New York: Plenum Press.

NOTES

1. At one level, the U.S. Air Force has a very different perspective on combat stress than the Army. The Air Force combat mission is focused on the deployment of combat pilots and combat support aircrews. As D. R. Jones notes (1995, p. 179) "at a 3,000-person airbase, only 300 or so fliers might be exposed to combat." For fliers and flight crews, first-level mental health care is provided by the unit flight surgeon. As was seen in the Gulf War, modern forward-deployed air bases are potential targets and all base members are exposed to attack. Unlike the Army (and Marine Corps) in which all military members (even those in support roles) are theoretically trained and equipped as combat soldiers, in the Air Force nonflyers may have to suffer through an attack in a passive role, waiting for other military services (or their own security police) to provide a defense. This potential, and the stress associated with victimization, provides an important role for Air Force mental health

personnel. In most cases, at the base level, a mental health team consisting of a psychiatrist, psychologist, social worker, and typically two enlisted specialists will provide this first level of support (in the overall Air Force model of medical care this is a second-level response that follows first-level "self-care"). Doctrine calls for augmentation by a fifty-bed Air Transportable Hospital, which includes a similar mental health team to provide some short-term psychiatric holding capacity and the use of combat stress treatment principles that reflect Army doctrine (Jones, D. R., 1995, pp. 196-206).

2. Navy Critical Incident Stress Intervention Teams (SPRINT) were developed after the peacetime sinking of the USS *Cuyahoga* in the Chesapeake Bay in 1978. Since their formal adoption as a part of the Navy's Mobile Medical Augmentation Readiness Teams in 1983, the Navy has deployed SPRINT to a number of sea accidents and natural disasters (Mateczun, 1995, pp. 234-240). While Navy social work officers are not included as one of the specialties that make up these teams, Navy social work officers have deployed as team members, and there is every reason to believe that they will continue to deploy in the future. Navy social work officers were assigned to the two hospital ships deployed to the Persian Gulf during the Persian Gulf War and to each of the four combat stress centers operated by the Navy in the Gulf combat theater (Mateczun, 1995, p. 231). While Navy social work officers are no longer designated as hospital ship members, it is also likely that they would be part of any future ship deployment. Navy social workers serve in family advocacy roles in Marine Corps communities and would likely play an important role in any major mobilization.

REFERENCES

Artis, K.L. (1963). "Human behavior under stress: From combat to social psychiatry." *Military Medicine*, 128(10): 1011-1015.

Belenky, G., Martin, J.A., and Marcey, S.C. (1996). "After-action critical incident stress debriefings and battle reconstitutions following combat." In Martin, J.A., Sparacino, L.R., and Belenky, G. (Eds.). *The Gulf War and Mental Health*. Westport, CT: Praeger, pp. 105-114.

Copp, T. and McAndrew, B. (1990). *Battle Exhaustion: Soldiers and Psychiatrists in the Canadian Army, 1939-1945*. Montreal: McGill Queen's University Press.

Ginn, R.V.N. (1997). *The History of the U.S. Army Medical Service Corps*. Washington, DC: Office of the Surgeon General and Center of Military History, U.S. Army.

Glass, A.J. (Ed.) (1966). *Neuropsychiatry in World War II. Volume I*. Washington, DC: Office of the Surgeon General, U.S. Army.

Glass, A.J. (Ed.) (1973). *Neuropsychiatry in World War II. Volume II*. Washington, DC: Office of the Surgeon General, U.S. Army.

Holmes, R. (1985). *Acts of War: The Behavior of Men in Battle*. New York: The Free Press.

Holsenbeck, S.L. (1996). "Psych Force 90." In Martin, J.A., Sparacino, L.R., and Belenky, G. (Eds.), *The Gulf War and Mental Health*. Westport, CT: Praeger, pp. 39-58.

Jones, D.R. (1995). "U.S. Air Force combat psychiatry." In Jones, F. D., Sparacino, L.R., Wilcox, V.L., Rothberg, J.M., and Stokes, J.W. (Eds.), *War Psychiatry*. Washington, DC: Office of the Surgeon General of the Army and The Borden Institute, pp. 177-210.

Jones, F.D. (1995a). "Psychiatric Lessons of War." In Jones, F. D., Sparacino, L.R., Wilcox, V.L., Rothberg, J.M., and Stokes, J.W. (Eds.), *War Psychiatry*. Washington, DC: Office of the Surgeon General of the Army and The Borden Institute, pp. 1-29.

Jones, F.D. (1995b). "Traditional Warfare Combat Stress Cassalties." In Jones, F. D., Sparacino, L.R., Wilcox, V.L., Rothberg, J.M., and Stokes, J.W. (Eds.), *War Psychiatry*. Washington, DC: Office of the Surgeon General of the Army and The Borden Institute, pp. 35-61.

Koshes, R.J., Young, S.A., and Stokes, J.W. (1995). "Debriefing Following Combat." In Jones, F. D., Sparacino, L.R., Wilcox, V.L., Rothberg, J.M., and Stokes, J.W. (Eds.), *War Psychiatry*. Washington, DC: Office of the Surgeon General of the Army and The Borden Institute, pp. 271-290.

Marmar, C.R. and Horowitz, M.J. (1988). "Diagnosis and phase-oriented treatment of post-traumatic stress disorder." In Wilson, J., Harel, Z., and Kahana, B. (Eds.), *Human Adaptation to Extreme Stress*. New York: Plenum Press, pp. 81-103.

Marshall, S.L.A. (1947). *Men Against Fire*. New York: William Morrow.

Marshall, S.L.A. (1956). *Pork Chop Hill*. New York: William Morrow.

Martin, J.A. and Cline, W.R. (1996). "Mental health lessons from the Persian Gulf War." In Martin, J.A., Sparacino, L.R., and Belenky, G. (Eds.), *The Gulf War and Mental Health*. Westport, CT: Praeger, pp. 161-178.

Martin, J.A. and Fagan, J. (1996). "Army Mental Health Units in the Theater of Operations: An Overview of the Gulf War." In Martin, J.A., Sparacino, L.R., and Belenky, G. (Eds.), *The Gulf War and Mental Health*. Westport, CT: Praeger, pp. 19-32.

Mateczun, J. (1995). "U.S. Naval combat psychiatry." In Jones, F. D., Sparacino, L.R., Wilcox, V.L., Rothberg, J.M., and Stokes, J.W. (Eds.), *War Psychiatry*. Washington, DC: Office of the Surgeon General of the Army and The Borden Institute, pp. 211-242.

Mitchell, J.T. (1991). "Demobilizations." *Life Net*. (Newsletter of the American Critical Incidents Stress Foundation), 2(1), pp. 8-9.

Naylor, S.D. (1996). "Next up: Looking beyond force XXI." *Army Times*, (June 10), p. 18.

Rock, N.L., Stokes, J.W., Koshes, R.J., Fagan, J., Cline, W.R., and Jones, F.D. (1995). "U.S. Army combat psychiatry." In Jones, F. D., Sparacino, L.R., Wilcox, V.L., Rothberg, J.M., and Stokes, J.W. (Eds.), *War Psychiatry*. Washington, DC: Office of the Surgeon General of the Army and The Borden Institute, pp. 149-175.

Shay, J. (1994). *Achilles in Vietnam: Combat Trauma and the Undoing of Character.* New York: Atheneum.

Stokes, J.W. and Jones, F.D. (1995). "Combat Stress Control in Joint Operations." In Jones, F. D., Sparacino, L.R., Wilcox, V.L., Rothberg, J.M., and Stokes, J.W. (Eds.), *War Psychiatry.* Washington, DC: Office of the Surgeon General of the Army and The Borden Institute, pp. 243-270.

Chapter 10

The Role of Social Work in Policy Practice

John Cox

INTRODUCTION

Social workers are major providers of health and mental health services within the Department of Defense and in the general population. Military social workers provide a broad range of services in both traditional and nontraditional settings and employ a wide array of interventions. In their work, military social workers utilize multimodal clinical approaches, conduct organizational and human resource consultation, perform program evaluation research, and administer an assortment of human service programs.

The number of military social workers and their roles have expanded over the past three decades (McNelis, 1987). Various authors have commented on the history and roles of social work in the military (Black, 1991; Hamlin et al., 1982). Social work in the military evolved from the early beginnings of the Home Service Bureau of the Department of Civilian Relief to the establishment in 1919 of the Bureau of Medical Social Work within the Public Health Service. The roots of Army social workers were psychiatric in nature and hospital or clinic based. In 1943, psychiatric social work became a military occupational specialty in the Army (Hamlin et al., 1982). McNelis (1987) traces military social work's long and distinguished record of service to military personnel in the Civil War. From its earliest beginnings during World War I, psychiatric social work served military personnel deemed the "neurotic casualties" of war (Black, 1991, p. 387). Military social workers, operating primarily in medical settings and employing quasi-psychiatric methodologies, established their legitimacy and military necessity. The emphasis during this gestation period was clearly on the *psychiatric* versus the *social work* functions.

The domestic turbulence of the 1960s and 1970s coupled with the strains of the Vietnam War led to some expansion of services beyond the medical setting. The development of Army Community Services, social work in corrections, addiction treatment, and family advocacy illustrate the expanding roles of military social work; a shift, albeit hesitant and modest, toward social action and advocacy. This shift toward social action reflected changes taking place in social work education programs (Hamlin et al., 1982).

Over time, the roles of the military social work officer have broadened from a clinical orientation with a micro focus to include policy practice activities. This expansion of social work first occurred within the medical/mental health setting. More recently, roles widened further to include policy consultation and program development functions on a macro-organizational scale. As military social workers developed experience with the organizational culture and attained senior leadership positions, they were able to establish their credibility in new and expanded roles. Increasingly, social work expertise turned its attention to the dual focus consistent with its value base: improving the response of the military institution to individual and family needs as well as the individual's adaptation to the demands of military life.

This chapter identifies the rationale for social work's policy practice role within the context of a rapidly changing United States armed forces, suggests a model for policy practice in the military, and explores the contributions, challenges, and opportunities of military social workers as policy practitioners.

THE CHANGING MILITARY

The mission, organization, and culture of the United States military are changing rapidly. These changes are profound and have wide-ranging implications for military personnel and their families. LaBerge (1993) documented the downsizing of the American army following the Civil War. Change, therefore, is not new to the military. While the U.S. military has always been a dynamic and changing organization, social forces over the past three decades have accelerated the pace and depth of changes faced by America's armed forces.

The end of the all-volunteer force (AVF) signaled a major new direction away from the traditional institutional military toward an occupational model (Moskos, 1983). With the AVF, the post-Vietnam era brought a Pentagon rapidly reinventing itself with business practices and a developing corporate culture; a culture increasingly responsive to and dependent upon market forces and changing social demographics. The metamorphosis of the U.S. armed forces from a predominantly single and conscript military to one composed of families, particularly families with children, began to transform long-held institutional values.

During this period, military family programs evolved from largely volunteer efforts to formal institutionalized responses to family needs. There was a growing recognition that morale, recruitment, retention, and combat readiness are linked to family support (Bowen, 1994; Wood, 1991; Segal, 1984). This recognition accelerated the establishment of Family Centers within each branch of the military. The Persian Gulf War demonstrated the critical contributions of Family Centers to combat readiness and highlighted the growing emphasis on the concept of *total force,* a reliance on Reserves and the National Guard to support active combat operations (Knox and Price, 1995).

Today's active duty American military is substantially smaller than that of the Cold War. The fiscal year (FY) 1998 strength was 1,431,000 versus 2,069,000 in FY 1990, a reduction of over 600,000 personnel (U.S. Department of Defense, 1996, 1997a).

The post-Cold War military, thus, finds itself downsized, right sized, and reorganized, with a vastly altered culture and redefined global responsibilities. Issues of gender integration and policies governing sexual orientation have shaken established norms of behavior. The combination of force reductions, heightened operational tempo, redefined missions, and organizational restructuring, coupled with shifting personnel demographics, has produced unprecedented force turbulence. This turbulence has shaken the foundations of long-cherished military values and traditions with consequences for the quality of life of military members and families.

PRACTICE IN THE CONTEXT OF THE MILITARY CULTURE POLICY

Understanding the environmental context within which military social workers practice establishes the rationale and functions of the policy practitioner. Social work values and professional education are consistent with the policy practitioner role. Effectiveness as a policy practitioner depends upon social workers who possess the attributes of loyalty, competence, and a core knowledge base coupled with a demonstrable understanding of the military institution, its cultural traditions, and organizational structures.

The United States military is a large and complex organization. Its history, traditions, and culture distinguish it in ways that significantly affect the lifestyle of its members and their families. The institutional military is further differentiated from other bureaucracies and exerts normative pressure on its members to conform to its unique institutional culture, a culture characterized by unconditional commitment to the mission, service before self, uncertainty and unpredictability in lifestyle, sometimes dangerous missions, frequent separations from family, and acceptance of a way of life without some of the constitutional protections commonly expected by American citizens.

The military is also differentiated from most other organizations by the imposition of these demands on the children and families of military members (Wood, 1988). Military personnel and their families are connected to the organization by a demanding social contract that places high expectations on each. Several authors (Hill, 1949; Martin, Sparacino, and Belenky, 1996; Balgopal, 1989) have examined the stress associated with the military lifestyle.

When the characteristics of a knowledge of the military system are combined with strong professional credibility, mastery of appropriate ecosystems theory, and political/interactional skills, the experienced military social worker has a powerful capacity to effect change at the institutional level. Military social workers in policy assignments are positioned to effectively advocate on behalf of military personnel and families. Social workers utilizing policy skills influence key policy decisions affecting quality of life, community resources, military readiness, recruitment, retention, human relations, and a host of human resource issues that can affect combat capabilities.

The military social worker practicing at the micro level must balance the constantly competing demands of combat readiness and individual/family well-being. Likewise, the policy practitioner recognizes that human resource and military operational policies should be complementary, or at least synchronous, in order to maintain the delicate balance between optimal readiness and individual and family needs.

FRAMEWORKS FOR POLICY PRACTICE IN THE MILITARY

The scope of military social work has evolved to include macro practice activities. This growth in the policy domain represents a natural extension of social work responsibilities. As military social work officers are promoted in grade, they occupy leadership positions where they may leverage power to bring about positive organizational change. However, no clearly articulated framework has been applied specifically to guide the military social work policy practitioner.

According to Jansson (1994, p. 8), policy practice involves "efforts to influence the development, enactment, implementation, or assessment of social policy." Policy practice for the social worker in a military setting is a legitimate service arena deserving equal import with clinical, community, and administrative social work intervention. Applied to the military social worker, policy practice involves a broad range of macro practice interventions. This systems-level involvement encompasses not only the more orthodox human service functions but also human resource consultation, organizational development, and program planning activities.

In many ways the U.S. military has been on the cutting edge of social services. Its uniqueness as an organization and the many demands placed on those who serve have required a significant investment in human service programs. The military social worker, grounded in ecological theory and equipped with an understanding of institutional and individual needs, is particularly well-positioned to engage in policy practice.

The stages of social services in the workplace proposed by Ozawa (1980), offers a useful model for tracing the development of social work's policy practice role. In this four-stage model, Stage 1 social services are narrowly focused on one or two discrete problem areas.

Services are essentially tertiary in nature and limited in scope. Early efforts by the Services in the areas of alcoholism treatment, drug rehabilitation, and short-term mental health interventions are examples of Stage 1 social services programs.

In Stage 2, the interconnectedness of problems is recognized. Social services expand to include a wider array of problems. Recognition of the role of prevention, education, and early intervention begins. The evolution within the military of a community-based approach to alcohol and drug awareness and prevention activities, Army Community Services, and expansion of child advocacy to family advocacy programs illustrate Stage 2 services.

In Stage 3, social service interventions are increasingly at the macro level, although the social worker remains involved in some micro-level activities. The organization is maturing and there is greater recognition of the impact of the work environment on worker well-being. Military social workers involved in Stage 3 interventions provide leadership consultation, conduct stress management training, engage in a broad array of health promotion activities, and design, implement, and manage programs focused on the human relations aspects of the organization.

In Stage 4, the focus shifts to systems-level services. The targets of such macro-level interventions are the institutional structures of the organization, the larger military community, and those aspects of the organizational milieu that shape the quality of life of its members. The challenges posed in this phase are complex and go far beyond the traditional boundaries of the medical or mental health setting. Social work interventions in Stage 4 encompass human resource development, strategic planning, identification of core values, program evaluation, team building, and community support activities. The overarching goal is to maximize personnel readiness through humanizing the organization and developing its system-level capacities. Military social work policy practitioners focus on issues such as work and family, expansion of family centers, community development, and human relations policy.

The four-stage model discussed here provides a useful framework for understanding the progression of social work interventions from a micro to macro focus. Military social workers initially engaged in clinical practice develop a knowledge base of the organization that helps to prepare them for the larger policy practice tasks. These include advocacy, mediation, organizational development, and program planning and management.

U.S. NAVY SOCIAL WORK AND POLICY PRACTICE

The distribution of uniformed social workers across the military branches is uneven, and the historical development of social work in the armed forces varies. The Navy social work program is the youngest of the military social work programs. Although the program is small and relatively young compared to those of the Army and Air Force, it is, nevertheless, vibrant. There are some thirty Navy social work officers (personal communication with U.S. Navy Captain Dave Kennedy, March 1998). One officer is presently serving at the O-6 (Captain) level; therefore, senior policy leadership opportunities are limited. There is one military social work authorization at the Bureau of Medicine and Surgery. In this policy position, the Navy social worker provides policy guidance and policy development services to TRICARE, Utilization Management, managed care, and case management activities. In this capacity, the policy practitioner's role has important implications for one of the most challenging dilemmas facing today's military; the provision of adequate and accessible health care to active duty and retired personnel and their families.

The Bureau of Naval Personnel (BUPERS) also has a social work billet in charge of its Sexual Assault Victim Intervention Program (SAVI). In this position, the social worker plans programs, writes policy, and develops intervention and training guidelines. Within BUPERS, a navy social worker also provides policy guidance for the Family Advocacy Program (FAP). Navy social workers selected for O-6 have opportunities to command a Navy medical clinic, naval hospital, or regional medical center. The specialty leader for social work is a member of the Medical Service Corps' Executive Planning Committee and in this role provides consultation on the corps strategic plan, annual plan, and establishes direction for the Medical Service Corps. Clearly, as the Navy social work program matures, social workers will attain senior officer standing, thus permitting a substantially larger role in the policy practice arena.

U.S. ARMY SOCIAL WORK AND POLICY PRACTICE

The Army's uniformed social work program is the oldest and, in terms of authorization, the largest of the military services. Policy practice by Army social work officers is advanced and extensive. Social work policy authorizations may be found in a wide array of positions.

Social work is represented on the staff of the Army surgeon general; chief, Army community services division in the department of community and family support center; Army center for health promotion and preventive medicine (CHPPM); behavioral health; and chief of the alcohol and drug policy branch. The Army has made extensive use of social work expertise in the policy arena. This is particularly shown by the contributions of Army social workers to policies regarding support to families during combat deployments and progressive planning in support of the Army Family Action Plan. Through representation in the senior ranks, Army social workers are especially well positioned to design, implement, and evaluate Army initiatives aimed at improving the quality of life for Army families and communities. Army social workers are involved in health policy practice within such organizational settings as the Uniform Health Services University of Health Sciences Family Practice Department, the Office of the Secretary of Defense for Legislative Affairs, the Office of Family Policy and Support Services Family Advocacy Program, health care studies and clinical investigation activity, and chief of Soldier and Family Support Branch.

With the restructuring of the Army medical departments into six regional medical commands (RMCs), senior social workers are actively engaged in policy practice. These social workers develop medical social service policy, plan and monitor service delivery, manage programs, and address issues related to the health and welfare of personnel and families throughout their respective regions (personal communication with U.S. Army Colonel E. Hamlin, March 1998). The positions identified above are not exhaustive but reveal the breadth and depth of the roles played by Army social workers in the policy arena. In these positions, social workers in the Army carry out a diverse spectrum of policy practice tasks that include work and family support, child care, race and gender relations, health policy, health promotion and fitness, youth services, community development, housing, quality of life, and combat support.

U.S. AIR FORCE SOCIAL WORK AND POLICY PRACTICE

The role of Air Force social work in policy practice has developed along the continuum outlined by Ozawa's four-stage model. For most of its history, Air Force social workers performed conventional clinical functions within the mental health setting. As the Air Force itself changed, the roles and functions of Air Force social work developed to respond to the changes.

Today, the Air Force reports that approximately thirty uniformed social work positions are considered as predominantly policy in nature (personal communication with U.S. Air Force Colonel Alice Tarpley, March 1998). These include a broad range of assignments related to health, mental health, personnel, force management, and readiness.

Air Force social workers have contributed to policies that established Family Support Centers, developed the Transition Assistance and Relocation Assistance programs, redesigned and strengthened the Family Advocacy Program, assessed the extent of sexual harassment incidents, strengthened equal opportunity and sexual harassment education and training, and restructured the Social Actions programs.

When the Air Force Chief of Staff directed a review of the Family Support Center program in 1988, Air Force social workers were key participants on the review panel. Because of social work contributions, the design of the centers was modernized to be community based, staffed with human service professionals and with programming that focused on prevention, education, and early intervention. Air Force social workers continue to provide important policy and program guidance in support of spouse employment, family readiness, and advanced telecommunications initiatives.

In 1990, Congress passed the Defense Base Closure and Realignment Act. By 1995, 250 installations had been closed or reduced in size. Air Force social workers contributed to strengthening the model Base Realignment and Closure (BRAC) process. Because of congressional interest in the impact of base closures on quality of life, the Services were required to measure this impact. Social workers at the Air Staff developed a measurement tool that became part of the base closure survey protocol.

In 1994, in response to congressional interest, the Secretary of Defense asked for a full report on the Services' gender and race relations programs. The Secretary of the Air Force and Undersecretary of Defense for Personnel and Readiness co-chaired the Defense Equal Opportunity Council Task Force on Discrimination and Sexual Harassment. An Air Force social worker was selected to serve as executive assistant to the Secretary of the Air Force to provide subject matter expertise in evaluating and recommending improvements to strengthen the Services' programs. This nine-month effort produced a report to Congress that detailed forty-eight improvements in the manner in which the armed services respond to discrimination and sexual harassment (Defense Equal Opportunity Council, 1995). Social work leadership was instrumental in providing the policy guidance contained in the report and led to the most sweeping changes to the equal opportunity programs in two decades.

Today, Air Force social workers may be found assigned to such varied policy activities as psychological operations, developing career instructor opportunities and providing consultation services; the Readiness Directorate in the Air Force Surgeon's office, managing global readiness responsibilities; developing recruitment policy; serving as a group commander; and in several major air command mental health positions.

CONCLUSION

The United States military of the future will face increasing challenges from the rapidly changing geopolitical and economic realities of a post-Cold War world. Advances in technology are bringing about a revolution in the nature of warfare. Continual pressure from downsizing, new and unfamiliar missions, operational tempo, and emerging market forces will place ever-increasing strains on the military's human resources. In addition to continued access to professional mental health services, military personnel and their families will increasingly require assistance in the areas of life skills development, child care, relocation, retirement planning, readiness, and family separation. To meet these and other challenges of the twenty-first century, the armed forces will continue to benefit from social work expertise in human relations, family support, combat readiness, and psychiatric casualty management.

The uniformed social worker, with an ecological systems perspective, dual client focus, military experience, and policy skills will play an even more critical role in assisting the nation's armed services to meet the changing demands of future military operations.

BIBLIOGRAPHY

American Forces Information Services (1997). *Defense 97: Almanac issue.* Alexandria, VA: American Forces Information Services.

Balgopal, P.R. (1989). Occupational social work: An expanded clinical perspective. *Social Work,* 24(5), 437-442.

Black, W.G. Jr. (1991). Social work in world war I: A method lost. *Social Service Review,* (September), 380-398.

Bowen, G.L. (1994). Effects of leader support in the work unit on the relationship between work spillover and family adaptation. *ARI technical report 1019.* Alexandria, VA: U.S. Army Research Institute for the Behavioral and Social Sciences.

Defense Equal Opportunity Council (May 1995). *Report of the task force on discrimination and sexual harassment, volumes I and II.* Washington, DC: Department of Defense.

Garbarino, J. (1992). *Children and families in the social environment,* Second edition. New York: Aldine de Gruyter.

Hamlin, E.R. II, Timberlake, E.M., Jentsch, D.P., and VanVrankin, E.W. (1982). *U.S. Army social work in the 1980s.* Washington, DC: U.S. Government Printing Office.

Harris, J. (1993). Military social work as occupational practice. In P.A. Kurzman and S.H. Akabas (Eds.), *Work and well-being: The occupational social work advantage* (pp. 276 290). Washington, DC: NASW Press.

Hill, J. (1949). *Families under stress: adjustment to the crisis of war separation and reunion.* New York: Harper and Brothers.

Hunter, D.J. (1982). *Families under the flag: A review of military family literature.* New York: Praeger.

Jansson, B.S. (1994). *Social policy from theory to policy practice,* Second edition. Pacific Grove, CA: Brooks/Cole Publishing Company.

Jones, S.J. (1998). Professional development in the human services: Implications for the 21st century. In S.J. Jones and J.L. Zlotnik (Eds.), *Preparing helping professionals to meet community needs: Generalizing from the rural experience* (pp. 3-13). Alexandria, VA: Council on Social Work Education.

Knox, J. and Price, D.I. (1995). The changing American military family: Opportunities for social work. *Social Service Review,* 69(3), 479-497.

LaBerge, W. (1993). Dangerous downsizing. *Armed Forces Journal International*, 131(3), 30-34.

Martin, J.A., Sparacino, I.R., and Belenky, G. (1996). *The Gulf War and mental health: A comprehensive guide*. Westport, CT: Praeger.

McNelis, P. (1987). Military social work. In A. Minhan (Ed-in-chief), *Encyclopedia of social work,* Eighteenth edition, volume II (pp. 154-161). Silver Spring, MD: National Association of Social Workers.

Moskos, C. (1983). The all volunteer force. In M. Janowitz and S.D. Westbrook (Eds.), *The political education of soldiers* (pp. 307-322). Beverly Hills, CA: Sage.

Ozawa, M.M. (1980). Development of social services in industry: Why and how? *Social Work*, 25(6), 464-470.

Richards, K.B. and Bowen, G.L. (1993). Military downsizing and its potential implications for Hispanic, black, and white soldiers. *The Journal of Primary Prevention*, 14(1), 73-90.

Segal, M.W. (1984). Conflict and competition between service members and family. *Armed Forces and Society*, 13(1), 9-38.

Segal, M.W. (1988). The military and the family as greedy institutions. In C.C. Moskos and F.R. Woods (Eds.), *The military: More than just a job* (pp. 79-96). Washington, DC: Pergamon-Brassey's International Defense Publishers, Inc.

Smith, M.L. and Gould, G.M. (1993). A profession at the crossroads: Occupational social work—present and future. In P.A. Kurzman and S.H. Akabas (Eds.), *Work and well-being: The occupational social work advantage* (pp. 7-12). Washington, DC: NASW Press.

U.S. Department of Defense, Defense Manpower Data Center (September 1996). *Military personnel by branch of service.* Washington, DC: Department of Defense.

U.S. Department of Defense, Defense Manpower Data Center (September 1997a). *Military personnel by branch of service.* Washington, DC: Department of Defense.

U.S. Department of Defense, Defense Manpower Data Center (1997b). *Report of the secretary of the Air Force*. Washington, DC: Department of Defense.

Wood, F.R. (1988). At the cutting edge of institutional and occupational trends: The U.S. Air Force officer corps. In C.C. Moskos and F.R. Woods (Eds.), *The military: More than just a job* (pp. 27-37). Washington, DC: Pergamon-Brassey's International Defense Publishers, Inc.

Wood, L.L. (1991). Family factors and the reenlistment intentions of Army enlisted personnel, *Interfaces*, 21(1), 92-110.

PART III: UNIQUE ISSUES OF MILITARY SOCIAL WORK

Chapter 11

Common and Unique Ethical Dilemmas Encountered by Military Social Workers

Steven H. Tallant
Richard A. Ryberg

INTRODUCTION

The purpose of this chapter is to identify and discuss ethical dilemmas both unique and common to all active duty military social workers regardless of branch of service or practice setting. The intention of this chapter is not to identify, discuss, and resolve all possible ethical dilemmas faced by military social workers. This would be both unrealistic and impossible. The purpose is, however, to help generate awareness and discussion of these dilemmas and the unique military factors that help to create them. Finally, a suggested outline for resolving ethical dilemmas is presented.

ETHICAL DILEMMAS IN SOCIAL WORK

Ethical dilemmas are neither new nor unique to military social workers. The issues of ethics and values are well documented in the literature (Reamer, 1995). Historically, social workers in all occupational settings have been faced with daily ethical problems. The earliest known attempts to formulate a way of dealing with ethical dilemmas can be traced back to the 1920s and attributed to Mary Richmond (Pumphrey, 1959). While the nature and complexity of these dilemmas have changed over time, contemporary social workers continue to grapple with difficult ethical questions, as do military social workers.

In fact, all professionals, regardless of their profession, face ethical dilemmas. As a result, over time, each profession (e.g., social work, law, medicine, military) has developed a method for dealing with dilemmas unique to their expertise. The most common and accepted method is the development and implementation of a professional code of ethics. A code of ethics is instrumental in the development and recognition of a profession by the larger society.

The National Association of Social Workers (NASW) developed the *NASW Code of Ethics* (1996) for the social work profession. However, before we discuss the development and use of this code of ethics, we need to define the term "ethical dilemma" and identify situations that create ethical dilemmas for social workers.

The term "ethics" comes from the Greek root *ethos*, which means custom, usage, or habit. But contemporary ethics goes far beyond mere custom or habit, dealing with professional performance and sanctions. Professional ethics are concerned with the correct course of professional actions. Social work ethics are designed to help social workers decide which of two or more competing goals is the correct one for the given situational context (Loewenberg and Dolgoff, 1996).

According to Loewenberg and Dolgoff, a dilemma is a problem, situation, or predicament that seems to defy a satisfactory solution. The word "dilemma" comes from two Greek roots: *di* (double) and *lemma* (propositions). Therefore, a dilemma is a predicament in which the decision maker must choose between two options of near or equal value. In addition, the dilemmas that confront modern professionals may result from options which are not well defined, or from solutions which create additional possible or known problems and harm for the problem carrier or for others.

Therefore, an ethical dilemma can be created because of several different types of situations. First, an ethical dilemma occurs in a situation where the social worker must choose the best moral course of action in a predicament in which there are two competing and equal moral choices. However, these moral choices may be based upon two different moral philosophies and they conflict with one another. Second, an ethical dilemma is encountered when the decision maker must choose the best moral course of action without knowing in advance the outcome of the decision. In the long run, the chosen course of action may not be beneficial for all parties involved or may even harm a party. The final ethical dilemma is encountered when the best moral choice may not be best for all the individuals involved in the predicament and, in fact, knowingly cause harm to one of the individuals. Each of these situations can create countless ethical dilemmas for a social worker.

DEVELOPMENT AND OVERVIEW OF THE NASW CODE OF ETHICS

The National Association of Social Workers adopted its first code of ethics in 1960. Since that time there have been two major revisions of the code. The first took place in 1979, and the current *NASW Code of Ethics* was approved by the 1996 NASW Delegate Assembly. The *NASW Code of Ethics* presents the ethical standards (both general principles and specific rules) that professional social workers are expected to follow.

"The *NASW Code of Ethics* is intended to serve as a guide to the everyday professional conduct of social workers" (National Association of Social Workers, 1996, p. 1). This code includes four sections. The first section summarizes the social work profession's mission and core values. Values include service, social justice, dignity and worth of the person, importance of human relationships, integrity, and competence. The second section provides an overview of the code's main functions and a brief guide for dealing with ethical issues or dilemmas in social work practice. The third section presents broad ethical principles, based on social work's core values, that inform social work practice. These ethical principles include the following: social workers' primary goal is to help people in need and to address social problems; to challenge social injustice; to respect the inherent dignity and worth of the person; to recognize the central importance of human relationships; to behave in a trustworthy manner; to practice within their areas of competence; and to develop and enhance their professional expertise (National Association of Social Workers, 1996).

The final section includes specific ethical standards to guide social workers' conduct and to provide a basis for adjudication. These standards concern social workers' ethical responsibilities (1) to clients,

(2) to colleagues, (3) in practice settings, (4) as professionals, (5) to the social work profession, and (6) to the broader society. Later in this chapter, we will refer to these values, principles, and ethical standards when discussing the unique and common ethical dilemmas encountered by military social workers.

When discussing the purpose of the *NASW Code of Ethics*, the code points out the complexity of resolving ethical dilemmas. For example, no set of rules prescribes how a social worker should act in all situations and the code does not specify which values, principles, and standards are most important. In fact, the code realizes that reasonable differences of opinion can and do exist among social workers with respect to the ways in which values, ethical principles, and ethical standards should be rank ordered when they conflict. Finally, the code notes that there are other sources of information about ethical thinking that may be useful, but notes that social workers should consider the *NASW Code of Ethics* as their primary source.

The majority of daily ethical dilemmas are no different for military social workers than for civilian social workers. All social workers, military and civilian alike, need to be familiar with the *NASW Code of Ethics* and use it for its intended purposes. In addition, numerous books on the subject can aid the professional social worker in the resolution of ethical dilemmas (Pumphrey, 1959; Loewenberg and Dolgoff, 1996; Rhodes, 1991; Reamer, 1982). Another excellent resource in helping resolve ethical dilemmas is *Social Work Speaks: NASW Policy Statement* (National Association of Social Workers, 1994). However, none of these resources discusses ethical dilemmas unique to military social work.

DISTINGUISHING MILITARY FACTORS CONTRIBUTING TO ETHICAL DILEMMAS

Five factors inherent in military life contribute to the development of ethical dilemmas for military social workers. These factors must be clearly understood to appreciate the complexity and uniqueness of the many ethical dilemmas confronted by military social workers. It should be noted that these issues are not independent of one another. In fact, sometimes the combination or the interaction of these factors increases the possibility of ethical dilemmas occurring. However, for the purposes of this chapter, each will be discussed independently. These factors include the dual profession of the military social worker, the multipurpose role of the social worker as a human service provider, hierarchical structure governed by military law (Uniform Code of Military Justice), dual clients (active duty and civilians), and geographic and professional isolation. Following a discussion and explanation of each factor, specific examples of ethical dilemmas related to each military factor are presented. In addition, each ethical dilemma is discussed with regards to the ethical standard prescribed by the *NASW Code of Ethics*.

While is it not the intent of this chapter to resolve the identified dilemmas, several of them are so germane to the everyday practice of military social work that they are labeled core ethical dilemmas. These core ethical dilemmas must be both clearly understood and resolved by all military social workers. If not, they can and often do lead to significant stress and eventual burnout for military social workers. The stress and burnout can lead to both an unproductive and unhappy military career. Therefore, these core ethical dilemmas must be identified and resolved prior to or shortly after a social worker enters active duty. Not everyone will be able to resolve these dilemmas in a personally and professionally satisfactory resolution. This does not imply that the individual is a poor problem solver, a poor social worker, unethical, or unpatriotic. However, it does imply that he or she may not be suited for a military career.

The Dual Profession of the Military Social Worker

The military social worker is both a professional social worker and a professional officer. While other social work settings may and often do create role conflict for the social worker, no setting is more prone to role conflict than the military setting.

As professional social workers, military social workers receive the same education as their civilian counterparts. They support and believe in the primary mission of the social work profession: to enhance human well-being and help meet the basic human needs of all people, with particular attention to the needs and empowerment of people who are vulnerable, oppressed, and living in poverty (National Association of Social Workers, 1996). Furthermore, military social workers focus on individual well-being in a social context and the well-being of society. They are concerned with and pay attention to the environmental forces that create and contribute to problems in living. Finally, military social workers support and use the *NASW Code of Ethics* in resolving ethical dilemmas and are held accountable to the social work profession for their professional actions. However, they are also held accountable to another profession: the military profession.

Upon entering the Service, military social workers are commissioned as officers. They are sworn to support the Constitution of the United States, defend the United States against all enemies foreign and domestic, and to follow the orders of their superiors.

As with all recognized professions, the military has both a moral base and an ethical base for the practice of arms (DeGeorge, 1987; Brown and Collins, 1981; Smith, 1988; Watkin, 1979). In addition, Huntington proposed a Code of Military Ethics including the following:

1. To prefer peace to war, and realize that the military serves most effectively when it deters and so prevents war rather than when it engages in war.
2. To use the utmost restraint in the use of force, using only as much as necessary to fulfill my mission.
3. To obey all legitimate orders, but only legitimate orders.
4. To remember that those beneath me are moral beings worthy of respect and I shall never command them to do what is immoral.
5. To be responsible for what I command and for how my orders are carried out.
6. To never order those under me to do what I would not myself be willing to do in a like situation. (Huntington, 1979)

As Davenport notes, "the modern officer corps is a professional body and the modern military officer a professional man [or woman]. The paramount duty of the military professional is to promote the safety and welfare of humanity and this duty, according to military law, takes precedence over duties to clients, who as his fellow citizens are but a particular portion of the human race" (Davenport, 1987, p. 5).

It is obvious that role conflict will develop for the military social worker. The military social worker is both a professional social worker and professional officer. Each profession has its own set of morals, values, and ethics. Each has it own purpose or mission. This role conflict will create core ethical dilemmas for the military social worker. The question is often asked: Can one be both an officer and a social worker? If so, which takes precedence? Are there different times or situations when one role takes precedence over the other?

Interestingly, this core conflict can be discerned in the article "Military Social Work," written by David Garber and Peter McNelis and published in *The Encyclopedia of Social Work* (nineteenth edition, 1995). In the article active duty social workers are referred to as both military social workers and social work officers. In the first description, the proper noun is social workers. In the second description, the proper noun is officers.

The Multipurpose Role of Military Social Work

For the most part, the individual unit where the military social worker provides services can be conceptualized as a human service organization (mental health, family support center, family advocacy, alcohol and drug unit, etc.). One of the hallmarks of modern society has been the vast proliferation of formal organizations explicitly designed to process and change people. Hasenfeld and English note that human service organizations accomplish their mission by three distinct strategies. First, human service organizations assume the responsibility of socialization by socializing individuals for the roles they will play in society (e.g., basic training, social and recreational centers). Second, human service organizations assume the responsibility of social control by identifying and removing individuals from their roles in society who fail to conform to role expectations (e.g., law enforcement, legal, medical, social service agencies). Finally, human service organizations assume the role of social integration by providing the means and resources to help individuals become integrated into the various social units (e.g., counseling, therapy, financial support, family support) (Hasenfeld and English, 1974).

Because of inherent conflicts of interest, most human service organizations are developed and organized according to only one of these strategies. Very seldom in the civilian world does one find a human service organization in which professional social workers engage in socialization, social control, and social integration. However, both social control and social integration are inherent in the role of the military social worker. Regardless of unit, the military social worker is often faced with providing treatment for the individual and, at the same time, providing assessments, recommendations, testimony, and so on, for administrative discharge or other forms of administrative action. A prime example is a social worker in the substance abuse field. In addition, on occasion, military social workers will be called upon to provide socialization activities such as working with juvenile defenders in coordination with local law enforcement agencies. These multiple purposes will create ethical dilemmas for the military social worker.

Hierarchical Structure Governed by Military Law (Uniform Code of Military Justice)

The military is organized as a classical bureaucratic organization with a rigid hierarchical structure. Two of the most distinguishing characteristics of the military are a clear chain of command and rank. A chain of command places each organization and its leaders in hierarchical order. Therefore, all organizations and leaders are clearly subordinate or superior to other organizations and their leaders.

In addition to a clear chain of command, all military members have rank. The rank structure of the military is divided by officers and enlisted members. Each officer and enlisted individual (noncommissioned officer) is distinguished by rank. Therefore, every military individual is either subordinate or superior to all other individuals regardless of organizational unit.

Military rules, regulations, and policies are established to ensure good order and discipline within the military. Furthermore, to ensure compliance with these rules, regulations, and policies all military members are subject to the Uniform Code of Military Justice (UCMJ). The military justice system is one tool used to correct breaches of discipline; it protects the rights of both the institution and the individual service member. Punishment may be rendered through nonjudicial punishment (Article 15) or judicial punishment (court-martial). According to the UCMJ, military service members do not lie, cheat, steal, or engage in activities that bring discredit upon the service, nor do they tolerate those who do. In addition, the UCMJ specifically states that all officers must become involved when breaches of discipline occur in their presence and report all such violations to the proper authorities within their chain of command.

The chain of command, rank, and the UCMJ all have significant implications for military social workers. While most civilian social workers are subjected to a chain of command and hierarchical leadership, there are several important and distinguishing differences. First, military social workers can and often are ordered to perform a task by either a nonsocial worker or an individual within the chain of command who is not their immediate supervisor. Second, military social workers are held responsible and punished for not following legal orders. Third, military social workers must work within the boundaries of both civilian and military law. Finally, military social workers cannot quit their jobs because they disagree with their immediate boss or with the chain of command. These factors often lead to ethical dilemmas for military social workers that are unique to the military context.

The Dual Population of Clients Served by Military Social Workers

Another unique factor faced by military social workers is the dual population served. Social workers serve both active duty and nonactive duty clients. Although most of the population served by military social workers is active duty service members and their families, social work practice may also include military retirees and their eligible family members as well as certain civilian populations (Garber and McNelis, 1995).

Civilians do not have to follow orders and are not held accountable to the UCMJ. However, family members are part of a family system. From a systems perspective it is impossible to separate the active duty family member from the civilian family member. In addition, it is sometimes difficult, if not impossible, to separate the family from the larger military system of which it is an integral part. These two realities create ethical dilemmas for the military social worker.

Geographic and Professional Isolation

The last factor is not unique to military social work. However, when combined with the other factors, the result can be an environment conducive to the development of ethical dilemmas for the military social worker. As Garber and McNelis note, "at some point in a military career, nearly all social work officers serve in an isolated or overseas tour of duty" (1995, p. 1726). In many of these assignments there will be only one social worker working with a limited number of helping professionals. At other locations the social worker may be the only provider. In the United States Air Force these assignments are referred to as "lone ranger" assignments and are usually staffed by junior officers. In almost all overseas locations, the military social worker is isolated from the civilian community and social work colleagues.

In both isolated and overseas assignments, "the limited availability of resources in these assignments requires the individual practitioner to develop and provide a broad range of services" (Garber and McNelis, 1995, p. 1726). While this situation allows professional growth and development, it can also create a host of ethical dilemmas for the military social worker.

DISCUSSION OF SELECTED ETHICAL DILEMMAS FOR MILITARY SOCIAL WORKERS

As previously noted, each of the five factors inherent in military life contributes to the development of ethical dilemmas for military social workers. Most of the ethical dilemmas are due to a combination or interaction of these five military factors. However, for the purposes of this chapter, specific ethical dilemmas are presented according to military factor. It would be impossible to generate a list of all possible ethical dilemmas. Therefore, a few examples are presented to highlight the issues confronted by military social workers. In addition, while the scenarios reflect the authors' specific experience with one branch of the military, the dilemmas presented by each scenario can be generalized to all branches of the military.

Scenarios Representing Dual Profession Dilemmas

Scenario One

You are a military social worker assigned to a battlefield unit during Desert Storm. You work in a mental health unit that treats casualties with battlefield stress. Your primary duties include assessment, treatment, and recommendations for disposition of these soldiers. You must make the choice of returning your patients either to their unit or to the States for further treatment.

One of your patients is a twenty-four-year-old noncommissioned officer (NCO) (E-5) who has been involved in numerous battlefield encounters. He has received several superficial wounds in the past and has been awarded several battlefield commendations. In addition, he has experienced all the horrors of war including the loss of several close friends.

He presents with recurring nightmares, intrusive thoughts, sleep disorder, and survivor guilt. These symptoms have become progressively worse during the past two weeks. After two days of rest and relaxed general duties he responds well and many of his symptoms have diminished.

He tells you his wife is expecting their second child within a couple of weeks and she is having complications with her pregnancy. Furthermore, he tells you that they lost their first child last year to leukemia. His wife is still dealing with the death of their first child and wants her husband home. Because of the soldier's battlefield experience, he believes he has "done his duty." He asks you to send him home.

You receive a call from his commander. His unit sustained heavy casualties that morning in a firefight. He needs this NCO returned to the unit as soon as possible. You must make your decision today. On one hand, you know he is ready to return to his unit. On the other hand, as a trained social worker, you want to promote his right of self-determination.

This is a core dilemma, created because of two competing moral choices. This scenario clearly illustrates the conflict between the competing missions of the military and social work. The military social worker must make a decision between mission and client. The duty of the military professional is to promote the safety and welfare of humanity through the mission and this takes precedence over the individual client. Therefore, as an officer, you need to return him to duty; his unit desperately needs him. However, as a social worker, you know it is in his best personal interest to go home and support his wife.

Ethical standard 1.01 notes that social workers' primary responsibility is to promote the well-being of clients. In general, clients are primary. This is one of the most important ethical standards in social work practice today. Social workers are taught that their primary responsibility is to their client. Social workers advocate and support what is best for the client.

However, ethical standard 1.01 also notes that the social workers' responsibility to the larger society or specific legal obligations may on limited occasions supersede the loyalty owed to clients. In addition, ethical standard 3.09 (a) states that social workers generally should adhere to commitments made to employers and employing organizations. As a military social worker, how will you resolve this core ethical dilemma—mission or client?

Scenario Two

You are a social worker working in an outpatient mental health clinic. A young, junior enlisted woman comes to your office stating she is agitated, angry, and scared. She is the mother of two small children, ages three years and seven months, and the spouse of a non-active duty member. She is a member of a unit scheduled to deploy on a six-month tour of duty in three weeks. She holds a high-level security clearance. She tells you that her husband abandoned her last week and nobody is available to watch her children during her six-month absence. Her Personal Readiness Plan has not been modified to reflect the husband's abandonment.

While in the military only for several years, she has an excellent record and plans on making the military a career. She wants to talk with somebody about the situation and has come to you for help and guidance. She does not want to turn to her family for help because they disapprove of her interracial marriage. She is not sure what you can do for her but feels desperate. She states that with your help, she can resolve the issue herself. She is looking forward to the upcoming mission and does not want to be left behind. Finally, she asks you not to tell her unit, because she is afraid it will hurt her career. She says her commanding officer is not flexible and will be angry with her.

You are faced with the dilemma of honoring her request for privacy and confidentiality or reporting the situation to her unit. Again, you are faced with conflicting moral choices: mission or client? In addition, because you have not worked with this unit before, you do not know how the unit commander will handle the issue. Therefore, this magnifies your dilemma because you must choose the best moral course of action without knowing in advance the outcome of the decision for your client.

The right to privacy and confidentiality are hallmark social work values. Ethical standard 1.07 (a) (*NASW Code of Ethics*) notes that social workers should respect clients' right to privacy, and ethical standard 1.07 (b) notes that social workers should protect the confidentiality of all information obtained in the course of professional service, except for compelling professional reasons. Ethical standard 1.07 (c) notes that a social worker may breach confidentiality when disclosure is necessary to prevent serious, foreseeable, and imminent harm to a client or other identifiable person or when laws or regulations require disclosure without a client's consent. In all instances the social worker should disclose the smallest amount of confidential information that is directly relevant to the purpose for which the disclosure is made. Finally, ethical standard 1.07 (d) notes that social workers should inform clients, to the extent possible, about the disclosure of confidential information and the potential consequences, when feasible before the disclosure is made.

The *NASW Code of Ethics* gives good direction for this scenario. First, a military social worker should always address the limitations surrounding the issue of privacy and confidentiality before meeting with an active duty member. However, does the social worker in this scenario have compelling professional reasons to breach privacy and confidentiality? If so, what are those compelling reasons? Is there a regulation requiring disclosure of this information? Is there serious, foreseeable, or imminent harm? Is it because of the mission? Is it because of the children? Is it because of her security clearance? Does age, gender, or rank make a difference in the decision? If confidentiality is broken, how much information does the commander need to know to make a decision regarding the individual?

Scenario Representing Multipurpose Role Dilemmas

Scenario Three

This scenario deals with ethical issues related to the multiple purposes of social work in the military. It reflects the dilemma of having to choose between the goals of social integration (by providing therapy) and social control (by identifying and removing individuals from their roles in society who fail to conform to role expectations). The same issues of privacy and confidentiality discussed in Scenario Two apply to this scenario. In addition, this scenario involves the ethical issue of self-determination. However, the situation is markedly different than that presented in the previous scenario.

You are a social worker in an inpatient treatment center for alcoholism. In addition to providing therapy for the inpatients, you are responsible for conducting weekly drug and alcohol assessments.

For the sake of discussion, the same individual in Scenario Two is a patient in your treatment center. The situation for the client is the same except for three factors. First, she is not scheduled for deployment. Second, she does not hold a security clearance. Finally, following her spouse's abandonment, she received a driving under the influence (DUI) arrest (blood alcohol test results were .195) and was diagnosed as an alcoholic. She was referred to your center for treatment.

She has responded remarkably well to treatment. Self-disclosure, participation, honesty, and openness to treatment characterize her progress. She has become actively involved in Alcoholics Anonymous (AA). Her prognosis is excellent. She is looking forward to returning to her family and job.

During treatment, she denied the use of illegal drugs. However, during her last week of treatment she tells members of AA that she used multiple drugs prior to treatment. In fact, she reported using marijuana regularly and abusing prescribed medication. She tells the AA members she is confident that she will remain clean when she returns to her unit.

One of the AA members is a recovering alcoholic and a member of your staff. She tells you about the client's self-disclosure. You ask the client about her remarks and she confirms her previous drug history. She said she lied because she feared she would lose her career. As with the AA members, she tells you she wants to be clean and believes she is well on her way to recovery. You believe her.

Current regulations prohibit marijuana users from remaining on active duty. If you report this to her commander she will be administratively discharged.

Again, this time you must choose between two competing and equally moral choices: social integration and social control. To complicate the decision, selection of the correct moral choice may cause harm to one of the individuals involved. For example, if she is discharged from the military, what will she do and what effect will this have upon her children? Do you follow the regulations and report her past drug usage or do you honor privacy, confidentiality, and self-determination?

The same issues of privacy and confidentiality discussed in the second scenario must be applied to this scenario. In addition, the issue of self-determination must be confronted.

As with privacy and confidentiality, social work has long valued the concept of self-determination. As ethical standard 1.02 (*NASW Code of Ethics*) notes, social workers respect and promote the right of clients to self-determination and assist clients in their efforts to identify and clarify their goals. Clients must have the freedom and power to change their lives as they see fit. However, ethical standard 1.02 does note that social workers may limit the client's right to self-determination when, in the social workers' professional judgment, clients' actions or potential actions pose a serious, foreseeable, and imminent risk to themselves or others.

How does the social worker resolve this dilemma? Since treatment appears to be effective, is there a need to discharge this individual? In other words, is social control needed after social integration appears effective? Who should make that decision, the commander or the social worker? More importantly, does the social worker have merit to limit the client's right to self-determination? Is there enough data to suggest serious, foreseeable, and imminent risk to her or others? If so, what is that data? Do you believe she will relapse and harm herself, her children, or the mission? Does the client have the right to prove herself? Should her commander be involved in this decision?

If you choose to inform her commander, what and when will you tell the client? What and how much will you disclose to her commander? If you choose self-determination, and keep this information to yourself, how will the military be able to monitor her aftercare?

Scenario Representing Hierarchical Structure Governed by Military Law

Scenario Four

You are a family advocacy officer dealing with issues of family violence. As the base family advocacy officer, you know the wing commander (O-7) very well. In fact, he has written you several key endorsements on your yearly officer performance report. Your are a captain (O-3) up for promotion this year and you believe the general will support you for promotion.

The general calls you at home on a Saturday evening around 11:30 p.m. and tells you that he and his wife just hosted a party for several couples at their home. During the course of the evening, his executive officer (O-6) became drunk and verbally abusive to his own wife. The couple left the commander's house in an argument. An hour later the general's wife telephoned the executive's wife to see if everything had settled down. The executive's wife was crying and clearly upset. She reported that her husband had hit her several times and had left the house for the rest of the evening. She did not know where he had gone.

The general orders you to do the following: first, he orders you to go to the home of the executive officer to check on the condition of the wife. Second, he tells you to conduct an assessment on Sunday morning with the executive officer to determine if this situation is abusive. Third, he tells you to not talk to anybody about the situation. Finally, he tells you to phone him Sunday afternoon with an update.

As ordered, you go to the executive's house. The wife has been hit several times in the face, but refuses to go to the hospital. She reports that the abuse has gone on for years and she wants her husband to get help. She asks for your help.

The next morning, you meet with the executive officer and he admits he hit his wife, but denies he "has a problem" with abusive behavior. He blames the incident on having too much to drink. He refuses treatment and says, "Captain, I am a colonel—get out of my life!"

After conducting your assessment, you come to the conclusion that this couple needs immediate help. You believe the incident should be opened as an active family advocacy case. You report this recommendation to the wing commander. He orders you to keep this case "off the record" and not to discuss the situation with anyone. The general says he will take care of the situation. He assures you that he will get this couple some help. In fact, he tells you that he will "order" his executive officer to get help. What will you do? How will you handle this situation?

While this scenario deals with the nature of the dual profession, it highlights the issue of power as it relates to chain of command, rank, and military justice. Some individuals may use their position within the chain of command and their rank to try to influence you in your decisions as a professional social worker. Will you be an officer and follow orders or will you be a social worker and report the incident so you can get help for this couple?

Regardless of the legality of the order, the dilemma occurs because the chosen course of action may, in the long run, not be beneficial for all parties involved in the decision or may even harm a party. If you ignore the situation, there may be additional harm to the wife—she may be killed or seriously harmed in the future! If you report the incident, there may be harm to your career—you may be passed over for promotion.

With regard to social work, there is good support for reporting the incident. As mentioned previously, ethical standard 1.01 (*NASW Code of Ethics*) says your primary responsibility is to promote the well-being of clients. Reporting the incident is best for your client (the wife). Furthermore, as a professional social worker, you have an ethical responsibility to the social work profession. Ethical standard 4.04 says social workers should not participate in, condone, or be associated with dishonesty, fraud, or deception. One could easily argue that by following the general's orders you would be participating, at minimum, in deception. Finally, ethical standard 3.09 (c) notes that social workers should take reasonable steps to ensure that employers are aware of the social worker's ethical obligations as set forth in the *NASW Code of Ethics* and of the implications of those obligations for social work practice. You could inform the general of your dilemma and tell him why you must report the incident.

However, officers are sworn to follow the legal orders of their commanders. Orders can be legal, but unethical. This may well be one of those cases. How will you handle the dilemma? Would your decision be different if you were not up for promotion? Would your decision be different if a squadron commander with the rank of major (O-4) gave the same order?

Scenario Representing Dual Population of Clients

Scenario Five

You are a social worker in an outpatient mental health clinic. For the past three months, you have been providing therapy to a thirty-six-year-old spouse of an active duty noncommissioned officer (E-7). She initially presented with complaints of anxiety and insomnia. Over the past several months, you have gained her trust and confidence.

During your last visit with the client, she reported the following facts to you. Her husband works in the intelligence field and has a high-level security clearance. She said that her husband is a "heavy drinker," drinking alcohol three to four times per week and consuming approximately fifteen to eighteen beers per occasion. He has maintained this drinking pattern for "years" and she says he is "just one of the guys." She does not believe he is an alcoholic.

However, she is concerned because he has recently begun discussing classified material when he drinks. Lately, the amount of disclosure has increased. She is not sure, but believes he has disclosed classified material on occasion to his friends while they were at the NCO Club. She is more concerned about the disclosure of classified material than his drinking. She is concerned about his career and how these disclosures could affect "their retirement." She confronted her husband regarding his disclosures. He reports blackouts and does not remember discussing any classified material. He says he will cut back on his drinking. She believes him. She wants to know how she can help him cut back on his drinking. She wants to know about blackouts. What causes them? Is there any way to prevent them?

Your client has not requested help for her husband. When you share your concerns regarding her husband she points out that she is the client and he does not need professional help. All she wanted was information and advice. She believed she could trust you with this information. He can retire in one year and *she* does not want to get him in trouble. You tell her you need to inform his commander about her husband's behavior. She becomes extremely upset, anxious, and pleads with you not to report the situation.

This scenario is indicative of problems often encountered when working with both civilian and active duty populations. The problem arises when a civilian spouse discloses information regarding the active duty member. The social worker must decide what to do with the information. The dilemma arises because the chosen best moral choice for the social worker may not be best for all individuals involved in the predicament, and, in fact, may knowingly cause harm to one or all of the individuals.

On one hand, according to the *NASW Code of Ethics* the social worker should respect the privacy, confidentiality, and self-determination requested by the client. The arguments for respecting these issues were presented in Scenarios Two and Three. On the other hand, the husband has engaged in serious misconduct. Disclosure of classified information could cause direct harm to the military mission and is in violation of military law. As noted previously, as an officer, the UCMJ specifically states that you must become involved when breaches of discipline occur in your presence and report all such violations to the proper authorities within your chain of command. Does secondhand information learned in therapy constitute "in your presence"? If so, does this information take priority over the issues of privacy, confidentiality, and self-determination? Finally, ethical standard 1.07 (c) notes that a social worker may breach confidentiality when disclosure is necessary to prevent serious, foreseeable, and imminent harm to a client or other identifiable person or when laws or regulations require disclosure without a client's consent.

What would you do in this situation? Would your decision be different if disclosure of classified material were not the case, but the client told you her husband was having a sexual affair, which is also punishable under the UCMJ? What if the husband were not taking official leave for days he did not work? Does the severity of the crime make a difference? If so, how does one measure severity and who has the authority to determine the severity it?

Scenarios Representing Geographic and Professional Isolation

Scenario Six

You are stationed on a small, isolated island in the middle of the Atlantic Ocean. You are the director of an Air Force family support center. Within your center a total of five individuals deliver a wide range of programs aimed at helping family members cope and adjust to both military life and the overseas environment. Air Force regulations allow personnel in your center to provide counseling services. However, the direct provision of therapy is strictly forbidden by regulation. In fact, headquarters recently relieved the director of a family support center from her duties for providing direct therapy to clients. Interestingly, prior to this assignment you were a clinical social worker providing treatment in an outpatient mental health clinic. Your areas of expertise include both family therapy and crisis intervention.

The installation hospital is located next door to the family support center. Another Air Force social worker, a close personal friend and colleague, is serving in a lone ranger billet as chief of the mental health clinic. There is no other mental health provider in the hospital. In fact, the only two social workers on the entire island are you and your colleague. By regulation, the mental health clinic is mandated to provide therapy to both active duty members and their families.

Due to organizational mission and geographical isolation, family members experience a high level of stress at this installation. As a result, family dysfunction, separation, and divorce run high. Families are begging for help. Your colleague at the mental health clinic works twelve-hour days to meet the overflowing demand for family therapy. He provides excellent service, but just cannot accomodate all the families requesting help. Because active duty members have priority in the mental health clinic, there is a one-month waiting list for couples.

It is a very small installation. There are only ninety-seven commissioned officers. As a result, you personally know every officer on the island. In addition, you personally know about one-quarter of the enlisted personnel. Everybody lives, works, and recreates together.

It is a Friday morning. You receive two phone calls within forty-five minutes of each other. The first call is from the squadron commander (O-4) of the transportation squadron. One of her key noncommissioned officers got into an argument with her husband the previous night. The husband is threatening to return to the States with their two children. He is not active duty and cannot be forced to stay on the island. In addition, the military cannot prohibit him from taking his children. After meeting with the squadron commander and the first sergeant, the husband agrees to stay, if and only if they can receive marital therapy. He wants therapy to start immediately. They cannot get into the mental health clinic for one month. The squadron commander asks you to see the couple. She says that everybody on the island knows the regulation, could care less about it, and nobody will ever report this to headquarters. She is doing her very best to take care of her troops.

What will you do? Will you provide therapy regardless of the regulation?

Scenario Seven

The next call comes from the first sergeant of the supply squadron. One of his troops is also having marital problems. He is a young, recently married airman. The husband is twenty and the wife is nineteen years old. They have no children and she wants children "now." She has been on the island only four months. The first sergeant found out that the couple is having acute sexual problems. They have requested sexual therapy to enrich their marriage and, hopefully, have children. Nobody on the island provides this service and you are neither qualified nor licensed to provide sexual therapy. However, you are well-read on the subject matter and your last supervisor was a licensed sexual therapist. The first sergeant asks you to work with this couple. You inform him you are not licensed to provide sexual therapy. He becomes upset with you. He says, "If you don't provide this service then nobody will." He questions your commitment to people and the mission. He asks you why you chose social work as a profession, "but won't help people when they ask for your help." The first sergeant ends by saying, "You can help this couple!"

What will you do? Will you provide sexual therapy regardless of licensure and professional competency?

Both scenarios are indicative of the remote assignment. Tremendous pressure is often placed on social workers to provide services they are prohibited from delivering. The dilemma arises because the social worker must choose between two moral choices that conflict with each other. The choice is to obey the law or regulation or provide much-needed services. In addition, choosing to obey the regulation/law may cause harm to the clients, because their needs will go unmet. However, while these two scenarios are similar, they are also quite different in nature. Scenario Six deals with ethical issues related to commitments to employers. Scenario Seven deals with ethical issues related to competency.

Scenario Six asks the social worker to perform a duty that he or she is quite capable of performing. In fact, the social worker in the scenario has training and experience in providing marital therapy. It is a question of disobeying a regulation. The ethical standards conflict with each other on this issue. Ethical standard 3.09 (a) (*NASW Code of Ethics*) states that the social worker should generally adhere to commitments made to employers and employing organizations. You have made a commitment not to provide therapy and, therefore, should adhere to your commitment. However, ethical standard 3.09 (d) states that social workers should not allow an employing organization's policies, procedures, regulations, or administrative orders to interfere with their ethical practice of social work. One could argue that under the circumstances, this regulation is unethical because it prohibits the social worker from his or her primary responsibility and commitment to clients. However, should an officer ever willingly violate a regulation?

Scenario Seven asks the social worker to perform a duty that he or she is not trained to perform. The *NASW Code of Ethics* is much clearer on this issue. Ethical standard 1.04 (a) states that social workers should provide services and represent themselves as competent only within the boundaries of their education, training, license, certification, consultation received, supervised experience, or other relevant professional experience. However, because of the unique conditions creating this dilemma, could a social worker justify providing this service?

SUGGESTED GUIDELINES FOR RESOLUTION OF ETHICAL DILEMMAS

There are many approaches to dealing with the above scenarios. Other axiologists have developed paradigms and models to guide the helping professional in deciding which course of action to take when resolving ethical dilemmas (Levy, 1993; Loewenberg and Dolgoff, 1996; Reamer, 1982). Established practices include using professional codes of ethics, laws, and decision-making models based upon a hierarchical order of values. Each of these is an important tool for the military social worker.

NASW Code of Ethics

The NASW Code of Ethics is the recognized and accepted code of ethics for professional social workers in the United States. All military social workers should be familiar with and use the NASW Code of Ethics as a guideline for resolving ethical issues. First, it is an insightful and invaluable tool. Most of the ethical dilemmas facing military social workers can be resolved by using the NASW Code of Ethics. Second, regardless of membership in the NASW, most states use the NASW Code of Ethics in holding social workers accountable for their practice decisions. It is the standard of the social work profession. Even though the code may on occasion complicate the decision-making process, being a military officer does not absolve one from professional social work obligations.

Laws

Social workers must be familiar with local and state laws pertaining to the practice of social work. Law affects social work practice in many ways. For instance, laws direct that certain social services be provided for those who need them, they authorize professional social workers to engage in some activities but prohibit them from others, and they require social workers to report certain information to government agencies (Loewenberg and Dolgoff, 1996). For example, most states require the mandatory reporting of suspected child neglect and abuse. It is important to realize a legal act may be unethical and an ethical act may be illegal! Therefore, it is important to know both the law and legal consequences for your chosen ethical decisions.

Decision-Making Model

Familiarization with both the law and NASW Code of Ethics does not guarantee an easy or uncomplicated resolution of an ethical dilemma. Therefore, models have been developed to assist the social worker. The model presented by Loewenberg and Dolgoff has been useful and offers a straightforward mechanism for decision making.

Their Ethical Principles Screen consists of seven ethical principles rank ordered from most to least important value. The reader is referred to Chapter 3 in Loewenberg and Dolgoff's *Ethical Decisions for Social Work Practice* (1996) for an in-depth discussion regarding each ethical principle. The principles are as follows:

Ethical Principle 1	The protection of life
Ethical Principle 2	Equality and inequality
Ethical Principle 3	Autonomy and freedom
Ethical Principle 4	Least harm
Ethical Principle 5	Quality of life
Ethical Principle 6	Privacy and confidentiality
Ethical Principle 7	Truthfulness and full disclosure

If a dilemma arises during an intervention, the social worker identifies the ethical principles defining the dilemma. The social worker must compare the principles and decide which is of higher value according to the Ethical Principles Screen. The social worker selects the highest valued principle in resolving the ethical dilemma.

As discussed previously, the military is unique in that everyone involved is working toward the mission. The mission comes first. Military social workers must always support the mission. It is your sworn duty as an officer and your commitment to the armed forces in general and your military organization in specific. Furthermore, the NASW Code of Ethics supports commitment to the mission because social work officers have responsibilities to both the organization (ethical standard 3.09) and the broader society (ethical standards 1.01 and 6).

Therefore, a modification to the Ethical Principles Screen is needed for military social workers in the resolution of core dilemmas. Since military social workers are sworn to support the mission, and the mission is the primary means of protection of life for humanity (Davenport, 1987), Ethical Principle 1, the protection of life, must incorporate the military mission. Our model is modified to reflect mission:

Ethical Principle 1	The protection of life/**military mission**
Ethical Principle 2	Equality and inequality
Ethical Principle 3	Autonomy and freedom
Ethical Principle 4	Least harm
Ethical Principle 5	Quality of life
Ethical Principle 6	Privacy and confidentiality
Ethical Principle 7	Truthfulness and full disclosure

The modified model can be applied to each of the scenarios in this chapter. For example, Scenario One, the battlefield stress scenario, highlights the ethical dilemma of choosing between military mission and autonomy and freedom of the individual. Based upon our modified model the social worker would return the soldier to his unit. The same is true for Scenario Five. Self-disclosure of classified material threatens the accomplishment of the military mission. Since the principle of the protection of life/military mission is paramount to the principle of privacy and confidentiality, the social worker would take appropriate action to inform the proper authorities of the alleged security violation.

While the Ethical Principles Screen will help in the resolution of many ethical dilemmas, it will not resolve all dilemmas. The social work officer works in an environment conducive to many complex and conflicting situations. It is characteristic of social work in the military, and the successful social work officer will become proficient, if not completely satisfied, in resolving these ethical dilemmas.

CONCLUSION

This chapter identified and discussed ethical dilemmas both unique and common to all social work officers. Contributing unique factors related to the military were identified and discussed. Scenarios representing the interaction of these factors were presented. While it is impossible to discuss and resolve all possible ethical dilemmas, a guideline was presented to aid the social work officer when dealing with core and complex dilemmas. This guideline included the use of the NASW Code of Ethics, the understanding of laws, and the application of a decision-making model.

REFERENCES

Brown, J. and Collins, M. J. (Eds.) (1981). *Military ethics and professionalism: A collection of essays*. Washington, DC: National Defense University Press.

Davenport, M. M. (1987). Professionals or hired guns? Loyalties are the difference. In *Military ethics: Reflections on principles* (pp. 5-12). Washington, DC: National Defense University Press.

DeGeorge, R. T. (1987). A code of ethics for officers. In *Military ethics: Reflections on principles* (pp. 13-32). Washington, DC: National Defense University Press.

Garber, D. L. and McNelis, P. J. (1995). Military social work. In R. L. Edwards (Ed.), *Encyclopedia of social work* (Nineteenth edition, Vol. 2, pp. 1726-1736). Washington, DC: National Association of Social Workers.

Hasenfeld, Y. and English, R. A. (1974). Human service organizations: A conceptual overview. In Hasenfeld, Y. and English, R. A. (Eds.), *Human service organizations* (pp. 1-23). Ann Arbor, MI: The University of Michigan Press.

Huntington, S. P. (1979). Officership as a profession. In Wakin, M. M. (Ed.), *War, morality, and the military profession* (pp. 11-24). Boulder, CO: Westview Press.

Levy, C. S. (1993). *Social work ethics on the line.* Binghamton, NY: The Haworth Press.

Loewenberg, F. M. and Dolgoff, R. (1996). *Ethical decisions for social work practice* (Fifth edition). Itasca, IL: F. E. Peacock.

National Association of Social Workers (1994). *Social work speaks: NASW policy statements* (Third edition). Washington, DC: Author.

National Association of Social Workers (1996). *NASW code of ethics*. Washington, DC: Author.

Pumphrey, M.W. (1959). *The teaching of values and ethics in social work education*. New York: Council on Social Work Education.

Reamer, F. G. (1982). *Ethical dilemmas in social service*. New York: Columbia University Press.

Reamer, F. G. (1995). Ethics and values. In R. L. Edwards (Ed.), *Encyclopedia of social work* (Nineteenth edition, Vol. 2, pp. 893-902). Washington, DC: National Association of Social Workers.

Rhodes, M. L. (1991). *Ethical dilemmas in social work practice*. Milwaukee, WI: Family Service America.

Smith, P. M. (1988). Leadership and ethics: A practitioner's view. In P. M. Smith (Ed.), *Moral obligation and the military: Collected essays* (pp. 129-140). Washington, DC: National Defense University Press.

Watkin, M. M. (Ed.) (1979). *War, morality, and the military profession*. Boulder, CO: Westview Press.

Wells, C. and Masch, K. (1991). *Social work ethics day to day: Guidelines for professional practice* (Revised edition). Prospect Heights, IL: Waveland Press.

Chapter 12

Career Progression and Grooming

James G. Daley

Joining the military as a social worker extends far beyond getting hired for a job. The military social worker has entered a path, potentially lasting twenty or more years, which is exciting, treacherous, and often defined by choices made early in the career. Ideally, the naive junior officer is embraced by a mentoring network of seasoned senior social work officers who guide and protect the new person as he or she orients to the new setting. The reality is that the successful new officer is sometimes adrift, does not even know what questions to ask or dangers to protect against, and the network is not aware of his or her existence. This chapter seeks to discuss some of the key issues a new military social worker should consider in building a successful career. For the nonmilitary reader, this chapter can hopefully help you better understand why the military social worker is so focused on issues that seem irrelevant or silly to you.

THE SUCCESSFUL CAREER: AN OVERVIEW

Regardless of service, the whole career of the military social worker is defined by proving potential, having a spectacular record of achievements, and achieving a growing span of leadership skills. The triad of "worthiness" is intertwined. For example, solidly achieving today's job proves potential and adds to the span of leadership skills.

A key factor to keep in mind is that each promotion is contingent on scoring high enough on the ranking by the promotion board. The rankings are increasingly competitive the higher the rank for which you are being considered. The promotion board will only be reviewing your personnel folder, a summary composite of your career achievements to date. Typically, each promotion board member will only review your folder for less than ten minutes to achieve your ranking against the other officers being considered for the next rank. And the competitors are not just social workers but can include many diverse professions (e.g., optometrists, psychologists, public health officers, dietitians). When reviewing your folder, the board members are looking for specific items and statements such as service school completion, span of job responsibility, impact of service provided, increasing and varied leadership positions. The slightest noncompetitive issue (e.g., not having completed the appropriate service school) can eliminate you from consideration. Nonpromotion equals the image of a less competitive officer and can lead to not continuing in the Service.

Notice that I have not mentioned clinical skills, client satisfaction with service, or ability to turn a highly dysfunctional family into a happily stable unit. Prospering in the military is not based on clinical success. You can be the most wonderful, effective clinician and be "passed over" for the next rank. The military (and most people beyond your co-workers and direct supervisor) assume that you are capable, successful, and a wonderful clinician. Otherwise, your supervisor should bring your skills up to standard or work to have you leave the Service. Only the most junior ranking officers focus on solidifying their skills (though we all continue to advance our skills throughout our careers).

Proving Potential

Proving potential consists of showing that you can provide solid service and are eager for added and expanded responsibilities. Developing new services, volunteering for community activities (e.g., chairing a blood drive, chairing local NASW projects, serving on special project teams), and seeking to demonstrate that you are more than just a clinician are all invaluable proof that you have "potential." Being a military social worker is not for the timid, hesitant, unsure person. As soon as you are sworn in, you (and all your competitors for future ranks) out the "starting gate." Recognition of this fact often seems to be forgotten by the new military social worker, who is overwhelmed by the new culture, heavy caseload, and span of clinical demands for expertise. Every step is a proving ground and the more aggressively successful player wins. Potential is based on assuming that you are ready for bigger and more responsibility. Achieving the next rank is based on the belief that you have potential for the next level of demands, not what you have already achieved. If what you have achieved is spectacular, the assumption is that you would be capable of more responsibility.

A Spectacular Record of Achievements

Social workers seem to have a strong self-effacing trait that helps us immensely in the office but can be deadly in our career paths. One of the most significant building blocks of your career is the annual performance reports (every six months for brand new officers), which succinctly summarizes what you have done and how your supervisory chain view your potential. All year long, you should be collating materials that can be included in the annual report (called the Officers Performance Report or OPR), and being meek or embarrassed to call attention to yourself hampers your competitiveness. You should be thinking of ways to spotlight your achievements. Some examples might include "maintains the heaviest caseload in the clinic," "increased the clients seen by 30 percent through implementing a new intake procedure," "commander lauded me as the best social worker he has ever worked with," "served as coordinator of blood drive which achieved 120 percent of its goal." Every task, job, or interaction you have can lead to a highly useful bullet statement in your OPR—but only if you are successful and remember to collect the data or personal reactions which you can then use in the OPR. Keep a folder throughout the year and place each event's key achievements in the folder.

Growing Span of Leadership Skills

Each promotion board for junior officers (O-1 through O-3) is basically looking for the colonel or Navy captain (O-6) hiding within the new officer. Your job is to let them see that inner skill. How do you do it? By showing a successful and broadening span of leadership efforts, you illustrate your "colonel" skills. Each assignment should add a new or different job experience. If you were in a clinic at your first assignment, you should strive to go to a different job (e.g., medical center, family support center, substance abuse treatment program) for the next job. Recycling through the same kind of job from assignment to assignment is the kiss of career death. For example, my assignments included sequentially being a clinical social worker in a clinic, director of a student outreach program, student in a PhD program, chief of a mental health clinic overseas, director of an alcoholism treatment program, faculty in a family practice residency program, and command consultant at a command surgeon's office. Each assignment added a different aspect of military social work. Each assignment built to a higher span of leadership. When I became the command consultant, I oversaw mental health, family advocacy, and substance abuse programs and responded to a very diverse series of "hot" issues erupting at the Pentagon and Command levels. The promotion board is looking to see if you are increasing your span of expertise throughout your career.

One issue that should come up early in your career is "career broadening" assignments (CBA) such as recruiter, teaching at a service academy, or serving as a squadron commander. There are a myriad of assignment choices and some social workers have actually made a whole career out of career-broadening assignments. The key issue is that the assignment is not because you are a social worker, it is available to many professions and is due to being an Air Force officer. The timing of the assignment is critical because you do not want to be in a CBA at the time of promotion unless it enhances your chances (e.g., a squadron commander position). Most CBAs are controlled tours (a fixed amount of time) and are highly competitive. Usually you have little say about where you will go with a CBA. The assumption is that the prestige of the CBA is enough of an incentive. CBAs are excellent opportunities to prove your potential. But check it out first by talking to a social worker (or at least a person) who is in the job before volunteering. The official description often is quite different from the reality of the job.

Besides carefully choosing assignments and demonstrating highly effective accomplishments with whatever you do, the military social worker must be aggressive in seeking out professional military education (PME) opportunities at the earliest possible time. Regardless of service, the military officer is expected to complete PME at the appropriate time within his or her career path. For example, in the Air Force a captain should achieve Squadron Officers School (SOS) either by correspondence, seminar, or in residence. The major completes Air Command and Staff College (ACSC). There is a limited window of opportunity to complete SOS or ACSC according to your date of rank. Every promotion board member knows what those dates are and will know if you completed the right school for the right rank. Not doing PME is an easy path to losing competitiveness.

CONTRASTING THE IDEAL PATH WITH THE REALITIES OF LIFE'S DEMANDS

The above description of successful progression to higher rank is repeated in any mentoring efforts by senior social workers. The reality is often more of a struggle. Picking the right assignment is a tug of war between what is available and when you are due to rotate. And the assignment choice gets thinner and thinner as you increase in rank. In addition, the right assignment is not always the right choice for the family. Finally, the right assignment is not always a choice that interests you professionally. It is a delicate balance between where to go and with what you can live. For example, an assignment on the Inspector General's team (which inspects all hospitals in the military) routinely ends up going to a nonvolunteer because of the frequent travel (50 percent plus on the road), some Pentagon jobs are dreaded due to the viciousness of the staff demands, and some overseas locations prompt family difficulties. In addition, your spouse might need one more year to finish his or her master's degree or have an excellent career-enhancing job at your present location. In short, the realities surrounding career-enhancing options are always balanced with the impact on self and significant others.

So what can you do if you don't want to move? (The exception is the Navy, which designates home ports where a person could stay for his or her whole career.) You have to demonstrate your potential by targeted efforts such as servicewide task forces, base or post additional duties that supersede typical medical duties, or creating service unique model programs. How do you find out about such opportunities? By networking! Periodic discussions with your command consultant or letting your service chief for social work know of your willingness to help are some useful ways.

In addition to military opportunities, you can seek out professional or community opportunities. Serve on the planning committee for the state NASW annual conference. Serve as co-chairperson for your local NASW unit. Publish in professional journals and build a national reputation. Volunteer to help run the United Way campaign for the base or post. Serve on the board of directors of a local social service agency. There are numerous ways to demonstrate that you are capable of leadership of large projects.

Regardless of your potential proving activity, the military social worker should keep a key issue as paramount: combat readiness. The military social worker routinely is involved in readiness exercises, can serve on deployment teams, and generally has periodic times when all typical work stops and combat readiness takes precedence. Taking a leadership role in readiness activity is a solid decision. Be a team leader. Design a combat stress briefing for the next readiness exercise. Volunteer for combat stress teams who are deployed to real operational events. The point is that your primary mission, regardless of your current job, is to serve in a wartime scenario. Any activity which confirms that skill enhances your promotion capability and, frankly, better prepares you for the real likelihood that wartime situations will occur and you will use those skills. The down side is all the early morning recalls, the separation from family, and the real fear of coming in harm's way. But if given the chance, grab it!

SURVIVAL TIPS FOR A SUCCESSFUL CAREER

There are many high-risk events that can torpedo a career. It is inevitable that you will be exposed to them. A vindictive boss, inappropriate demands on you, unethical or awkward requests, pressure to do it "the Air Force way," and threats of administrative action are just a small sampling of possible scenarios. The military is an excellent way of life, but it is like living on a beautiful beach. You swim every day in the balmy sunshine but there is always a shark circling. You might go a whole career without being bitten, or you might get attacked today. And the military has very real teeth when it wants to use them! There are no guarantees of success or protection. But there are some common sense tips that increase your likelihood of success.

Get a Senior Social Work Mentor

The first thing any military social worker should do is make contact and develop a health network with the closest senior (O-4 and above) social worker. If you are at a small base or post, contact the nearest major medical center. Once you have developed a healthy relationship with the senior social worker, you can continue that link throughout your career (and remember to reciprocate when you become a senior social worker). Your discussions with him or her should not be about issues that you can and should resolve yourself. Your discussions should be about macro events (OPR rough drafts, assignment choices, picking career-enhancing tasks) or significant crises (ethical dilemmas, interprofessional clashes, chain of command decisions). Do not bother lamenting to the mentor about heavy workload, clinical decisions, or how tired you are of being called at 3 a.m. for a telephone recall exercise. The mentor knows the realities of military social work. Focus on what is fixable or unique to the military experience. *Always* process significant action with the mentor before storming off to the hospital commander to argue some supervisor's decision. The mentor is a gentle guiding force but will rarely step in directly and intervene (first of all, the mentor is not in your direct chain of command). The mentor knows the system, but you have to fight the battles.

Choose Your Battles Wisely

I vividly remember being a junior captain, the only social worker at a small isolated base and at my first duty station. One of my first efforts was to contact a senior social worker at a medical center on the nearest large base and develop a mentoring relationship with him. When the inevitable crisis occurred, I called him and he listened as I raved. Then he said, "The thing you have to remember is to choose your battles wisely. Sometimes you have an issue for which you should fall on your sword, but you choose it rather than have it choose you." Great advice was given and I rethought the issue and chose to wait it out (good decision as it turned out). Every professional faces different moments when something offends, jeopardizes, or terrifies him or her. Many times, decisions made by others will be different than you would make. The key decision is to choose carefully and infrequently to challenge the issue directly. Once you have decided that the battle should be entered, be aggressive in resolving it in your favor. Usually you want to choose a battle you have a good chance of winning, but not always. The most important result is to develop a reputation that you are flexible generally but, if you object, people had better listen because you will push the issue to the highest levels if need be. This is great advice which I pass on to future generations.

Use Rather Than Abuse Your Chain of Command

A common error made by new military social work officers is to violate the chain of command. Don't do it! The chain of command is one of the oldest and most venerable traditions within the military and should not be taken lightly. Some tips on the chain can be helpful. First, you can use the chain to your advantage through escalating a decision or issue higher than your supervisor or department head. But do it rarely because the supervisor will not be happy. You use an "in turn" letter, which lists all the chain links (supervisor, department head, flight leader, hospital commander) and outlines the issue. Make sure you have all your homework done and can defend your position effectively. Second, there are many forums (e.g., commander's call, commander walk-through, suggestion box) by which you are directly invited or asked for suggestions or concerns. A commander will always say that he or she has an "open door" policy. Do not broach a subject no one in your chain is aware of because the first thing that commander is likely to do after leaving you is call the head of your chain and blindside that person with the issue. Then the issue will ripple down and you will be in deep trouble by the time you mention it to your supervisor. When the top brass direct scenario inevitably occurs, the key action is to immediately brief your direct supervisor of the issue discussed and the setting. Your supervisor will quickly run the issue up the chain and prepare the head of the chain for when the commander calls. Likewise, when confronted with queries from high-ranking officers outside the hospital, you should do the same rapid briefing of your supervisor, as the hospital commander is likely to be blindsided. No one is trying to hide any issue, they all just want to appear prepared when asked a question about any topic. Third, do not bury a time-bomb issue or go along with your supervisor burying the issue. The chain of command serves to ensure that everyone has the right to appeal any decision so that no high-risk decisions are made by any one person. Your commander is responsible for everything that happens, whether the commander knows about it or not. Use the chain when needed. Fourth, the chain of command includes organizations that are officially not in the chain (e.g., inspector general, legal services) but accepted as an appropriate place to appeal if the formal chain does not respond appropriately. Or if key members are the problem (e.g., sexual harassment), you can skip them and report the issue to that person's boss. Or if you are uncertain of how to navigate a high-risk event, you can talk to a military attorney before escalating the issue. The point is that the chain of command is a potent resource if used properly and a deadly enemy if abused.

Document, Document, Document!!

If it is not on paper, it did not happen. Though not literally true, the military is a strong advocate of the "paper trail" and it behooves any military social worker to put in writing any issue that might become or is high risk (and save a copy for yourself!). You can do a memo for record (for yourself or addressed to the appropriate person), or document the issue in a formal letter or (if appropriate) within the client's medical record. Do not just talk about it; write down what you talked about with the person. I cannot stress this issue strongly enough as issues can reemerge months or years later, and having a written record can keep you out of significant trouble. The memo for record should include facts, quotations of significant statements made, and action taken. It should not include speculation or hearsay. Inevitably the issue about which you wondered, "Should I make a memo on this?" will be the issue that erupts. So write it down and save your career.

Advocate for Yourself

You should be your best advocate. When OPR time arrives, put together a rough draft of the OPR or a well-crafted list of achievements for your supervisor. When a recipient of quality service lauds your skills, ask him or her to write a letter of appreciation. When a top-quality project is mentioned in commander's call, seek to be a part of the project if not in charge of it. When you see a better way to provide service, provide a written outline of the idea to your supervisor. Your abilities remain dormant until flexed. You are hopefully surrounded by a group of highly talented folks, so assert yourself. Every experience expands your talent. Use the opportunities available. If you hear about other military social workers achieving laudable feats, call them and ask how they went from desire to achievement. In short, you should advocate for your chance to prove yourself. You are not being boastful or pompous, you are being assertive and effective. The risk you always take is failing at the task. But you are talented and the challenges get tougher as you increase in rank. So get the experience while you are junior enough in rank that episodic ineptness is excused and eagerness is expected.

SOME INSIGHTS FOR OUR CIVILIAN COLLEAGUES

If you have read the chapter to this point, I commend you. What you have learned is that military social workers are take-charge, competent clinicians who are open to volunteer and leadership opportunities. Further, they exist in an environment that thrives on excellence and initiative. They will absorb all the knowledge you can share and strive to make the situation better. In short, they are wonderful additions to steering committees, task forces, special projects, or as consultants. Add them to your organizational efforts. You won't regret it!

However, there is a negative side to working with the military social worker. They can be deployed (as an exercise or for real) with very little notice. They are very busy and often have low tolerance for unproductive meetings. They have a very realistic concern about image and credibility in any task in which they are involved. Remember, they are accountable to the military twenty-four hours a day regardless of where they are or what they are doing. They have little knowledge of the local politics or milieu (which sometimes is a real advantage) but are eager to learn. And they will only be in your location for a short time (so grab them quickly to maximize their potential utility). The average military social worker (except Navy) moves every three years. So you have a maximum of two years of usefulness (a very long time from a military perspective). Almost all military social workers are replaced when they transfer, so you can keep up with who is coming and plan accordingly.

Civilian colleagues should learn the different ranks and understand the significance in value to your local professional community. Mistaking a colonel for a captain in skill level is a significant error and could lead to resistance to being involved in your project.

Understanding that there is a chain of command, a clear mechanism for communicating about change, can help the civilian social worker to navigate the system when seeking new or revised services. Military social workers can often be helpful translators of the military culture and strategies for getting your project moving. A joint effort between military and civilian social workers is an ideal vehicle for advocacy.

From reading the earlier sections of this chapter, you recognize that the junior military social worker is under intense stress to succeed and has a myriad of duties that would not be common civilian social work tasks. Use that drive to your advantage. But when you do involve a military social worker in a project, please ensure that you write a highly laudatory letter to his or her commander. A letter to the social worker is nice. A letter to the commander is better because it ensures a cover letter or comments from each level of the chain of command. It helps keep the higher levels of command aware of the talented social worker they have working for them.

Finally, I hope that our civilian colleagues reach out to military social workers for friendship and social interaction. Being in a very closed society, the military social worker needs to be reminded of the larger social context and have someone who is not within the environment. We can get quite myopic about issues if not reminded periodically of other perspectives. Your interaction offers diversity and a refreshing span of concerns contrasting with ours. Sharing and caring expands both sides.

SOME FINAL IDEAS

This chapter sought to provide some thoughts on how to have a successful career as a military social worker, what career-ending dangers can emerge, and how to successfully navigate those barriers. Realistically, every person will navigate a somewhat different path as he or she struggles to balance opportunities with potential personal hardships. Promotion chances are sometimes reduced due to staffing cutbacks, rather than to the sterling quality of your record. Sometimes opportunities are less available because of your location. A myriad of unique events can affect your career progression. But the successful military social worker must be a wind surfer of change. Learn as much as possible, develop an effective network of mentors quickly, and advocate throughout your career for yourself and your skills. The military is a fruitful and rewarding place for a person with vision and drive. Embrace the best aspects, and grit your teeth and endure the worst aspects. Being a social worker and military officer is a dual career. Bloom in both fields and savor the cross-fertilization!

Chapter 13

Understanding Life in the Army: Military Life from a Service Member and Family Member Perspective

Rachel Henry
Rene J. Robichaux

The intent of this chapter is to paint an overall picture of what life in the Army is like. We begin with a general discussion of living the Army life. Then we describe some of the stresses and issues affecting the new recruit, the newly forming Army family, and unique conditions affecting dual military families. We conclude with an overview of common adjustment tasks or problems experienced by military families including risk of injury or death, frequent relocation, separation, overseas assignments, and intercultural/interracial marriages. Our hope is that the reader will gain a deeper understanding of what Army life entails. Many Army families savor the positives, survive the hardships, and blossom into resilient families within an often demanding environment. Some families, especially young families, are bombarded by stressors that overwhelm already meager personal resources. We hope to illustrate the environment that nurtures some and capsizes others. Come join us on our journey through Army territory.

LIVING THE ARMY LIFE

TDY, FAP, CCC, ACS, BSB, FMW, PRP, ASG! Imagine waking up one morning and realizing that while you were sleeping, your

---

Opinions in this chapter are the authors' and do not represent the opinions or policies of the U.S. Army.

everyday language had been reconfigured into some kind of foreign alphabet soup that made no sense to you at all. Also, your world had become one of ranks, titles, uniforms, orders, pamphlets, regulations, and numbers. Though the adjustment is somewhat more gradual than overnight for most individuals, every service member has to come to terms with these changes when enlisting or being commissioned into the Army. But it does not end there. If the service member is married, or marries after joining the military, the family members are also thrown into an adjustment process—a process that could determine the outcome of a soldier's career in the military as well as the quality of his or her personal and family life. The family's level of maturity, the ability to acculturate to an unfamiliar environment (especially if the marriage is intercultural or interracial), and the sophistication of the existing support systems (both their availability and their utilization) greatly affect this process.

The U.S. Army continues to be a primarily married force, with 79 percent of officers and 62 percent of enlisted soldiers married as of September 1997. Commanders and Army leaders have long understood the importance of family issues in personnel retention. Over 100 scientific and applied documents and briefings have helped to understand the relationship between the Army and its families (Segal and Harris, 1993). What the research has found is that the variable with the strongest impact on unit readiness is the soldier's perceptions of the amount of support that the unit leaders give soldiers and their families. Further, there is a positive link between the quality of partner support for a soldier making a career in the Army and the soldier's intent to remain in the Army. Finally, there is a strong relationship between the degree of problems experienced during relocation and overall family adaptation to the Army (Segal and Harris, 1993).

This research highlights the value of social workers as a significant part of the Army's response to the challenges associated with life in the Army. Their understanding of family systems and emphasis on the biopsychosocial functioning of family members places them in a unique position to advocate for families within a military setting. Social workers are renowned for their understanding of human behavior under crisis conditions as well as their ability to provide crisis intervention services that assist the individual and family in the reestablishment of emotional balance. The stresses associated with military lifestyles overseas are more intense and varied than the adjustments imposed on service members and their families who are assigned within the United States. Of course, there can be significant stresses within the United States if the soldier's spouse is a foreign national, especially if the spouse's native country has drastically different languages, cultural norms, and traditions than the United States.

The acculturation of an individual from a civilian to a military lifestyle is riddled with complexities, both positive and negative. Even individuals who take a position as a civil service employee or a contractor working for the Department of Defense have less stress than the new military person. A civil servant or a contractor has a life separate and apart from the expectations of "Uncle Sam," whereas a soldier, sailor, or airman literally belongs to the military, as they say, "24/7," meaning twenty-four hours a day, seven days a week. This total commitment by the military member clearly affects family members, often resulting in an emotional tug-of-war for the soldier between his or her professional and personal goals and obligations. The military has adopted a belief that if a soldier has a happy home life, free of complexities and problems, she or he will then be "mission ready." Mission readiness is the ultimate goal of all Army units. In reality, very few units have the resources to maintain the highest level of readiness. Similarly, the majority of families struggle with life's challenges and very few are problem free.

Many positive benefits are frequently associated with being in the military. There is usually stable job security. With acceptable job performance, the successful soldier can advance within a "company" that will allow very diverse job settings and responsibilities and retirement at a relatively young age (twenty years of service). There are financial benefits beyond a soldier's basic pay, such as housing allowances or housing on post, and access to lower priced grocery stores (called commissaries) and department stores (called post exchanges). In fact, most posts are designed to function as nearly self-contained communities with most services available. Medical care is usually free or at least significantly less expensive than a civilian counterpart. The soldier gets educational training, often of a caliber as high or higher than most civilian training settings. Travel to diverse locations, including overseas sites, offers the ability to broaden one's cultural horizons. The Army is a built-in social and professional system, at least for the service member, where the soldier and often the family are embraced by a community that prides itself on the ability to "take care of our own." Army families often interact with and support each other through hardships.

Hardships are inherent with Army life. Though we will discuss many of the hardships later in this chapter, the Army family copes with frequent relocation and limited choice of where they are transferred. The Army community has a small-town atmosphere, which can feel intrusive at times. Financial support (especially for lower ranking enlisted soldiers) is sometimes lower than financial need. There is an inherent risk of death for every soldier, who could be deployed at a moment's notice to a myriad of high-risk scenarios. The rather rigid hierarchy (enlisted versus officer) can negatively affect you choice of associates.

Besides the typical hardships, there are current national uncertainties that enhance the stress levels of many Army families. The downsizing efforts increase uncertainty about job security or career potential. Changing health care systems (see Chapter 5 for more details) sometimes reduce traditional "free" medical care resources. Limiting or reducing military benefits exacerbate fiscal strain on Army families. Privatization of services reduces the closed-society status of the Army and increases the likelihood that service providers will have less identification with the Army. In sum, the rapidly changing external environment sometimes contributes to the hardships experienced by Army families.

Civilian occupations such as missionaries or foreign service share the stresses or hardships often associated with a military lifestyle. However, it is the authors' belief that there are few, if any, which have so many of the stress factors combined in one occupation. The successfully coping Army family is truly a resilient unit engulfed in an environment ripe with stressors!

ADAPTING TO ARMY LIFE

The average enlistment age of a soldier in the United States Army is approximately eighteen to twenty years. Occasionally a soldier may be as young as seventeen if parents or legal guardians have signed a document giving the individual permission to enlist in the Army.

Many young enlisted soldiers come from middle- to lower-class families. They often view the Army as an opportunity to leave their limiting surroundings and establish a career for themselves without the expense of college, or as an opportunity to obtain an education by utilizing the various educational benefits provided for service members.

There are highly successful, capable people who join the Army. But the Army makes intense demands and is not for the meek or fragile. Some individuals come into the Army with numerous unresolved issues from their families of origin and are often unable to adjust to the rigorous demands of the military. Still others are drawn to the structure and external controls exerted by the organization. They may have come from chaotic, abusive homes with parents who were neglectful and unpredictable. They generally do quite well during basic training, advanced individual training, and the period of time they live in the barracks. They find comfort in knowing what the rules are and what they must do to receive recognition. It is only later when they are married, living off post, and starting a family that the rules are not as clear and their capacity to succeed is called into question. Many of these soldiers are either administratively separated from the military or receive criminal punishment and discharge. Occasionally they may come under the protective guidance of a moncommissioned officer who may mentor them and continue to provide enough external structure to allow them to have a full career. In addition, some young soldiers, faced with being alone in a strange environment, choose to marry even younger wives who are either pregnant or who have also never been away from home (some are as young as sixteen or seventeen years old). It is not unusual for a soldier who is perhaps twenty or twenty-one years old, with a wife who is nineteen or twenty years old, to have two to three children under the ages of three or four years.

With all of these responsibilities thrust upon them, many soldiers never realize their dream of going to college. Instead they become further burdened, discouraged, and oftentimes depressed. They inherently lack the life experience and maturity required to deal effectively with the difficult demands life has placed on them. For those who came from dysfunctional homes, good role models and adequate problem-solving skills are nearly nonexistent. Thus their ability to cope with all of their problems is compromised from the very beginning. Add to this the issues of alcohol and drug abuse, financial problems, relationship problems and conflicts at work, and one can begin to understand why some soldiers are in urgent need of military social work services.

THE DUAL MILITARY FAMILY

Another situation occurring in the Army is the "dual military family," in which both spouses are in the military. There are 6,750 family units identified as dual career in the Army. The dual military family has unique stressors affecting its stability. On the positive side, the dual military family has better financial stability with dual incomes and housing benefits, an ability for clear understanding and acceptance by both of the Army lifestyle, and the capability of both partners to advance in military careers. On the negative side, both partners are at risk of rapid military deployment, there is high likelihood of some assignments at different posts during their careers, and they must deal with the added stress of managing a household while both are working long hours. For example, what happens to their children when both soldiers are required to go TDY (temporary duty) or go to the field? It is not unusual for a couple to belong to the same unit. Oftentimes, these two young people meet in a military training school and therefore have the same military occupational specialty (MOS). When their unit deploys, both parents are scheduled to go and the question of child care becomes an issue. Occasionally, a couple will be blessed with a good care plan (which is especially required for single-parent soldiers), and this is not a problem. However, there are instances when this is, indeed, a real issue with no quick or easy solution. The unit may assist in the development of a sound and dependable care plan for a soldier and his or her family but, ultimately, the responsibility rests squarely on the service member's shoulders.

Another tough decision point for dual military families is the choice of giving up one's career to stay at home with the children. Who, then will make this sacrifice and at what cost? In an organization that is steeped in tradition and continues to be male dominated with an emphasis on mission readiness and a certain "male bravado," the majority of the time the female military member gives up her career. This may ultimately lead to resentment and discontent and, again, the quality of this family's life is compromised, both personally and professionally.

COMMON ADJUSTMENT TASKS AND PROBLEMS EXPERIENCED BY MILITARY FAMILIES

Risk of Injury or Death

The dangers associated with combat operations are known to most through film or published accounts. While the percentage of the active force and reserves who actually are placed in harm's way is relatively small, families perceive that there is a chance that their soldier will be placed in a dangerous situation, and that danger remains real for them. Actual risk factors vary from operation to operation and from unit to unit.

Even when not engaged in hostile operations, unit training for such operations can present significant dangers. Aircraft collide, crash upon take off and landing, spray fuel over hundreds of assembled soldiers, and leave much death and destruction in their wake. Munitions fall short of their intended targets, maiming or killing trainees and their instructors. Vehicles crush and roll over soldiers both in combat and in peacetime. What is significant is not the actual risk factors associated with a particular military occupational specialty, but the perception that being in uniform carries a certain amount of danger and risk of injury.

Family members are aware of the dangers and live with the added stress of knowing that their soldier is deploying again or going to the field for training. Most commonly, families will distract themselves from the dangers and behave as if they are not concerned about the risk. Their denial operates fairly well until a training accident occurs on their post or is reported in the national media. Suddenly, the reality of the dangers may overwhelm their previously effective use of denial and force them to confront their fears and worries. Eventually the threat will subside and families are able to reestablish a degree of comfort.

Critical event and critical incident debriefings are part of Army doctrine designed to assist small groups and units to recover from loss. Similar group support has been used with entire communities when the loss has been so overwhelming in size or quality that recovery might be expected to be problematic.

Men and women in uniform present attractive targets for terrorists who wish to exploit them as representatives of their government and abuse them in a symbolic act of protest against U.S. government policies. As terrorism increases throughout the world, the danger for soldiers increases and so does the stress associated with heightened vigilance.

Frequent Relocation

Frequent relocations are the most stressful adjustment associated with a military lifestyle. The Army moves and relocates soldiers and their families on an average of every two to three years. For example, findings from a U.S. Army Research Institutes study indicated that roughly 33 percent of all soldiers surveyed experienced problems with moving, finding permanent housing, and/or setting up a new household; almost 50 percent of the soldiers surveyed reported problems with costs incurred; and 33 percent reported waiting five months or longer for permanent housing (Bowen et al., 1992). In sum, relocations equal disruption, fiscal strain, and delays in stability.

Frequent moves require adaptation to the change associated with leaving all that is familiar and routine and the challenges of making all that is now unfamiliar become familiar. Among the most common problems associated with frequent relocation are spouse unemployment, financial setbacks, and difficulty in acquiring adequate housing in a timely manner. Disruption of routine begins three to four months prior to the actual move or reassignment date. It continues at least until permanent housing is found and most often months beyond that time. In the worst cases, families may experience up to ten months of total additional stress because of a particular move.

The impact of frequent moves is felt most profoundly in its association with spouse unemployment and underemployment. Employers are reluctant to invest time and training dollars in an employee whom they know will not be available in twenty-four months or less. Frequent moves also prevent employees from moving up the career ladder, having to start over each time they leave a position and begin a new job with a new employer. There are obvious exceptions, such as when the employer has locations in many states or when the spouse is a Department of Defense civilian employee. When the family has relied on the spouse's income to meet many of their basic expenses, the entire period of unemployment takes on enormous significance.

Credit card debt has often been the way that families compensate for the loss of income during a relocation move.

The Army has attempted to minimize the out-of-pocket expenses associated with a move by providing dislocation allowance, individual and household goods transportation expenses, and per diem for a short period of time before permanent housing is available. Despite these significant efforts, most families experience these moves as depleting their savings and increasing their indebtedness. Costs that must be covered from the dislocation allowance include car repairs if driving, additional eating out expenses on both ends of a move, utility and security deposits, and a considerable amount of household cleaning, gardening, and repair items that cannot be shipped due to spillage or their corrosive nature (often given away or discarded). Frequently these items must be purchased again at the next location. Another added expense occurs when property is damaged or lost during a move. The government acknowledges that one in every four moves results in a claim for loss or damage. The DoD pays the service member a depreciated allowance for loss or damage. The individual must then replace the item by providing the difference between the allowance and current price.

Many of these out-of-pocket expenses are kept to a minimum when on-post government quarters are available. Unfortunately, most installations have a severe shortage of family quarters. The waiting list may vary from six months to one year. Affordable housing may be in such short supply that families are forced to locate a considerable distance from the installation. Commuting times of forty-five minutes to ninety minutes are not rare.

Another significant issue related to frequent moves is the amount of adaptation required of the children. Past research has been quick to identify the impact of military relocations on a child's adaptability. Specifically, some children easily adapt to new surroundings and new adventures while others withdraw and resist adapting (Marsh, 1976; Rodriguez, 1984; Wertsch, 1991). The universal problem appears to be the teenager who may always be counted on to resent efforts to move him or her during the critical high school years.

Much less attention has been given to the special needs child who finds safety and comfort in routine. These children do best in an environment where there is predictable structure. Frequent moves challenge the parents of these children to work extra hard to reestablish patterns previously familiar to their child. There are so many variables that cannot be controlled during a move that parents of special needs children are doubly challenged. One could easily argue that the military lifestyle is a poor fit for many special needs children; however, it is the access to medical care and the fear of catastrophic medical costs that encourage so many families to remain in the Service and tolerate the frequent changes.

It is an accepted axiom in the helping profession that some amount of stress is healthy and produces growth. Excessive stress is seen as unhealthy and debilitating. In 1967, Holmes and Raye developed an instrument for the self-assessment of change experienced over the previous twelve months. High socres on this instrument (>300) have been associated with a greater risk for accidents and illness. An Army chaplain in Germany who used the stress inventory for a number of years determined that when he administered the instrument to groups of soldiers at Stateside locations he could expect that 25 percent of the soldiers would report or achieve total scores of 300 or greater (personal communication, Major John Sumner, August 1991). In contrast, groups of soldiers in Germany reported total scores in excess of 300 at a rate of between 40 percent and 50 percent. Using the same instrument, parents of newborns hospitalized in the intensive care unit in Germany were asked about their levels of adjustment. The average scores reported on the Holmes and Raye Social Readjustment Rating Scale were in the 800 range. Clearly, these families were under enormous stress and required all of the additional support and services that could be made available to them. Additional challenges associated with overseas assignments will be addressed in a later section.

It is not unusual to hear a military family member say: "This is the fifth move in six years"; or "We have moved twelve times in the past twenty years." What these few words mean, literally, is that the family has had to re-create its life that many times in so many years. It means leaving a home that was carefully decorated and enjoyed, cherished friends and oftentimes family members, a comfortable church, a school in which the children have become intimately involved, and the knowledge of "where to go" to get shoes repaired, clothes altered, that certain type of ethnic food, or your favorite sandwich. Some of these losses may seem insignificant; however, it is the little things in our day-to-day lives that bring us comfort, that remove some of the stress and nurture us. Perhaps some of these losses are even taken for granted in our daily lives. But when they are taken away, these little things may create just enough of an edge to create an unspoken, unacknowledged stress or tension, a lack of security or confidence. People are, for the most part, very adaptable beings. However, when this pattern of "re-creation" is too frequent, a certain relocation overload may set in. This chronic spending of one's self may have a cumulative effect on a family's emotional "budget," causing a recession in the family members' ability to nurture, care, and be supportive. At some point, each family and each individual must decide how they wish to spend their "coin of life," that is, the time, energy, and resources allotted to us from beginning to end. It must seem at times, to these young families, that what is continually demanded of them puts them on the edge of emotional bankruptcy.

Separation

To reduce the negative impact of additional moves on family members, soldiers frequently volunteer for unaccompanied assignments. Such separations can vary from one year in Korea, to two years in Germany, and three years Stateside. While this prevents many changes for family members, the soldier is often required to absorb the bulk of the stress without family support. Also, the spouse is left to perform both roles previously shared with a partner. Couples must adjust to the loneliness and then readjust often to reunion.

In today's smaller Army, committed to worldwide stability and support operations, families are experiencing more separations. Short deployments and training rotations are at times more stressful than the longer term, planned, unaccompanied tour. They introduce the same sense of loneliness, stress of sole parenting, and reunion challenges as the planned separation. They allow for less preparation and often do not begin with a clear end date.

The familiar tune, all too well-known in most families, "You just wait until your father comes home!" is also rehearsed and sung in many military families. But what happens when the "head" of the household is deployed for three weeks, three months, or even six months? By default, the primary role of decision maker, bill payer, disciplinarian, and entertainment committee rests squarely on the shoulders of, generally speaking, the wife. Johnny becomes accustomed (hopefully) to Mom making all of the decisions for the family. Mom learns that even though checking the oil in the car is not in her marriage vows, it might be in her best interest to do so occasionally. Thus, the family adjusts to functioning without the service member, which is analogous to a four-legged animal learning to walk on three legs. After all, it is a form of amputation in the family when a key player is temporarily removed. Then two, four, or six months later: Enter the service member! Remember, when he or she departed the home front, so many months ago, the service member was the "head of the household." Now, Johnny is asking Mom if he can spend the night at David's. The garage is calling Mrs. Blair to tell her the parts she ordered for the Volvo are in. And so it goes. Rather than feeling like a hero returning from the war, the service member begins to feel like superfluous, excess baggage, or worse yet, threatened in his role as the head of the household. This, too, is a recurring cause of stress and conflict, especially in younger families who have not yet settled into comfortable roles with one another. Roles in a family, just like any other organizational unit, are the basis for homeostasis; they provide relative stability among the interdependent actors. Remove one of the actors or change one of the roles and homeostasis is compromised. The extent of the compromise, as discussed in previous pages, depends on the maturity of the individuals, the support systems in place, and the frequency of the disruption. Certainly, if this occurs once every two years, the family has the opportunity to restore stability and gain strength. However, if it occurs on a monthly basis, as is often the case with soldiers in the European theater of operations, the cycle of deployment is so frequent and erratic that the completion of an adjustment cycle is seldom realized. This is but another characteristic of military life that most civilians do not have to cope with and that makes being part of a military family the challenge that it is.

Reunions are extremely stressful. Expectations by all family members are frequently not realistic and are seldom articulated. There are great opportunities for disappointment and hurt feelings, followed by anger and withdrawal. Family violence reports have always experienced a significant surge following unit homecomings. The conflict associated with loyalty issues, financial overspending, and the transition from single to couple status always has produced a potential for expression in the form of domestic violence.

Overseas Assignments

Overseas assignments separate young families from their families of origin. Most young military families, with all due respect, are similar to an infant who is just beginning to walk. The infant has the will to walk, but the belief that it can is still not deeply ingrained. Consequently, it teeters unsteadily between determination and fear, heading doggedly to its nurturing parents when it stumbles or falls. And so it is with young families. They know that they want to strike out on their own and create a life for themselves, and they set out to do so. However, when the first strong winds of life blow problems their way, they do not have the life experience behind them to know that they can succeed. They do not yet know that there are many challenges to overcome on their journey through life; that pain is inherent to growth, and that this is an integral part of the maturation process. Those who are fortunate enough to have family close by may draw on their family's wisdom, guidance, and support. With every challenge and, consequently, with every success, the individuals/families grow stronger, begin building their reserves and feeling more confident. This is not the case for many military families. Rarely are they in close proximity to their family of origin. Not only are they most probably not in the same state, but oftentimes they are not even in the same country. This fact, compounded by the numerous characteristics already discussed in this chapter, can have a devastating impact on young families in times of difficulty. It can be extremely lonely and frightening for a young wife whose husband is in the field, coping with two or three children under the age of four, with no telephone, no car, or worse yet, no driver's license, and who has to depend on neighbors she hardly knows.

For many, this experience is their first time away from the family of origin and, as mentioned above, their first instinct is to run home to the comfort of their parents, siblings, or friends. Learning to endure the pain of separation, loneliness, and sometimes depression is all part of being married to a soldier in the Army. It is literally, for some, "baptism by fire." Rather than growing up and then embarking on life's difficult journey, these families are often challenged to endure life's greatest hardships without the maturity and skills required. Some young family members require counseling, antidepressants, and occasionally may request an early return of dependents (EROD) to their home of origin.

Intercultural/Interracial Marriages

Although the authors recognize that the topic of intercultural/interracial marriages could fill a book in itself, and certainly deserves one, due to space limitations this chapter can only highlight some key elements of the military intercultural/interracial marriage. This topic is vital to the understanding of what many military families experience in all facets of their lives.

Due to the effects of mass media, affordable international transportation, and World War II, there are more similarities now among world cultures than ever before. And in spite of the definite trend toward military "right-sizing" mentioned earlier, American soldiers continue to be stationed in foreign countries and, accordingly, continue to marry natives of these countries. Most often the soldier is male and the native is female, so it will be discussed in those terms. These intercultural and interracial relationships bring with them a myriad of new problems and challenges above and beyond those already discussed as unique to military families. People in such relationships must face the difficulties that stem from basic cultural differences, including the occasional disapproval of the woman's family for marrying an American soldier, the differences in child-rearing beliefs, and the differences in financial, religious, and basic family values. This transition may prove to be more challenging in an Asian community than in a European community due to strong Eastern definitions of cultural roles and expected behaviors. However, regardless of the variables, additional difficulties will arise and a voluntary or command-directed visit to an Army social worker or chaplain may well be in the couple's future.

While the couple continues to reside in the woman's native country, little or no adjustment may be needed. The service member continues to work on an American post and legalization of the relationship lends an aura of stability. The new wife continues to enjoy the comfort and support of living in close proximity to her family, and her social life is expanded through her husband's circle of friends. For the most part, there are initially fewer problems than if a young American wife accompanies a service member to a foreign country.

Although many of these couples end up seeking help for marital problems, as many couples do, their more serious problems begin when it is time for the soldier to return to the United States. It is not uncommon at this point, especially if the relationship is going well and the service member has fewer than eight to ten years of time in the military, for a service member to consider separating from the Army in order to avoid the major separation that moving to the United States would cause. In Germany, for instance, where families continue to live together in the same building, with the parents living in the main part of the home and the offspring living either in the basement apartment or the upstairs apartment, it can be enticing to accept the available home, the security of a ready-made social system, and the convenience of live-in baby-sitters for the children. Germany has not yet caught up with the independent lifestyle of the average American family. They continue to be interdependent, relying largely on family members to provide what they need.

However, if the couple decides to stay in the military and return to the United States, the compatibility of the marriage is severely tested. Regardless of how supportive and helpful the service member is, most women who come from close-knit communities and families will have an extremely difficult time adjusting, not so much to moving to the United States, as to moving away from their own families and support systems. Homesickness and even depression are almost certain to occur during the first year. This is when a couple really begins to notice that the "opposites" that initially attracted them to each other are now becoming a source of conflict. They are more apt to have arguments and disagreements. The difficulty of the adaptation process of this couple is, again, directly proportionate to their level of maturity, problem-solving skills, and support systems.

Some service members lack the maturity and sensitivity to understand and are not supportive. They do not understand why their spouses are having such a difficult time adjusting. After all, they manage to adapt to foreign countries. They do not recognize the subtle, and not so subtle, differences. When they are assigned overseas, they are stationed on an American post. They continue to eat American food and to have American friends. They do not have to learn a new language as many wives are forced to do. And yet, even when service members do have some understanding of the problems their family members are experiencing, they often feel helpless in comforting their wives and are unable to mobilize the appropriate resources.

There is also an element of ethnocentricity involved in this lack of compassion and understanding. Many service member husbands expect their wives to adapt to the American way of life and to forsake their own culture once the family returns to the United States. And, although most wives do not mind becoming "bicultural," it is a process that will require time, support, and a great deal of patience and understanding. However, the service member's genuine attempt to learn his spouse's language is equally important. Being able to converse in her native language may alleviate some of the homesickness as well as indicate to her that her husband is willing to meet her half way.

The adjustment task in an intercultural/interracial marriage is tremendous. Plus, when the couple begins to have children, child-rearing conflicts are often the norm, and the biracial offspring of this family are caught in the middle of a cultural conflict. Besides the management of homesickness and loneliness, a lack of empathy and understanding, unrealistic expectations, poor communication, and role confusion, the intercultural family also has the same financial, professional, and personal issues all of us must deal with. Though it may be true that "opposites attract," in the long run it is the similarities that provide the most understanding, support, and longevity in a marriage.

CONCLUSION

Being a family in today's Army, in spite of the lack of any major conflict or war, is more demanding and difficult than it has ever been in the past. Just as everyone is being asked to do more with less, so these young families are expected to do the same. The family system as we knew it during World War II is slowly but surely becoming a thing of the past. Even though communication with families, especially overseas, is more accessible, the quality of this exchange may be greatly diminished. Rather than having the support of a letter or phone call from home, young families often are asked to support, both emotionally and sometimes financially, their own mother who is a single parent of siblings, who is disabled and cannot work, or who is dealing with teenagers involved in gangs, drugs, and pregnancies.

Being a social worker in a military environment necessitates that the clinician become parent, counselor, teacher, cheerleader, and advocate all rolled into one talented, insightful, compassionate, mindful individual. It involves the reparenting of a young couple without causing them to become dependent on the system. It is the role modeling of how to solve communication issues, how to manage anger and other confusing emotions, how to implement effective parenting skills, and how to manage on the limited resources most young couples have at their disposal.

REFERENCES

Bowen, G.L., Orthner, D.K., Zimmerman L.I., and Meechan, T. (1992). *Family Patterns and Adaptation in the U.S. Army* (Technical Report 966). Alexandria, VA: U.S. Army Research Institute for the Behavioral and Social Sciences.

Marsh, R.M. (1976). Mobility in the military: Its effects on the family system. In McCubbin, H.I., Dahl, B.B., and Hunter, E.J. (Eds.), *Families in the Military System.* Beverly Hills, CA: Sage, pp. 92-111.

Rodriguez, A.R. (1984). Special treatment needs of children of military families. In Kaslow, F.W. and Ridenour, R.I. (Eds.), *The Military Family.* New York: Guilford Press, pp. 46-72.

Segal, M.E. and Harris, J.J. (1993). *What We Know About Army Families* (Special Report 21). Alexandria, VA: U.S. Army Research Institute for the Behavioral and Social Sciences.

Wertsch, M.E. (1991). *Military Brats: Legacies of Childhood Inside the Fortress.* New York: Harmony Books.

Chapter 14

Understanding Life in the Navy

Glenna L. Tinney
Lawrence L. Zoeller
Janet Cochran
Steve Bromberek

The role of the U.S. Navy is to control the seas during periods of conflict and maintain freedom of the seas in peacetime. The United States Navy was born on October 13, 1775, when Congress first authorized a naval committee and then ordered the purchase and fitting of several ships. The Navy has fought in many wars over time and has been influenced by many people. It has changed from sail to steam, from coal to fuel oil, and then to nuclear power. Evolution has brought the corps from wood to steel, from only surface ships to submarines and aircraft, and from a Navy of just men to one of both men and women. The fascination and intrigue of the ocean and the irresistible urge to explore over the horizon has beckoned many to risk the unknown and seek adventure. Even though the smell of tar and linseed oil is all but gone, this sense of adventure still calls to the men and women who join the ranks of the Navy today.

The United States Navy is an elite force of highly trained professionals dedicated to protecting our freedom and ensuring a secure future for America. For more than 200 years, in war and in peacetime, at home and around the world, Navy men and women have stood tall for principles that make America the greatest nation on earth. In the Navy, these unchanging principles, honor, courage, and commitment

---

Opinions are those of the chapter authors and do not reflect the policy or the opinions of the U.S. Navy.

are known as core values. To know, understand, and faithfully live by them is the duty of all Navy people.

Life in the Navy is not for the fainthearted. Isolated duty stations, long deployments, separation from family and friends, and frequent relocations are stresses that must be framed within the context of service to country. The unique aspect of naval service is in the area of deployment. While other branches of military service also deploy, the Navy is the only service that goes to sea. However, some Navy service members are shore-based and will never go to sea for the duration of their careers. To understand life in the Navy is to understand what sailors go through on a daily basis. Although there are many universal aspects of being in the Navy, the day-to-day experience is affected by several factors. These factors include rank/rate, the community to which one belongs (e.g., surface, aviation, submarine), the location to which one is assigned (e.g., outside of the United States, ashore or afloat), and whether one is serving in a combat zone or in a peacekeeping mission.

To deploy means to be directly engaged in the operational activities of the Navy, to protect and defend the waterways and coastal borders of the United States and other agreed-upon world territories. In recent times, Navy ships have also deployed to assist with humanitarian and peacekeeping missions throughout the world. Most deployments have both diplomatic and operational aspects. Whenever a Navy ship enters a foreign port, the ship is representing the United States. Each crew member acts as an ambassador. This is a responsibility that is taken seriously by the commanding officer and every crew member. Whether enlisted, warrant, or commissioned officer, the Navy prepares its members well and ensures they know the job to which they are assigned. Life at sea has challenges above and beyond the professional requirements of the enlisted rate or commissioned rank of a person in the Navy. Some professions take their members into specific job environments that are unique, stressful, dangerous, require personal sacrifice, and have demanding physical requirements. When sailors deploy to a location during a time of conflict or increased threat conditions, the sailors, family, and friends all share feelings of anxiety and fear about a safe homecoming.

Deployment aboard a Navy ship requires being away from home for extended periods. It is an environment that requires living in close quarters with other people for months at a time. The ship is both home and workplace while deployed. Sailors have quarters on the ship, eat on the ship, and have most of their needs taken care of on the ship. The ship is their home and running it and keeping it afloat is a twenty-four-hour-a-day job! While deployed, sailors must find ways to stay in touch with family and friends back home. There must be a commitment to hard, intense work followed by periods of relative inactivity. This lifestyle can be very enjoyable and exciting with opportunity for travel to many interesting sites throughout the world. An "esprit de corps" develops from these experiences which is a unique life experience that few ever forget and most cherish for a lifetime.

Danger is the constant companion of personnel living and working aboard a ship. Navy ships are inherently more dangerous than other ships because of the nature of their missions. Crowded living conditions, confined working spaces, and combat necessities (e.g., guns, ammunition, aircraft) all make life at sea hazardous under any circumstances. Going to sea involves working with powerful machinery, high-speed equipment, intense high-temperature-pressure steam, volatile exotic fuels and propellants, heavy lifts, high explosives, stepped-up electrical voltages, and the unpredictable forces of wind and waves. In foul weather and times of stress, the danger increases. A comprehensive shipboard safety program greatly reduces the chance for accidents, actually making Navy ships among the safest afloat. Constant awareness of the hazards involved is required of all hands to prevent accidents and to minimize the effects of accidents that happen.

To understand life in the Navy, we must look at the various communities to which a person can be assigned. Since the unique aspect of Navy life is going to sea, this chapter focuses on communities that deploy on Navy ships.

SURFACE COMMUNITY

The surface community is the most visible within the Navy. It is also the most diverse. It includes every size ship ranging from tugboats to aircraft carriers and everything in between. These ships, whether carrying a crew of 4 or 5,000, are integral parts of the Navy's surface community. Each ship prepares for deployment in the same manner, taking on supplies and checking the ship's functioning to make sure it is ready for the mission. Yet, since their missions are different, this preparation may be where the similarities end. Before the junior sailor, newly commissioned officer, or any other newly assigned sailor steps onto a ship for the first time, there are feelings of anxiety, excitement, and anticipation.

While deployment is generally referred to as a "cruise," this should not be mistaken for a vacation for the ship's crew. When the ship leaves the pier, it is part of a battle group but in essence becomes an independent community under the direction of the captain (commanding officer). It is now the responsibility of all hands onboard to meet the ship's mission. Each ship's deployment schedule varies according to the classification and mission of the ship. An auxiliary ship (AE), for example, may have a higher operational tempo (schedule) than other types of ships. An AE is responsible for providing fuel and ammunition to other ships while at sea. So if the ship is responsible for replenishing the rest of the fleet, it may be in transit more than some other ships. Some surface ships are designated amphibious ships. They transport marines to land on foreign shores. Hospital ships provide medical care to the wounded and/or the critically ill. These ships are part of the Military Sealift Command and generally consist of a civilian crew with a small cadre of military personnel onboard. If ordered to full operational status, this cadre crew will be augmented to approximately 1,200 as operational requirements dictate.

An experience universal to all Navy ships is General Quarters (GQ) drills. GQ means "prepare to fight." Crew members report to their stations to await further instructions. Each sailor has a role to play. The reality of life at sea is that the crew must fight fires, repair structural damage, and defend against enemies while meeting the ship's mission. Another aspect of life at sea is the ever-present danger of "man overboard." There is always a risk that a crew member could fall overboard during a cruise. All hands work together to recover a shipmate from the water. Time is a critical element in a "man overboard" situation. The amount of time a ship has to safely recover a crew member depends on many variables, including water temperature and depth. These variables affect the likelihood of survival. For example, if the water temperature is low enough to cause hypothermia, the individidual's likelihood of survival decreases as the recovery time increases. The priority is the safety of the crew member.

SUBMARINE COMMUNITY

Where the surface community is the most visible, the submarine community may be the least visible. The operations and uniqueness of the environment can be very demanding. Operating a submarine continuously submerged for more than seventy days is not uncommon. Privacy is a luxury that typically exists only for the commanding officer and executive officer. Everything that crew members own is stored in or under their bunks.

One unique aspect of the submarine community is the "two-crew" concept. On the ballistic missile submarines (boomers), there are two crews that alternate, the blue crew and the gold crew. Each crew deploys for 180 days per year. Their mission is part of the strategic defense of our nation should a nuclear weapons attack occur. While the blue crew is onboard, the gold crew will take their leave, undergo training, etc., before deploying again. These are considered the most stable commands in the submarine community because of the set deployment schedule. The deployment schedule and operational tempo are conducive for service members to spend time with family and friends.

The fast attack submarines vary dramatically from the boomers. They are assigned one permanent crew and have a very high operational tempo. One of these submarines can be away from home port up to 265 days per year. The mission of the fast attack is different from its ballistic missile submarine counterpart. The fast attack submarine is used to hunt other submarines and support battle group operations. Also, fast attack submarines support classified missions vital to national security. Fast attack submarines are smaller than the ballistic missile submarines. Sometimes two crew members may be required to share one rack (bed). This requires what is called "hot racking." Two crew members with alternate watches share the same rack. The mission and operations of the fast attack submarine are quite exciting; however, the schedule can be very demanding on sailors and their families.

On both types of submarines, the crew has three rotating shifts called watches. Each crew member stands watch for six hours and then trains or performs maintenance. This leaves approximately six hours for sleep, relaxation, or personal pursuits before they go back on watch again. The crew of a submarine must also respond to any emergency. The vulnerable position of a submarine beneath the ocean surface places additional stress and pressure on the damage control team and allows no room for mistakes.

When a submarine is underway, the lighting system adds to the sense of confinement. Because of rotating shifts, someone is always sleeping. Therefore, the lights in the berthing area are always off. The only exception is on field days when the areas are being cleaned. As a result, on a submarine, it is easy to lose track of night and day. Without the sun and the moon as a reference, the days seem to run together. Each evening following dinner a movie is shown in the crew's mess. These types of activities help the crew members maintain some semblance of closure to the day. Mealtimes are another means of setting the time of day for the sailors. Meals are social times where the crew has the chance to unwind and talk with their friends. Unfortunately, due to the small size of the mess decks (seating approximately twenty-five people) meals have to be eaten rather quickly (fifteen to twenty minutes) to make room for other shipmates. When a submarine is at periscope depth, a pick-me-up for the crew is periscope liberty. While it may appear to be a small thing, the ability to see beyond the confines of the submarine means a great deal to the crew members.

AVIATION COMMUNITY

An aircraft carrier is best described as a floating city that never sleeps. The carrier includes every aspect of life in a small city except that most small cities do not have F-18 fighter jets at their airports. The carrier environment is loud, continuously busy, and potentially dangerous. The initial sight of a carrier in port is incredible. The length of the ship is equal to five continuous football fields. Its height from top to deck is twenty stories. Each link in the anchor chain weights over 300 pounds, and the chain is over 2,000 feet long. When entering a carrier, you walk through the hangar deck where the aircraft are housed and maintained in top mechanical condition. The initial feeling upon seeing a carrier is to wonder how anything so gigantic can stay afloat. Its mammoth size allows the carrier to house over 6,000 crew members.

A perpetual smell of jet fuel permeates the air and blends with whatever happens to be served in the kitchen that day. Add to this the smell of propane used to fuel utility vehicles on the hangar deck and the smell of burning rubber from the tires of jets hitting the deck at over 180 miles per hour. All of these odors combined with the smells of the ocean remind you that you are on a Navy aircraft carrier.

A carrier environment can be dangerous. The danger certainly includes the possibility of war but also involves more mundane everyday risks. It is easy to be injured just moving around the ship accomplishing daily tasks. Moving through the various passageways can be dangerous because it is easy to bump your head on the steel-encased ladder wells between each level of the ship. A fall on the hangar deck could result in a serious laceration. crew members constantly have to watch out for the small utility vehicles on the flight and hangar decks. Fire is a constant danger given the flammable materials (e.g., chemicals, fuel, weapons, etc.) on a carrier. High winds and heavy seas can cause accidents as they destabilize the internal environment of the ship. The dangers of carrier life are brought home when the announcement comes over the public address system saying, "Medical emergency, medical emergency." Another announcement that is often heard is, "Attention: all nonessential personnel clear the flight deck due to high winds and heavy seas." The winds become so high and the sea so heavy that a crew member could easily be swept overboard, so the "man overboard" drill is repeated often during deployments. Even though a carrier is large, high winds and heavy seas provide numerous challenges, including keeping your food on the table and not in your lap when you eat.

Another risk on a carrier is hearing loss. A carrier is a very loud environment. The noise level is high for the obvious reason—aircraft are taking off and landing. Each plane is catapulted off the ship by a steam-powered piston that runs below the flight deck. The steam-powered piston with the plane attached above it travels down the length of the runway at 180 miles per hour and then slams into a brake at the end of the runway that launches the aircraft. The noise of the piston slamming into the brake is incredible. It is as if a race car going 180 miles per hour suddenly slams into a steel wall. This process is repeated each time aircraft takes off from the flight deck. These flight operations take place both night and day. Ear protection is a must to ensure safety.

Additional risk factors include fatigue and monotony. Difficulty establishing a regular pattern of sleep can result in fatigue. Fatigue coupled with an environment of high-powered sophisticated machinery can double the jeopardy. Crew leaders, to ensure that crew members are able to perform their jobs safely, must constantly assess personal fatigue. The work on a carrier never stops, even in port. There are necessary functions that must be performed at all times. After a few weeks at sea, the daily routine can begin to wear on the crew, especially those in highly focused jobs. Being out to sea is a time-warp experience. Days run upon days, week upon week. Being out to sea is the unusual experience of having no reference point; all you can see for miles is blue water with no idea of where you are or how far you have traveled. This time-warp experience can increase the danger and enhances the overall stress of the carrier environment.

Sailors endure these hardships and dangers because there is excitement and comfort in being part of an elite and powerful force unparalleled in the rest of the world. Deployments create challenges for people on a personal level, but quality of life has improved on carriers in recent years. Involvement in physical activity and health promotion is encouraged and supported by the chain of command. Recreation facilities, movies, and access to e-mail and telephones help to enhance and maintain a positive attitude when deployed.

Deployed sailors find creative ways to maintain their sense of psychological privacy. This is sometimes difficult for the enlisted sailor with six to eight sharing a small room. Junior officers often live three to a stateroom. Psychological space is most often sought on the decks. Sailors often retreat to the decks to enjoy the luxuries of fresh air, sunshine, a wide-open space, and the beauty of the ocean. Psychological space is an intangible that can never be fully appreciated until you have deployed on a Navy ship.

Although most sailors experience deployment on a ship or foreign shore at some time in their careers, the job, profession, or naval community to which one belongs will determine whether a sailor's job is afloat or shore-based. All seagoing sailors also spend time in jobs ashore on a sea/shore rotational basis. There has to be a break from going to sea. Deployment has a major impact on sailors and their families, requiring adjustments to the constant comings and goings.

The Navy recruits individuals but retains families, so it is critical to have support services available to sailors and family members to aid them in coping with a very stressful lifestyle. The Navy has developed and implemented a range of services at both the command and installation levels to support sailors and family members. These services include pre- and postdeployment briefs for sailors and family members. Family Service Centers (FSC) provide classes on stress management, parenting, financial management, anger management, and so on. FSCs also provide information and referral to appropriate base and civilian services, as well as transition, relocation, and counseling services. The Navy Family Advocacy Program (FAP) provides a range of services to both prevent and respond to family violence. Chaplains are available to provide spiritual support for sailors and family members. The Navy also has a range of programs to prevent and respond to substance abuse issues. This is not an all-inclusive list of available services but does illustrate that the Navy is committed to ensuring a positive quality of life for all sailors and family members. Social workers, as well as a variety of other professionals, play a key role in the provision of many of these services.

Overseas assignments, while sometimes posing challenges to activities of daily living, offer wonderful opportunities to explore a different culture and see the world. Overseas living has a big impact on sailors and families. When a ship is homeported overseas, the same lifestyle changes occur as for all deployed sailors. They are away from home for long periods of time with the ship as their primary home away from home. The family is left behind but is far away from their extended family support system in an alien culture. The Navy has expanded services and assistance for sailors and families living in a foreign culture to help make the experience more enjoyable and manageable.

Apart from the normal Navy requirement to stay within height and weight standards and to be physically fit, some jobs in the Navy require special physical and mental characteristics. At one end of the spectrum are the special warfare personnel known as the SEALS, who rely on their physical abilities and strenuous training to meet the requirements of a job that may send them into multiple wartime environments at any time. Naval aviators and their support crews also have rigid physical requirements because of the highly busy and active life on the decks of an aircraft carrier. Navy divers, submariners, and nuclear power personnel are pitted against the extremes of temperature, pressure, and radioactive hazards on a daily basis in performing their jobs. Each job in the Navy requires greater or lesser levels of physical activity and hence reliance on good health and physical fitness. Whatever the exposure, all sailors must be in excellent physical and mental condition to accomplish the Navy's mission safely. Any sailor can be called upon at any time to perform strenuous, stressful, and dangerous jobs on the sea, on the land, or in the air to defend the nation. Maintenance of these high standards by all service members is a requirement for the job, but it is the individuals and families who make the personal sacrifices.

Service, which is rooted in the time-honored traditions of this nation's first great military leaders, is to defend and protect. A great personal strength is to be able to stay afloat in times of change. Anchored between the boundaries of land and sea, stability and change, the Navy asks its members to journey to new horizons of personal growth and achievement within an environment of constant change. It takes special people to make this journey—these are the men and women of the United States Navy!

Chapter 15

Understanding Life in the Air Force

James G. Daley

As you approach an Air Force base, the first thing you notice is the guards at the gates. Crisp uniforms, highly shined boots, armed with sidearm or M-16 rifle, the guard is polite but clearly in charge. Millions of dollars in equipment, highly sensitive information, and some of the most sophisticated weaponry are protected behind those gates. But beyond the gates also exists a society called by Wertsch (1991) "America's most invisible minority," which is a "separate and distinctly different subculture from civilian America" and "exercises such a powerful influence on its children that for the rest of our lives we continue to bear its stamp" (pp. xii-xiii). I was born into this invisible society and grew up in a setting where combat uniforms (called BDUs), marching soldiers, and readiness for war were as common and normal as cornfields to a farming family in Iowa. I spent most of my adult life (eighteen years) serving in the Air Force, raised a family within its bosom, and retired into the netherland of obsolescence. This chapter is my effort to paint the portrait of my society. It is part of a triad of pictures of life in the military (see Chapter 13 for life in the Army and Chapter 14 for life in the Navy). My goal is to help the reader naive to the military to bridge the chasm and better understand what my life was like (also refer to Chapter 18, which describes the military as an ethnicity).

THE SOCIAL CLASSES WITHIN THE AIR FORCE

Aircrew As a Special Class

Equal opportunity is a high priority, but not equal status. Bias based on race or ethnicity is swiftly chastised. The basic principle is duty excellence, and personal drive warrants status, not cultural background. However, there are distinct status categories within the Air Force. *Aircrew,* especially pilots, are most prestigious. Aircrew have their own medical specialists (called flight surgeons) for themselves and their families. Their medical records include the big bold letters "*FLY*" so that no one mistakes them for other personnel. The specialty care is based primarily on the need to ensure flying capability, called "flying status," and the worst trauma to an aircrew member is to be declassified or disqualified (called DNIF) from flying status. The Air Force invests millions of dollars in training costs in each pilot, and the pilot routinely has control over millions of dollars worth of aircraft. Therefore, aircrew have priority, are called "mission essential," get quicker on-base housing at some bases, can have the base gymnasium opened just for them, and so forth. Families of aircrew form tighter social connections, though clearly keeping officer and enlisted separate. They get special pay, called flight pay, to supplement the pay of other military persons of the same rank. In fact, pilots are so significant that all nonpilots are called support officers.

Officers As a Class

The next significant class status is officer versus enlisted. The vast majority (over 80 percent) of the Air Force are enlisted and officers are by design in charge of all activity within the Air Force. Officers strive throughout their careers to gain larger and larger command responsibilities (e.g., moving from squadron commander to company commander to base commander).

Within the officer ranks, there are additional status hierarchies. *Company grade officers* are the newcomers (lieutenant and captain) who are expected to be naive to the military ethnicity. Company grade officers are to be mentored, challenged, held accountable, and given limited responsibility. They are still considered on "probation" to see if they fit in and successful promotion indicates further entry into the military society. New officers have a service commitment (usually three years) and the company grade officer is deciding whether to make a career of the Air Force. By the second year, the company grade officer must decide to apply for "indefinite reserve status" (IRS) or "regular," which would mean a date of separation in twenty or thirty years (though IRS is being phased out). The point is that the officer who applies for regular status at the earliest time and gets promoted to captain is a person who embraces the core elements of the Air Force.

The next step, *field grade officer* (major and lieutenant colonel), is a milestone. You are clearly a "lifer" (committed to a career) and have enough military experience to be a credible advocate on issues. The higher the rank, the more competitive and less likely it is that anyone will be promoted. Therefore, the field grade officer has shown that he or she has the "right stuff."

The next rung in the ladder is *colonel*, one of the most influential players in the Air Force. The colonel is a high-status individual. For example, many bases request to be notified when a colonel will be visiting, have a staff car with driver available, and ensure that a greeter meets the colonel as a distinguished visitor. The temporary living quarters are more plush, called VIP suites. The colonel is expected to be mentor and protector of the military way. Assignments become handpicked by the "colonels group" and a colonel is only placed in an assignment commensurate with his or her rank.

The final rung in the ladder is *general*. Generals have the ultimate status (though ironically the least freedom) of any Air Force person. They are status icons who maintain select leadership roles (e.g., wing commander, commander in chief). In sum, officers have their own status and then rankings depending on how high they are able to get promoted. The higher the rank, the more span of influence and responsibility the officer has to ensure that the military culture blossoms.

Enlisted As a Class

The relationship between officers and enlisted is one of distance and status deference. Officers are paid more than enlisted people. For example, a brand new lieutenant (the lowest officer rank) makes $1,774.20 per month as compared to a staff sergeant (E-5) with ten years service, who makes $1,685.70 per month (data obtained from the Internet at http://www.dfas.mil/money/milpay/98pay/98bp.htm). Officers are given respect and deference by the enlisted (e.g., calling the officer "sir," saluting when approaching an officer, and obeying the officer's directives as a "lawful order"). Fraternization ("being good friends" in civilian terms) between officer and enlisted is forbidden regardless of the person's marital status (e.g., single) or supervisory linkage. Cordial but separate interaction is expected and fraternization can lead to military trial and jail time. Obviously, sexual relationships between officer and enlisted are high offenses. Officers' housing is separate from enlisted housing, and officers' clubs are separate from enlisted clubs (though that policy is being reviewed at some locations). Even officers' children feel the social awkwardness of relationships when one is an officer's child and the other is an enlisted member's child (see Chapter 9 in Wertsch, 1991). Everyone knows his or her place and the society monitors the mores. An interesting paradox occurs when a married couple consists of an enlisted person and an officer (a common event). The society acknowledges their legality but frequent social awkwardness emerges. I once knew a couple (she was a nurse officer, he was enlisted in military intelligence) who were extremely secretive while dating (for good reason), got married, and then announced their relationship. The society grudgingly accepted the fait accompli and slowly began to socially engage. But the couple still had to downplay the rank contrast.

NCOs As Part of the Enlisted

A bridging rank structure are the noncommissioned officers (NCOs). However, they are not really officers. They are the senior enlisted persons (E-5 and above), called *sergeants* (except the highest rank, which is called *chief*). They are the standard bearers of military protocol and culture. If you want to know what ribbon goes where on your uniform, ask a sergeant. They are the backbone of the military and proud of it. Promotion is very competitive, with a combination of a service record (the personnel folder showing accomplishments), an elaborate system of points for a broad range of achievements (e.g., having attended military service schools, gotten medals, span of command responsibility), and a formal written test. The competition is so intense that gaining that next stripe can hinge on a quarter of a point difference (rather like Olympic competitions). It is common for NCOs to have to recompete for several times before achieving the next rank. And the higher the rank, the less chance of achieving it. For example, 50 percent of people competing for staff sergeant (E-5) achieve it, but only 20 percent achieve master sergeant (E-6), 2 percent achieve senior master sergeant (E-7), and 1 percent achieve chief master sergeant (E-8). The higher the rank, the greater span of leadership and command expected. Though an enlisted person will never move up in rank to officer (e.g., E-8 does not automatically lead to O-1) unless they reenter the Air Force as a new officer. The vast majority of senior enlisted have at least a bachelor's degree, but usually the switching of career paths to officer only occurs early in an enlisted person's career. It is very difficult to restart at the bottom officer rung as you go higher and higher up the enlisted ladder of success.

In reviewing the officer versus enlisted ranks, several common features are noted. The higher the rank, the more prestige and responsibilities. Both officer and enlisted promotion are highly competitive and drive a career-long push for the Right Job. Firmly established boundaries are respected by both sides and relationships unfold within those boundaries. Family members often pay a price of confusion and awkwardness in terms of relationship and intimacy boundaries between enlisted and officer.

Family Members As a Class

The final class status is *family member*, historically called the military member's "dependents" (a term loathed by some family members). Family members are essential but peripheral players within the military community. How can they be both essential and peripheral? Family members are show stoppers of combat readiness and even military careers. Family members, especially spouses, have informal clout (if they choose to use it) that remedies many awkward social scenarios (e.g., an isolated military family, inadequate or insensitive base programs, increasing stress levels in military personnel). Some examples of the use of such clout might be calling up a newly arrived military family and inviting the spouse to the NCO spouses club or officers' spouses club meetings, educating a newly married spouse about what resources are available, or hearing of a financially distraught family and working through the first sergeant to get financial counseling. Numerous studies have shown that one of the top reasons for military persons not remaining in the Air Force is family dissatisfaction with the military.

A multitude of social programs have been developed to preventively intervene to enhance family wellness (see Chapters 4 and 5). The Air Force learned many years ago that family stability is a force multiplier. Therefore many social structures are in place (see next section) to create a pleasing environment within which to raise a family. Housing allowances and other special pay supplements have been added to military base pay to alleviate fiscal stressors (though not enough according to many lower-ranking enlisted families). Social organizations such as officers' spouses clubs and enlisted spouses clubs are institutionalized at every base. Efforts are made to offer special briefings for family members when significant changes are occurring (such as TRICARE; see Chapter 5). Health care facilities provide pediatric, obstetric, and family practice for family members, and other specialty services for handicapped family members (see Chapter 4). Schools often are built on the base and, in overseas locations, school systems are managed by a military-affiliated organization (Department of Defense Dependents Schools). Family support centers offer prevention-oriented classes, relocation assistance for the next transfer, financial counseling, and many other family-focused efforts. Mental health and family advocacy programs offer a range of preventive and ameliorative family programs on issues ranging from parenting to depression to caretaker stress. In essence, the Air Force exerts massive effort to produce an environment that is family-friendly and an excellent location to raise a family. Families are essential to the "Air Force way of life" (though much is also offered for single military members too).

So why are they also peripheral? Families have specific status within the Air Force, especially at higher ranks. But the status is contingent on being stable, nondisruptive, and able to cope with whatever mission demands arise for the military member. Resilient and pleasant family members on the arm of a military member enhance status; acting-out adolescents picked up for the third shoplifting offense or defacing the base chapel can end careers. The more quietly supportive and helpful, the better the scenario. Families facilitate the mission by "carrying on" and not being demanding of the deployed personnel. Unexpected crises (sudden onset of labor in pregnant spouse, car accident, death in extended family) are acceptable and extraordinary efforts are made at times by the Air Force to expedite the military member arriving home. But chronic issues (fiscal crises, a spouse depressed or inebriated for the third time, a repeatedly runaway child) reflect an inability to "control" the family (see Chapter 20 for more on ethnic standards). A reasonable time is allotted to "fix" the issue and then the member begins to lose status and viability to remain in the Air

Force. In other words, the family should be highly visible as a nurturing support system but as peripheral as possible with any life crises.

I remember vividly a military client that I had who was repeatedly physically abused by his female spouse. After the third time that the military authorities responded to the house, the commander and first sergeant were sympathetic but also clearly asking for him to resolve the issue. The primary issue was not the abuse but the disruptiveness to the unit (though I know the commander would and did argue that his concern was with "one of my troops"). He eventually divorced the spouse primarily to salvage his career, as he had still not resolved his issues with his spouse.

The expectation is that military members seek help as soon as possible, resolve any issues quickly, and ensure readiness for the mission at all times. Families are essential to the social functioning of the military community but also resiliently peripheral when the mission calls.

A TOUR OF AN AIR FORCE BASE

An Air Force base is a combination of social community and organizational hub. Most bases have family housing, always separated by rank sections (enlisted, NCOs, company grade officers, field grade officers, generals' quarters, base commander, and wing commander). Each house has the rank and last name of the occupant listed on a plaque on the front door. Different ranks might be housed on different streets or even sections of a street. But the higher the rank, the nicer the house. Maintenance is provided by military repairmen (or on rare occasions, civilian contractors) but each family is expected to keep the house in excellent condition. Very thorough inspections occur when a family moves in or out. The inspections are true white-glove obsessions and have prompted a whole industry of cleaning services who specialize in guaranteeing your house will pass. Discrepancies in home condition (holes in wall, dirty floors, etc.) are charged to the military member unless he or she can prove the condition was pre-existing. The point is that the houses are well maintained, though sometimes quite old (e.g., built during World War II).

The social community goes beyond just housing. A typical base has a movie theater (or two), a gas station, a grocery store, a department store, a bowling alley, a golf course, arts and crafts center, automotive repair shop, child care center, youth center, elementary school (and, if large enough, a middle school and high school), a swimming pool (if large enough, an officers' pool and a general use pool), a post office, a furniture store, several churches (called chapels), a hospital, several fast food restaurants (e.g., Burger King, Baskin Robbins), two restaurants/bars (an officers' club and an enlisted club), a community center (called Family Support Center) that offers classes or helpful programs such as financial counseling, college sites offering a wide range of degree programs, commercial banks, and sometimes lakes and boating/camping spots. In essence, all the services needed to shop, entertain, worship, bank, educate, and recreate are all within this exclusive gated community. A military family could conceivably never leave a base while stationed there. In addition, the families surrounding you are quite homogeneous in interest, shared history, and often have neighborhood parties or other social events.

There is a sense of security, stability, and sameness to a base. But the base is also an ultimate "fishbowl" where gossip abounds, few secrets are truly secrets, and you see friends (or enemies) while you shop, eat, worship, swim, and so on. Of course, the larger the base, the less fishbowl-like the environment is. But military families quickly recognize that the price of being part of the community is social visibility.

Some military persons (especially single or troubled families) specifically chose to live off base to secure some privacy and distance from prying eyes. Mission-essential personnel do not have a choice. They must live on base or within a few miles. But for other families, the decision is based on a combination of privacy and finances. People who live on base pay no rent or utilities; people who live off base get a housing allowance that usually covers part of the costs. It is not unusual to wait a year to get into base housing. Families who seek separateness simply do not put their name on the waiting list to get on-base housing.

Besides the social community, an Air Force base is a thriving industry whose main product is airpower. Everything centers on the ability to launch aircraft and each base has a different combination of airpower (transports, fighter jets, tankers, etc.). Military squadrons are industrial organizations responsible for a component of that mission and all the squadrons must mesh together in a focused manner to get the mission done. Overseeing all the squadrons are groups, and all the groups report to a wing commander. Every component has a commander (squadron, group, wing), and all commanders report to the wing commander, who reports to the Numbered Air Force commander, and so forth. The chain of command is clear, unbroken, and must work smoothly in rapid, unpredictable, and chaotic times. The base commander is responsible for the smooth functioning of the base components (roads, services, security) but the most potent individual on the base is the wing commander.

Therefore, when you spend some time on a base, you observe a fascinating blend of industry and social community. Driving down the well-groomed landscaped roads, you might not notice the intensive activity occurring in the office buildings. While you are enjoying your ice cream cone on a bench, people across the street are in a top secret briefing on the latest international crisis and its impact on that base's mission.

An Air Force base is more than just leisure and job. It is a developmental way station in a continual life cycle for military member and family. Each base is both a place and a piece of a career. Air Force families blend the base into a component of a career. A combination of renewed old friends and new friends, a mixture of scars and joys, a stepping stone to advancement or the graveyard of a career, each base is part of the emotional scrapbook of an Air Force family. For example, Keesler Air Force Base is where my son was born, I was accepted into a PhD program, and my spouse got her master's degree. Travis Air Force Base is where my daughter was born, I decided to begin moving toward retirement, and we met dear friends. Lajes Field (Azores, Portugal) was the lowest emotional point in our career and is our standard for comparison (e.g., "It's not that bad, at least it's not the Azores"). Each Air Force base is both place and memory in a long journey. The Air Force has shaped us much more than we have shaped it. The base is the conduit, but the electricity flowing through it is the vitality and ethnicity of the military. The base is merely buildings. What brings it to life is what it represents: continuity, standards, purpose.

In today's base-closing, force-reducing, service-outsourcing, cost-reducing environment, the Air Force is going through an identity crisis.

The continuity is threatened and the mission will surely suffer. What I have described above is a rich, ancient heritage. How long it will last is hard to say. My "mission" is to capture the richness of the Air Force environment. I hope I have succeeded.

REFERENCE

Wertsch, M.E. (1991). *Military Brats: Legacies of Childhood Inside the Fortress.* New York: Harmony Books.

Chapter 16

Soldier and Family Wellness Across the Life Course: A Developing Role for Social Workers

Mike W. Parker
Vaughn R. A. Call
William F. Barko

> Youth is not a period of time. It is a state of mind, a result of the will, a quality of the imagination, a victory of courage over timidity, of the taste of adventure over the love of comfort. A man doesn't grow old because he has lived a certain number of years. A man grows old when he deserts his ideal. The years may wrinkle his skin, but deserting his ideal wrinkles his soul. Preoccupations, fears, doubts, and despair are the enemies which slowly bow us toward earth and turn us into dust before death. You will remain young as long as you are open to what is beautiful, good, and great; receptive to the messages of other men and women, of nature and of God. If one day you should become bitter, pessimistic, and gnawed by despair, may God have mercy on your old man's soul.
>
> General Douglas MacArthur

General Douglas MacArthur may be best remembered for his retirement message before Congress, in which he declared, "Old soldiers never die; they just fade away." Didactically more notable, however, may be the general's digest on the victuals of "youth" and his view

Opinions are those of the chapter authors and do not reflect the policy or opinions of the U.S. Army.

that age was not a vital variable in achieving and maintaining "youthfulness." Seminal reviews on successful human aging have argued similarly that the negative effects of the aging process itself have been exaggerated and suggested that change in lifestyle, diet, exercise, personal habits, and psychosocial factors can modify the vicissitudes of age (Rowe and Kahn, 1997, 1998; Parker et al., 1995). The current health promotion zeitgeist and its associated themes of exercise, diet, and increased awareness of at-risk behaviors, coupled with the highly touted cost savings associated with efficacious prevention programs, provide an opportunity for those concerned with successful aging and health promotion.

Military social workers and other behavioral scientists are playing an increasingly active role on multidisciplinary teams within the health promotion field because their expertise is needed in helping individuals change negative life styles and maintain positive behaviors (e.g., exercise, dietary habits). The purpose of this chapter is twofold: (1) to describe a new health promotion role for military social workers that is currently being established at the Army's premier leadership school and (2) to emphasize the efficacy of a life course perspective in the development of health promotion initiatives.

As the U.S. armed forces face "downsizing" of current medical resources, "partnering" individual responsibility with an effective, streamlined medical care system within an efficacious health promotion system remains a major challenge for the next decade. The fitness, health, and welfare of senior leaders and officers in the U.S. armed forces are of vital concern to the Department of Defense and to the security of our nation. Twentieth-century leaders must not only be increasingly health conscious, but also prime examples and promoters of healthy behaviors and programs. Historically, military medicine has pioneered the development and refinement of countless procedures, programs, and techniques (e.g., diagnosis and treatment of post-traumatic stress victims), but more recently has come under serious criticism and scrutiny.

ZEITGEIST

The American population is experiencing a demographic revolution that has important implications for the military. Gains in life expectancy, declining birth rates, increased female labor force participation, and more diverse, multigenerational family structures affect the active military, veterans, and their families. The number of U.S. veterans eighty-five years and over is expected to increase nearly 600 percent by 2010 (Parker et al., 1995). Retirees and their dependents will be an increasing proportion of patients in the military health care system in the near future. At present, these individuals account for more than half of all patients in the system. Active duty personnel account for only 18.9 percent of the consumers of DoD health care services. Age-related illnesses (cardiovascular disease, stroke, and Alzheimer's disease) will be an increasingly important factor driving DoD and DVA health care costs in the years ahead. Managed care approaches to health care will not reduce the overall cost without effective forms of primary, secondary, and tertiary prevention.

Significant progress in the field of aging is directly relevant to military leaders, medical practitioners, and policymakers who are concerned about successful aging and health promotion. In their initial, seminal review article on human aging, Rowe and Kahn (1987) argued that the negative effects of the aging process itself have been exaggerated, and suggested that changes in lifestyle, diet, exercise, personal habits, and psychosocial factors can modify the vicissitudes of age. Evans and Rosenberg (1991) suggested biointervention processes to postpone entry into the "disability zone." In more recent reviews, Rowe and Kahn (1997, 1998) have proposed a model that amplifies successful aging deductively constructed from the growing body of literature. They define successful aging as including three main components: low probability of disease and disease-related disability, high cognitive and physical functional capacity, and active engagement with life. Successful aging is more than the absence of disease and more than the maintenance of functional capacities in combination with active engagement with life that represents the concept of successful aging.

To enhance the total wellness and successful aging of officers, the U.S. Army War College is providing America's future senior military leaders the skills and information needed to maintain their own and their family's optimal health and well-being. Officers are provided fitness and health promotion programs that focus on life events associated with midlife and the officer's ability to cope with those events.

THE U.S. ARMY WAR COLLEGE

Since 1901 the U.S. Army War College has prepared highly selected military, civilian, and international leaders to assume strategic leadership responsibilities in military and national security organizations. Selected senior officers are identified through a formal selection process each year and represent the top 5 percent of their military service or government agency. The War College's purpose is "professional development in strategic leadership and strategic art; and personal development in the mental, physical, moral and spiritual attributes of character . . . the student development plan provides a process by which the student creates a personal road map to meet the organization's purpose" (U.S. Army War College, 1996, pp. 3-4).

ARMY PHYSICAL FITNESS RESEARCH INSTITUTE (APFRI)

The APFRI "prepares senior leaders to assume individual responsibility for optimum health and fitness. It educates on the biomarkers of aging, researches over 40 health and fitness issues and conducts outreach programs that benefit the Army and the nation" (U.S. Army War College, 1996). Since 1982 APFRI has conducted health and fitness assessment on over 6,000 students and faculty at the War College. The assessments include the physical, mental, and spiritual components of health.

Senior leaders face a unique set of extreme stressors. Like chief executive officers of major corporations, senior officers make command decisions affecting the daily lives of thousands of soldiers and their families. In contrast to civilian executives, senior military leaders are often responsible for the twenty-four-hour security of soldiers under their command and, in combat situations, may issue orders that result in the loss of life of many soldiers. In addition to the stress, hierarchical command structure and military traditions can produce a sense of isolation among senior military leaders. High stress and isolation can be linked to negative health outcomes and poor decision making. Descriptive studies of senior military officers have shown specifically that this group is at risk (Seigman, Franco, and Barko, 1998; Mitchell and Barko, in press; Wright et al., 1994; Labatte et al., 1995). In particular, an effort is being made to identify high-probability life events for this cohort group as a means of better understanding the stress situations they face and the developmental tasks related to health and family life that occur at this stage in the life course.

THE IMPORTANCE OF LIFE EVENTS

Historically, military families have had to cope with numerous high-stress events and transitions that are atypical for civilian counterparts (e.g., foreign assignments, command, dangerous frequent family relocations, midlife "retirement"). Military families simultaneously face demanding, often unanticipated life events associated with midlife such as parenting older children and elder care (see Parker et al., 1995; Parker, Harrig, and Martin, 1997). Family separations related to deployments, training, and tours of duty without the presence of family have been considered among the most difficult aspects of military life (Etheridge, 1989; Coolbaugh and Rosenthal, 1992; Segal and Harris, 1993). Overlapping life course transitions and events place senior leaders and their families at risk (e.g., women on active duty are particularly vulnerable to the demands of elder care (Parker, Harrig, and Martin, 1996). The linkages between life events and health behaviors for military personnel are not well known (see e.g., Gade, 1991; Elder, Pavalko, and Hastings, 1991), and little information is available on the mitigating effects of health promotion interventions on these factors. A life course perspective provides a useful framework for understanding the relationship between physical health, psychological well-being, and common life events that officers face with family and career.

THE LIFE COURSE PERSPECTIVE

The life course perspective emerged in the early 1960s out of life span developmental psychology, life cycle research, social relations (role theory), and social and developmental psychology of age (Elder, 1997). Unlike conceptualizations of the individual life cycle and the family cycle, life course theory is not concerned with a priori stages, but with life patterns. Life course theory emphasizes the transitions into and out of various roles and developmental tasks in relation to social and historical time. To understand individual development and change, we must take into account the social, family, institutional, and historical changes that are occurring. A person's trajectory is "a product of multiple histories, each defined by a particular timetable and event sequence-histories of education and work life, marriage and parenthood, residence and civic involvement" (Elder, 1977). The essence of the life course perspective is embodied in six basic principles:

1. Linkages between social and psychological states form trajectories
2. Life course trajectories are embedded in social contexts
3. Significant deviations from social pathways have negative consequences
4. Life course trajectories are shaped by historical events
5. Life course trajectories are interdependent
6. The impact of transitions is largely contingent on timing in the life course

Linkages Between Social and Psychological States Form Trajectories

As people make numerous role transitions across time a life pattern develops, and they experience numerous changes in social status and personal identity as a result of the pathway they follow (Glaser and Strauss, 1971). Many major transitions occur early in the life course as young people make decisions about education, marriage, military, and occupation roles in their late teens and early twenties (Call and Teachman, 1991). As they make these transitions, they establish a trajectory of choices that largely defines the pathways they will follow through life. We refer to these life patterns or pathways as trajectories. These trajectories are determined by the linkage of a person's social and psychological states across time and are largely constructed by the actions and role choices a person makes through his or her own personal agency.

Major turning points in life course trajectories frequently reflect involuntary role changes that occur due to biological, psychological, social, and historical events beyond the person's control. These major life course contingencies are quite common. For example, a heart attack or other serious illness, an accident that causes a severe injury, the death of a spouse, and company downsizing or an economic recession are just a few events that may cause a complete change in a person's life course trajectory. Military service is hazardous duty and places a soldier at increased risk of life course contingencies. These contingencies often invoke numerous, abrupt changes in soldiers' and their families' lives. The mobilization during Desert Storm, for example, caused family separation, significant disjunctures in occupational careers, and increased problems managing family finances (Bell, 1991).

Physical separation from family is a fact of life for most military personnel with field exercises, military courses, and unaccompanied tours as part of their jobs. Long-term separations are more common for enlisted personnel than officers (Coolbaugh and Rosenthal, 1992). Nonetheless, about two-thirds of the officers in the classes of 1997 and 1998 at the Army War College experienced at least one long-term separation from their families as the result of a deployment or duty assignment (see Table 16.1). These separations have negative impacts on families and their ability to adapt to military life (Segal and Harris, 1993) that military support systems attempt to ameliorate. This type of life course contingency is not present in the civilian workplace. About 70 percent of married, male civilian workers are never away from home overnight because of work-related travel and half of those who do travel averaged less than one night a month away from their families.

Once wars and long-term deployments end, lives have to be reconstructed. This reconstruction often involves a significant change in life course trajectories. At the end of the Civil War, Robert E. Lee simply stated, "I am a soldier no more" and, after thirty-nine years of military duty, made a significant break with his past trajectory to follow a new occupational, family, and social pathway (Parker et al., 1995).

TABLE 16.1. Percentage of Officers Who Had One or More Separations from Spouse

		Regular Army	Reserves/ National Guard	Other Armed Forces	War College Total
Separated from Spouse		67.7%	47.2%	60.3%	63.8%
	n=	291	53	68	412

Note: Officers were members of the Army War College classes of 1997 and 1998. Separations were caused by deployment or duty assignments that lasted three months or more.

Life Course Trajectories Are Embedded in Social Contexts

Life course trajectories are embedded in a social context that, to a certain degree, establishes the social pathways (role alternatives) available. These social pathways reflect (1) the proscriptive and prescriptive age norms and institutional requisites that structure the timing, spacing, sequencing, and duration of roles, and (2) the informal and formal social constraints that limit or prohibit access to certain pathways by a few, most, or all members of that society.

All major social institutions (government, military, religion, education, business, and family) establish and regulate the appropriate timing of life course transitions (Mayer, 1986; O'Rand, 1990). Age expectations regarding the appropriate timing of life course transitions operate as "prods and brakes upon behavior" (Neugarten, Moore, and Lowe, 1965). In some instances such as induction into the military, age norms are very rigid. Even though age norms provide a great deal of structure to life course options, there is considerable variation in the incidence and timing of many transitions (O'Rand, 1990; Elder, George, and Shanahan, 1996). People take these rules into account as they construct their own life courses (Elder, George, and Shanahan, 1996). As a result, people are able to determine if they are early, on time, or late relative to when transitions normally occur (Neugarten, Moore, and Lowe, 1965; Neugarten and Datan, 1973; Lawrence, 1984).

Rank advancement in the Army occurs at fixed time intervals in an officer's career. Officers passed over for promotion become worried about their military careers because they are not "on time" for a critical transition. Officers who receive early selection for advancement generally feel that their military career prospects are enhanced. Most officers attending the Army War College reported that their promotions occurred early or on schedule. Nonetheless, about 5 percent of the regular Army officers and over a fourth of the Reserve and National Guard officers at the War College had been passed over for promotion at some time in their careers (see Table 16.2). Conversely, about a third of the regular and a fourth of the Reserve/National Guard officers received early selection for promotion. Thus, there is some variation in the promotion process but most officers attending the Army War college were either on time with all their promotions (62 percent) or selected for early promotion one or more times.

TABLE 16.2. Percentage of Officers Passed Over for Promotion or Selected for Early Promotion

	Regular Army	Reserves/ National Guard	Other Armed Forces	War College Total
Passed over for promotion	4.6%	26.4%	2.9%	7.1%
Early selection for promotion	34.8	24.5	19.1	31.1
n=	305	53	68	425

Note: Officers were members of the Army War College classes of 1997 and 1998.

Significant Deviations from Social Pathways Have Negative Consequences

When a person has unusually early or late transitions, makes a transition out of sequence from the normative pattern, or stays in a role longer than normatively prescribed, this person may experience negative life course consequences. For example, those who marry early (in their teenage years) and those who marry late (over age thirty-five) have the highest rates of marital disruption (Sweet and Bumpass, 1987). Hogan and Astone (1986) suggest that many of these negative consequences occur because there is a poor fit between the demands of labor markets and schools and the needs of individuals. The lack of fit occurs because our educational and occupational institutions are organized to process age cohorts (Featherman and Carter, 1976).

After twenty or more years of military service, most soldiers face a very "off-time" transition back to the civilian labor market, particularly if the civilian economy is in a recession. Most soldiers are over age forty when they retire from the military and many have never held a full-time civilian job. Their nonveteran peers are midcareer and approaching the peak of their career advancement. With the increased technical requirements of military service, more soldiers find their military skills transferable to the civilian sector (Magnum and Ball, 1987, 1989) and, depending on the historical era, greater employer acceptance of military service as evidence of enhanced physical and mental capabilities (Teachman and Call, 1996). Many soldiers and NCOs, however, do not have transferable skills and all new veterans must compete with their nonveteran peers who have often have twenty years of direct civilian job experience within firms.

Age discrimination laws and government regulations and programs to facilitate access to the civilian labor market exist to alleviate difficulties that older people and veterans frequently face. Most people do not think about the effects of deviating from the normal pathways because any deviation is unanticipated (a layoff) or too far in the future to be salient (postmilitary plans). As a result, they often hold unrealistic assumptions about off-time transitions. Former Army War College officers, for example, may be somewhat overly optimistic about their transition into the civilian labor market, particularly with respect to salary. When compared to civilians who have the same level of education (a master's degree or higher) and the officers' expected age at military retirement, more officers anticipate being in the higher income groups than civilians actually obtain at that stage of their life course (see Table 16.3). While they have experience and leadership skills, these officers make an off-time entry into a civilian labor market where corporate downsizing and age discrimination take a severe toll on this age group, who generally are in middle management positions.

Almost half of the officers expect to have a civilian job within two months of leaving the military (see Table 16.4). Unless there is considerable advance preparation and negotiation prior to leaving the military, such a quick transition may be difficult to achieve, particularly if the officer's final assignment is overseas. The extent to which this off-time transition affects officers' reentry into the civilian labor force and the associated effects of this transition on other domains of the life course is not well-understood. Future follow-up research on these officers will directly address this issue.

If soldiers and officers experience negative consequences of their off-time transitions, there is evidence that suggests that the negative effects may be ameliorated—at least for soldiers. Recent research on one of the most socially sanctioned off-time transitions, a nonmarital birth, demonstrates that women avoid the long-term negative consequences of their off-time transition if they subsequently marry and reestablish the normal pathway (Hearne et al., 1996). This appears to apply to the workplace as well. Military service acts as a bridging environment that allows people who are not doing well in their educational and occupational roles to abruptly change to a new pathway that allows them to succeed. For example, Elder and Bailey (1988) found that middle-class men who had a poor academic record and little prospect of completing college were more likely to enter the military and, through World War II GI benefits, were able to obtain relatively high levels of educational attainment after the war. More recent data suggest that military service serves as a bridging environment for less advantaged whites (relative to less advantaged, nonveteran whites) but has only minimal effects for blacks, who tend to be among the more qualified blacks prior to entry into the military (Teachman and Call, 1996).

TABLE 16.3. Level of Salary Expected from Civilian Occupation After Retirement by Officers in Army War College Classes of 1997 and 1998

	Regular Army	Reserves/ National Guard	Other Armed Forces	War College Total	NSFH Civilian Peers
Less than $19,000	0.0%	5.1%	0.0%	0.6%	5.5%
$20,000-$39,000	24.0	33.3	19.3	24.3	20.3
$40,000-$59,000	25.2	35.9	42.1	29.1	39.1
$60,000-$79,000	26.4	18.0	24.6	25.1	21.6
$80,000-$99,000	14.6	0.0	8.8	12.0	9.0
$100,000 or more	9.8	7.7	5.2	8.9	4.4
	100.0%	100.0%	100.0%	100.0%	100.0%
n=	254	39	57	350	114

Note: Data for the civilian comparison comes from the National Survey of Families and Households (Sweet, Bumpass, and Call, 1998). The NSFH had 13,008 respondents in 1998. We used a subsample of males, age 45-54 (comparable to their retirement age), with at least a master's degree.

TABLE 16.4. Expected Length of Transition Time into Civilian Job After Retirement by Officers in Army War College Classes of 1997 and 1998

	Regular Army	Reserves/ National Guard	Other Armed Forces	War College Total
Job waiting for them	22.9%	30.2%	20.7%	23.4%
1-2 months	24.0	14.0	6.9	20.2
3-8 months	38.7	53.5	55.2	43.0
9-11 months	6.6	2.3	5.2	5.9
12+ months	7.8	0.0	12.0	7.5
	100.0%	100.0%	100.0%	100.0%
n=	271	43	58	372

Life Course Trajectories Are Shaped by Historical Events

Social pathways and individual life course trajectories are shaped by historical events that alter the set of pathways available within the society and the social context defining those pathways. Major historical events such as the Depression and wars can produce very different life course trajectories for those who experience the event and those who do not. The extent of difficulty people experience in dealing with events that can alter their trajectory depends upon their coping resources and the timing of those events in the life course. After World War I and World War II, for example, most veterans did not suffer adverse consequences from the disruption of their life courses because generous GI benefits permitted these soldiers to quickly reestablish themselves (Fligstein, 1976). Most Vietnam veterans entered the military at a young age and did not remain long. As a result, this historical event only had modest long-term negative consequences on these young men and, with respect to marriage, had no influence at all (Call and Teachman, 1991). Operation Desert Shield/Storm, however, resulted in numerous social and financial problems, particularly for reservists who tended to be older and more established in careers and self-employment (Bell, 1991; Segal and Harris, 1993).

Life Course Trajectories Are Interdependent

A person's life course trajectory is interdependent with the trajectories of other people in his or her social networks. As a person becomes more dependent upon other people, interlocking trajectories occur and personal trajectories become subject to the requisites of multiple pathways and a greater variety of life course contingencies.

Although most enlisted personnel and officers are not married when they enter the military, the longer people stay in the military the more likely they are to marry and have children. About 60 percent of soldiers and 80 percent of officers in the Army are married (Segal and Harris, 1993). Over 97 percent of the officers in the Army War College are currently married. Segal and Harris (1993) found that about 60 to 70 percent of Army spouses were employed and that about 7 to 10 percent of married military couples have dual military career marriages. The same pattern appears to hold for senior officers. Among Army War College officers, about 6 percent are dual career military families (see Table 16.5).

In addition to multiple career pathways, officers, particularly senior officers at the War College, face elder care issues that overlap with transitions into senior command positions. About half the officers still have both parents living and more than 80 percent have at least one parent still living (see Table 16.6). More than half the married officers still have both in-laws and over 80 percent have at least one living in-law (see Table 16.7).

The interlocking life course pathways with parents produce additional stress for these officers. About 30 percent of the officers stated that they were worried about the health of their parents (see Table 16.8). Much of this worry centers on the health of their parents and parents-in-law. Over 35 percent of the officers in the Army War College rated their parents' health from poor to very poor and 39 percent rated the health of their in-laws as poor or worse. About two-thirds of the officers have spoken to their parents about their parents' plans for the future as they age (see Table 16.9). About a third of these officers were not satisfied or were very unsatisfied with their parents' plans (see Table 16.10). These officers are beginning to feel the stress associated with elder care responsibilities. Inasmuch as women usually face the larger caregiving roles, the officers' wives will likely experience more stress than their husbands, particularly given overseas assignments and limited housing arrangements that reduce their options as they try to cope with their parents' failing health. As a result, we found that many officers resort to contributing cash toward their parents' care because other options are not viable.

TABLE 16.5. Percentage of Married Officers in Army War College Classes of 1997 and 1998 with a Spouse Currently Enlisted or an Officer in the Armed Forces

		Regular Army	Reserves/ National Guard	Other Armed Forces	War College Total
Dual Military Career Families		5.1%	9.6%	9.2%	6.3%
	n=	295	52	65	412

TABLE 16.6. Percentage of Officers Who Have Experienced the Death of One or More Parents

	Regular Army	Reserves/ National Guard	Other Armed Forces	War College Total
Both Parents Deceased	16.1%	16.1%	18.6%	16.5%
One Parent Deceased	36.5	39.3	22.9	34.6
Both Parents Alive	47.4	44.6	58.5	48.9
	100.0%	100.0%	100.0%	100.0%
n=	310	56	70	436

TABLE 16.7. Percentage of Officers Who Have Experienced the Death of One or More Parents-in-Law

	Regular Army	Reserves/ National Guard	Other Armed Forces	War College Total
Both Parents Deceased	17.7%	26.8%	18.6%	19.0%
One Parent Deceased	29.0	23.2	27.1	28.0
Both Parents Alive	53.3	50.0	54.3	53.0
	100.0%	100.0%	100.0%	100.0%
n=	303	55	67	425

TABLE 16.8. Percentage of Officers in Army War College Classes of 1997 and 1998 Who Worry About the Health and Fitness of Their Elderly Relatives

	Regular Army	Reserves/ National Guard	Other Armed Forces	War College Total
Yes, worry	28.4%	34.2%	22.9%	28.3%
n=	222	41	48	311

Note: The Class of 1997 was asked whether they worried or not; the Class of 1998 responded to a seven-point scale. We coded scores 5, 6, and 7 as "worried."

TABLE 16.9. Percentage of Officers in Army War College Classes of 1997 and 1998 Who Had Spoken with Their Elderly Parents About Their Parents' Future Plans

		Regular Army	Reserves/ National Guard	Other Armed Forces	War College Total
Yes, spoken to parents		66.9%	74.5%	66.7%	67.8%
	n=	284	51	63	398

TABLE 16.10. Degree of Officer Satisfaction with Parents' Plans for Their Future

		Regular Army	Reserves/ National Guard	Other Armed Forces	War College Total
Very satisfied		14.3%	13.2%	11.9%	13.8%
2		17.5	21.0	26.2	19.3
3		16.9	7.9	11.9	14.9
4		19.6	23.7	23.8	20.8
5		15.9	18.4	7.1	14.9
6		11.6	15.8	14.3	12.6
Very unsatisfied		4.2	0.0	4.8	3.7
		100.0%	100.0%	100.0%	100.0%
Mean Score		3.6	3.6	3.5	3.6
	n=	189	38	42	269

Compounding the stress associated with elder care is the financial and parenting stress associated with teenagers. The parent-adolescent child conflict over appropriate behavior as a child launches on his or her own life course pathways has been the subject of volumes of advice columns, books, and seminars. Almost half of the Army War College officers have teenagers at home (see Table 16.11). One fourth of these families also have one or more young adults (ages nineteen to twenty-three) as dependents. This is a considerable stress on the family unit as children seek their independence, go to college, or marry. Thus at the most critical, high-stress point in a military officer's career, the officer must also deal with interlocking family life course issues.

TABLE 16.11. Percentage of Officers in Army War College Classes of 1997 and 1998 Who Have Dependent Children Ages 13-18 and Ages 19-23

	Regular Army	Reserves/ National Guard	Other Armed Forces	War College Total
Ages 13-18				
One	28.4%	45.6%	24.3%	27.7%
Two or More	17.1	21.4	21.4	18.8
Ages 19-23				
One	9.4%	10.7%	5.7%	8.9%
Two or More	4.5	16.1	5.7	6.4
n=	310	56	70	436

The Impact of Transitions Is Largely Contingent on Timing in the Life Course

The developmental impact of voluntary and involuntary transitions in a person's trajectory is largely contingent on when that transition occurs, the social pathway the person is following, the salience of the role domain in which the transition takes place, and the degree to which the transition was anticipated. In their analysis of World War II veterans, Elder, Pavalko, and Hastings (1991) found that men who were older at mobilization experienced a greater risk of marital instability, family strain after the war, and substantial lifetime earnings losses (also see Elder and Bailey, 1988).

If a life course transition or contingency can be anticipated, people prepare to cope with the event and experience less stress or cope with the stress more adequately when the event does occur. For example, some literature suggests that adjustment to the death of a loved one is more difficult if it is sudden and unexpected (the death of a child in a traffic accident) in contrast with the death of an elderly parent who had been very ill for a long period of time and whose death was anticipated (Lund, Caserta, and Dimond, 1993).

SUMMARY: A FAMILY DIMENSION OF WELLNESS

A variety of components of the APFRI model are unique within the U.S. Army, and this uniqueness is largely due to the influence of behavioral and social scientists and social workers who have designed a program that broadens the concept of wellness. For example, the wellness model at APFRI includes family-related concerns or tasks. Utilizing life event survey data and data from follow-up surveys, it is possible to reliably predict high-probability life events (e.g., elder care, retirement) that are likely to occur within the next five years and to identify the coping strategies officers have used to successfully deal with those events. Once these common events and coping strategies are identified, programs can be designed to prepare other soldiers and their families for these future likely events (e.g., retirement), or, in some cases, to prevent the event from occurring (e.g., heart attack, stroke). For example, there is a growing body of evidence that links religious involvement and spirituality with positive health outcomes (see Matthews, Larson, and Barry, 1993; Matthews and Larson, 1995; Levin, 1994, 1996). By taking social and family events into account, the overall health promotion program becomes developmentally sensitive to the real experiences of military families across the life span. The program is dynamically self-monitoring in that evaluation data feeds program development. At the same time, the program utilizes state-of-the-art assessments and interventions to prepare military members and their families for the next five years. Programs are constantly being developed to help and to prepare for specific developmental tasks often associated with a particular age and life span period.

In summary, some life events are predictable for certain age groups (e.g., death of a parent, college attendance of children). Military families must cope with numerous high-stress events and transitions that are atypical for civilian counterparts (e.g., deployments, foreign assignments, command, extended work hours, dangerous assignments, frequent family locations, midlife retirement). The integration of phase of life or cohort-specific concerns with spiritual, familial, and physical health evaluations provides an effective approach to affect and understand overall body-mind-soul states of preparedness, readiness and fitness. Sociologists, psychologists, and social workers will play an increasing role in health prevention programs as these programs become more sensitive to the developmental tasks faced by soldiers and their families at different stages of the life course.

REFERENCES

Bell, D.B. (1991). The impact of Operation Desert Shield/Storm on Army families: A summary of findings to date. Paper presented at the Fifty-Third Annual Conference of the National Council on Family Relations, Denver, CO.

Call, V.R.A. and Teachman, J.D. (1991). Military service and disruption of the family life course. *Military Psychology* 3(4): 233-251.

Coolbaugh, K. and Rosenthal, A. (1992). *Family Separations in the Army.* Alexandria, VA: U.S. Army Research Institute for the Behavioral and Social Sciences.

Elder, G.H. Jr. (1977). Family history and the life course. *Journal of Family History* 2(6): 279-304.

Elder, G.H. Jr. (1997). The life course and human development. In R. M. Lerner (Ed.), *Handbook of Child Psychology. Volume 1: Theoretical Models of Human Development* (pp. 1194-1234). New York: Wiley.

Elder, G.H. and Bailey, S.L. (1988). The timing of military service in men's lives. In D.M. Klein and J. Aldous (Eds.), *Social Stress and Family Development* (pp. 157-174). New York: Guilford Press.

Elder, G. H. Jr., George, L.K., and Shanahan, M.J. (1996). Psychological stress over the life course. In H.B. Kaplan (Ed.), *Psychological Stress: Perspectives on Structure, Theory, Life-Course, and Methods* (pp. 247-292). New York: Academic Press.

Elder, G.H. Jr., Gimbel, C., and Ivie, R. (1991). Turning points in life: The case of military service and war. *Military Psychology* 3(4): 215-231.

Elder, G.H. Jr., Pavalko, E.K., and Hastings T.J. (1991). Talent, history and the fulfillment of promise. *Psychiatry* 54(3): 251-267.

Etheridge, R. (1989). *Family Factors Affecting Retention: A Review of the Literature.* Research Report 1511. Alexandria, VA: U.S. Army Research Institute for the Behavioral and Social Sciences.

Evans, W. and Rosenberg, I.H. (1991). *Biomarkers: The 10 Keys to Prolonging Vitality.* New York: Simon and Shuster.

Featherman, D.L. and Carter, T.M. (1976). Discontinuities in schooling and the socioeconomic life cycle. In W.H. Sewell, R.M. Hauser, and D.M. Featherman (Eds.), *Schooling and Achievement in American Society* (pp. 133-160). New York: Academic.

Fligstein, N. (1976). The G.I. Bill: Its effects on the educational and occupational attainments of U.S. males, 1940-1973. Center for Demography and Ecology Working Paper 76-9. Madison, WI: University of Wisconsin.

Gade, P. (1991). Military service and the life course perspective: A turning point for military personnel research. *Military Psychology* 3(4): 187-200.

Glaser, B.G. and Strauss, A.L. (1971). *Status Passage.* Chicago: Aldine.

Halle, J.S. (1997, April 23). Request for protocol modification: Risk factor modification and physiological responses in a group of senior Army officers following an educational and physical training program. Carlisle Barracks, PA: U.S. Army War College, Log Number A-4072.

Harig, P., Halle, J., Mosier, R., Reagan, J., and Richardson, M. (1995). *Wellness for Senior Leaders Taking Care of Yourself: A Proactive Approach.* Army Physical Fitness Research Institute, Carlisle Barracks, PA: U.S. Army War College.

Hearne, G.K., Evans, J.V., Driscoll, A.K., Moore, K.A., Sugland, B.W., and Call, V.R.A. (1996). The many faces of non-marital childbearing. Paper presented at the Annual Meetings of the Population Association of America, San Francisco.

Hogan, D.P. and Astone, N.M. (1986). The transition to adulthood. *Annual Review of Sociology* 12(2): 109-130.

Labatte, L.A., Fava, M., Oleshansky, M., Zoltick, J., Littman, A., and Harig, P. (1995). Physical fitness and perceived stress relationships with coronary artery disease risk factors. *Psychometrics* 36(4): 555-560.

Lawrence, B.S. (1984). Age grading: The implicit organizational timetable. *Journal of Occupational Behavior* 5(1): 23-35.

Levin, J.S. (1994). Religion and health: Is there an association, is it valid, and is it causal? *Social Science and Medicine* 38(11): 1475-1482.

Levin, J.S. (1996). How prayer heals: A theoretical model. *Alternative Therapeutic Health Medicine* 2(1): 66-73.

Lund, D.A., Caserta, M.S., and Dimond, M. (1993). The course of spousal bereavement in later life. In M. Stroebe, W. Stroebe, and R. Hanson (Eds.), *Handbook of Bereavement* (pp. 240-254). New York: Cambridge University Press.

Magnum, S. and Ball, D. (1987). Military skill training: Some evidence for transferability. *Armed Forces and Society* 5(2): 219-242.

Magnum, S. and Ball, D. (1989). The transferability of military-provided occupational training in the post-draft era. *Industrial and Labor Relations Review* 42, 230-245.

Matthews, D.A. and Larson, D.B. (1995). *The Faith Factor: An Annotated Bibliography of Clinical Research on Spiritual Subjects,* Volume III. Rockville, MD: National Institute for Healthcare Research.

Matthews, D.A., Larson, D.B., and Barry, C. (1993). *The Faith Factor: An Annotated Bibliography of Clinical Research on Spiritual Subjects,* Volume II. Rockville, MD: National Institute for Healthcare Research.

Mayer, K.U. (1986). Structural constraints on the life course. *Human Development* 29: 163-170.

Mitchell, G. and Barko, W.F. (in press). Health risk and physical fitness in senior Army leaders. Unpublished paper under review.

Neugarten, B.L. and Datan, N. (1973). Sociological perspectives on the life course. In P.B. Baltes and K.W. Schaie (Eds.), *Life-Span Developmental Psychology: Personality and Socialization.* New York: Academic Press.

Neugarten, B.L., Moore, J.W., and Lowe, J.C. (1965). Age norms, age constraints, and adult socialization. *American Journal of Sociology* 70(4): 710-717.

O'Rand, A.M. (1990). Stratification and the life course. In R.H. Binstock and L.K. George (Eds.), *Handbook on Aging and the Social Sciences,* Third Edition (pp. 130-148). New York: Academic Press.

Parker, M.W., Achenbaum, W.A., Fuller, G.F., and Fay, W.P. (1995). Aging successfully: The example of Robert E. Lee. *Parameters,* Winter, 1994-1995: 99-113.

Parker, M.W., Harrig, P., and Martin, S. (1996). Eldercare: An issue that's "come of age" for military families. *Military Family Research Digest* 2(3): 9-11.

Parker, M.W., Harrig, P., and Martin, S. (1997). Eldercare: The demographic imperative. Paper presented at the 1997 Tri-Service Medical Conference, Tampa, Florida.

Rowe, J.W. and Kahn, R.L. (1987). Human aging: Usual and successful. *Science* 237(1): 143-149.

Rowe, J.W. and Kahn, R.L. (1997). Successful aging. *The Gerontologist* 37(4): 433-440.

Rowe, J.W. and Kahn, R.L. (1998). *Successful Aging.* New York: Pantheon Books.

Segal, M.W. and Harris, J.J. (1993). *What We Know About Army Families* (Special Report 21). Alexandria, VA: U.S. Army Research Institute for the Behavioral and Social Sciences.

Seigman, A., Franco, E., and Barko, W. (1998). Lipid concentrations and glucose levels: Relationships with anger expression and physical fitness. Paper presented at the International Congress of Behavioral Medicine: Copenhagen.

Sweet, J.A. and Bumpass, L.L. (1987). *American Families and Households.* New York: Russell Sage Foundation.

Sweet, J.A., Bumpass, L.L., and Call, V.R.A. (1987). The Design and Content of the National Survey of Families and Households. Working Paper. Center for Demography and Ecology, University of Wisconsin.

Teachman, J.D. and Call, V.R.A. (1996). The Effect of Military Service on Educational, Occupational, and Income Attainments. *Social Science Research* 25(1): 1-31.

U.S. Army War College (1996). *Strategic guidance for the United States Army War College.* Carlisle, PA: U.S. Army War College.

Wright, D.A., Knapik, J.J., Bielanda, C.C., and Zoltick, J.M. (1994). Physical fitness and cardiovascular disease risk factors in senior military leaders. *Military Medicine* 159(1): 60-63.

Chapter 17

Working with Military Families During Deployments

David J. Westhuis

THE IMPACT OF MILITARY DEPLOYMENTS ON FAMILIES

The U.S. military has an extensive history of deployments in peacetime, wartime, and for training missions. These deployments have included wartime operations such as World War II, the Korean War, the Persian Gulf War, and the Grenada mission. Various units have also been deployed for extended periods for peacekeeping missions such as in Bosnia, Somalia, Kuwait, Haiti, and other areas of the world. Individual members of active duty units and U.S. Reserve units have also been deployed for various reasons such as the Vietnam War. Past researchers such as Hill (1949), McCubbin et al. (1975), Segal, Kammeyer, and Vuozzo (1987), Rosen et al. (1995), and others have studied the impact of these deployments on families and soldiers. These studies have found that families and soldiers varied in their adjustment to the deployments and later family reunifications subsequent to the deployments. The studies have also suggested various treatment and prevention strategies that social workers and other providers can utilize to assist families in these adjustments. This chapter will summarize the research done on family members and their reactions to deployments and make recommendations for various strategies and interventions that active duty and civilian social workers can then use to assist the families and soldiers.

Family reintegration following prolonged separation was first addressed by Hill (1949) following World War II. He focused primarily on the role of family background variables, family members' adjustment during the separation, and family dynamics at reunion. Medway et al. (1995) conducted two studies to examine the impact of Desert Storm separation disruption on spouses' personal distress. They found that separation was correlated with emotional distress for spouses and that maternal distress was highly related to children's behavior during the deployment. Pearlman (1970), Bey and Lange (1974), and Glisson, Melton, and Roggow (1984) also found that spouses experienced distress and depression associated with military separation. Pearlman (1970) attributed a portion of the depression to masochistic attitudes in the marital relationship and the belief that being a good wife meant never disagreeing with one's spouse. Bey and Lange (1974) found that wives were apprehensive about how they and their husbands would deal with changes that had occurred during a separation. The researcher found that irritation and disappointment often followed the return of the spouse, and flawed communications made it difficult for couples to share their individual experiences and thus reduced intimacy. Conflict areas for couples included discipline of children and the wife's unwillingness to relinquish the independent role she had assumed during the separation.

McCubbin et al. (1975) studied the impact of separation on families of Vietnam POWs. They found that the best predictors of reintegration among families of returned POWs were length of marriage before casualty, the wife's retrospective assessment of the quality of the marriage before her husband was deployed to Vietnam and became a POW, and her emotional dysfunction during the separation period (Rosen et al., 1995).

Studies of involuntary separation following routine military training exercises or planned peacetime deployments suggest that certain factors which may be associated with marital adaptation (Rosen et al., 1995). Patterson and McCubbin (1984) found the following four factors reduced the distress associated with long-term separation for wives of Navy aviators. Aviator wives who accepted the military lifestyle, who were optimistic, self-reliant, and had high self-esteem experienced less distress during a long-term separation. Segal, Kammeyer, and Vuozzo (1987) studied the adjustment of Army wives following a six-month deployment during peacetime. She found that the more wives changed during the separation, the more adjustment was needed after the return, and that younger wives were prone to change the most.

Various news reports following the return of soldiers from the Persian Gulf War indicated a high rate of ruined marriages and soaring divorce rates following the war. Teitelbaum (1992) found that divorce filings actually declined during the war, then rose steeply in the first two months after the soldiers returned, and finally fell back to predeployment levels after three months. He reported that the total number of divorces granted over the year in which the war occurred was not significantly different from previous years, which suggests no effect due to the war.

Raschman, Patterson, and Schofield (1990) reported that an Air Force pilot's extended separation from his or her family was the second most frequent cause of marital conflict (following poor communications). Bey and Lange (1974) suggest that marriages already in jeopardy prior to a separation were further weakened by the stress of this separation in some but not all situations.

Rosen et al.'s (1995) study on marital adjustment of Army spouses following the Persian Gulf War found that the following variables had a negative impact: problems in the couple's authority structure regarding children, feelings by the soldier of being left out of the family after reunion, mistrust of the spouse, and resentment by the spouses. It was suggested that the presence of these factors in the marriage following a reunion contributed to couples having difficulty in completing the reunification process. Rosen, Westhuis, and Teitelbaum (1994) also found that stressful events both during and after the Gulf War, along with consideration of divorce prior to the war had a negative effect on marital adjustment. They also found that increased emotional closeness and the soldier's satisfaction with the wife's management of the household finances during the war were positively associated with marital adjustment. It was also found that the patterns of increased dependency of the wife and withdrawal of the soldier were associated with negative marital adjustment. This was the same pattern described by Bey (1972), which was labeled "returning veteran's syndrome." Bey found that returning veterans exhibited depressive symptoms and irritation with any demands placed on them, while their wives felt let down by their husband's withdrawal.

Kelly (1994) studied the effects of peacetime versus wartime deployments on wives. She found that mothers of younger children reported lower self-esteem than did mothers of older children. Maternal depressive behavior significantly decreased over time during a routine separation. But she also found that maternal and child behavior differed for wartime and peacetime deployments. Women whose husbands had been deployed during the Persian Gulf War reported more dysphoria than did a matched sample of women from a peacetime deployment.

Other research during the Persian Gulf War also found that during the deployment phase, families experienced various stressors but that there were also stress mediators (Rosen, Teitelbaum, and Westhuis, 1993b). It was found that emotional stressors of the deployment were the greatest predictors of a wife's developing physical and emotional symptoms. These emotional stressors included feeling loss of support from the deployed soldier, concern for the safety of the soldier in the wartime environment, loneliness, and having to be a single parent. Deployment-related instrumental stressors such as having to manage the household budget alone, being confused about military entitlements, needing to get home and car repairs done, increased child care expenses, and problems exercising a power of attorney also had an impact on emotional and physical well-being. Stress prior to the deployment, lack of comfort in dealing with military agencies, and a poor postalert unit climate was associated with increased deployment stress. Other predictors of deployment stress included age of a wife, lack of support from the extended family, and the expectation that spouses deserved special treatment by the military. Lower levels of stress were reported if a spouse had prior experience with the military and deployments, her husband had a higher rank, and the unit's family support group and rear detachments were perceived as supportive.

In another study by Rosen, Westhuis, and Teitelbaum (1994) on patterns of adaptation among Army wives during Operation Desert Shield and Desert Storm it was also found that spouses who had the most difficulty coping tended to be younger and their soldiers tended to have lower ranks. But it was also found that this was not consistent among all younger and lower-ranking spouses. For example, Hispanic spouses who were younger tended to have more problems than non-Hispanic spouses. This could have been due to the primary role of the male in the Hispanic family and the stress the wife encounters when that male leaves the home. It was also found that younger spouses who moved in with or near extended family had lower levels of stress due to the increased emotional and physical support they received. But if these spouses had inappropriately high expectations of what the military would do to solve their problems, their levels of stress again increased. This study found one group of older spouses who were also experiencing high levels of reported stress. They tended to be employed full-time, were married to senior enlisted soldiers, and had inappropriately high expectations of what the military would do to solve their problems. The combined stress of having a full-time job, becoming a single parent, and not having their expectations met by military service agencies probably was instrumental in increasing their stress.

Rosen, Teitelbaum, and Westhuis (1994) also studied the children of deployed Gulf War soldiers and found they also reacted to the deployment and separation from the deployed parent. This study found that 55 to 64 percent of the girls between the ages of three and twelve experienced sadness and tearfulness. It was also found that sadness was a fairly widespread problem, 42 to 49 percent, for the boys. Discipline problems both at home and at school were low for girls, but home discipline was a frequent problem for boys. Demanding more attention was also a problem for both boys and girls. There were increased symptoms among children if other family members were experiencing an increased number of symptoms. This finding is similar to previous studies (Jensen, Traylor, and Xenakis, 1988; Kashani, Beck, and Burk, 1990) which found a relationship between parental psychopathology and the number of psychiatric symptoms reported for children. This could possibly occur because parents with psychiatric symptoms are also more intolerant of certain behaviors and report them as symptoms (Weissman et al., 1984), or because of shared environmental stressors or genetic factors (Wender, Kety, and Rosenthal, 1986). While the increased frequency of symptoms for children of Desert Storm tended to be common, there was little evidence that these symptoms were perceived as serious problems by the parent living with the children. Approximately 5 to 15 percent of the children were thought to need counseling, and 2 to 12 percent received counseling (Rosen, Teitelbaum, and Westhuis, 1994). The primary predictors of receiving counseling were being in counseling prior to the deployment and having problems in school performance before the war. This suggested that children who developed serious problems during Desert Storm had already displayed this tendency previously.

In a study by Jensen, Martin, and Watanabe (1996) on children's response to parental separation during Operation Desert Storm, it was found that children of deployed parents experienced elevated self-reported symptom levels of depression, as did their parents. However, it was also determined that the deployment rarely caused pathological levels of symptoms. They also found that boy and younger children appeared to be especially vulnerable to deployment effects.

The results of the Persian Gulf research by Rosen, Teitelbaum, and Westhuis (1994) also found that different problems were present in the family depending on the phase of the deployment. This is supported by a study by Blount and colleagues (1992), which also found that a military deployment entails stages of adaptation for families and each phase generates its own emotions and problems. The stages can include a predeployment phase, an adjustment phase directly after the actual deployment, a phase of stable functioning during the middle of the deployment, a preparation phase for the return of the deployed soldier, and then a family reunification phase after the soldier actually returns. During the predeployment phase families were dealing with separation issues, the stress of the soldier preparing for the deployment, and possible changes in family finances and daily schedules. The separation problems were complicated when the soldiers were given a specific deployment date which was later changed. In some situations families experienced the psychological stress of two or more separations before the soldiers actually deployed.

Another major issue during this phase was arranging for powers of attorney so that the remaining spouse could make financial decisions in the absence of the soldier. Often this had to be done just prior to the deployment, and couples did not have adequate time to discuss what issues needed to be considered in creating this power of attorney. Frequently the wife was not involved in the creation of the document.

Single-parent families in which the lone parent was deployed had other major issues during this predeployment phase such as finding a care provider for the children. The research indicated that many single parents had not developed viable family care plans that could meet long-term child care needs. Seventy-year-old grandparents were able to care for the children for one or two months, but when that was extended to six months or a year some of these family care plans became nonfunctional and other arrangements had to be made.

For the single-parent family, arrangements also had to be made to deliver the children to the deployment care provider. This had to occur while soldiers were preparing for a rapid deployment, which often required them to work extended hours to prepare military equipment, attend deployment briefings, make changes in their financial records, and receive the required medical exams and shots.

Once the soldiers actually deployed, the spouses and family members had to adjust to the soldier's absence. This adjustment included meeting household responsibilities alone, adjusting to the loss of companionship and another adult to talk to about decisions, adjusting to the multiple demands of the single-parent role, and taking over the instrumental roles in maintaining the car, the house, the yard, etc. It was during this postdeployment adjustment phase that many of the families had their most significant and frequent problems. Children and spouses were dealing with the loss of a significant adult and had the normal grief associated with this. Families had to adjust to unfamiliar roles and financial problems were at their most difficult point during the Desert Storm experience. Many families were unaware of what resources were available to cope with these difficulties. This included resources from the military, civilian sources, extended families, and friends.

Problems in communicating with the deployed soldier also made decision making more difficult. If a spouse had a problem she needed to discuss with her husband, it frequently took a week for her letter to get to the soldier and then a week for the soldier's response to be mailed back to her. Thus, if a spouse wanted to know what to do with a car that was nonfunctional, but yet her only form of transportation, it would take two weeks for her to receive her husband's input. The communication problems were more complicated for Reserve families because mailing addresses and units of assignment while in the Gulf were frequently changed.

The adjustment phase was also complicated if soldiers did not properly prepare their families with power of attorney. Occasionally soldiers provided no power of attorney or provided a restrictive one. They did not give the spouse the legal authority to make decisions on how to use money, sell a nonfunctioning car, or sign for and terminate apartment and home leases. Thus, during the initial postdeployment phase some wives were left with inadequate money and problems that they could not resolve, because they could not independently and quickly make decisions to deal with these issues.

Another complicating factor in this initial adjustment phase occurred when families and soldiers did not know how long the soldier would be deployed. Many families thought the Desert Shield deployment would last for one or two months and thus went into a "holding pattern," assuming the spouse would return soon and take care of certain duties. This "holding pattern" lengthened the adjustment phase because the family did not make the more significant family structural changes needed for a long-term deployment.

Once the families accepted that the soldier would be deployed for the entire Persian Gulf War they were able to complete the initial adjustment phase and progress to a phase of stable operation without the soldier. Spouses became more comfortable with making decisions about what to do with money and how to manage the children, and developed daily and weekly routines that provided the stability needed. Appropriate powers of attorney were in place. Spouses had developed support groups through unit family support groups, friends, churches, and extended families. Families knew what resources were available to them through the military and other agencies and generally knew how to access them appropriately. A significant number of the younger families who did not own homes, have children in school, and have emotional and logistical support in the military post area returned to their extended families. There were still significant concerns for the health and safety of the deployed soldier, but telephone networks had been set up that allowed the soldiers and family members to speak to one another when necessary. Many families ran up significant telephone bills that would later pose a problem. The times of greatest stress during this period occurred just prior to and during the actual war due to fears of the soldier being killed or injured.

After the war, the families quickly anticipated the return of the soldier. They were very relieved that few soldiers had been injured or killed. But there were concerns that the soldiers might have changed due to the deployment experience. There was also awareness that the spouses had changed and that they could function more independently if needed. Family members were concerned about how they would react to each other when they once again became a family unit. Other couples were cognizant that they did not want their relationship to return to its predeployment status. These couples were confused about how to address these issues and then move the relationship and family to a new structure comfortable for all involved. Briefings were provided to soldiers and spouses on what to expect and how to deal with the reunion. This helped to answer some questions and alleviate anxiety.

Once the soldiers returned home, the families went through a "honeymoon period" of excitement and happiness due to being together again. After several weeks the couples and family members began the arduous task of readapting the structure of the family to accommodate the returning soldier. For most family members this was not problematic because they wanted to return to previous structures. In other families where the spouse found she enjoyed her new independence, more challenging structural changes needed to be made. Teitelbaum (1992) found that some couples had unresolved marital issues that had originated before the Persian Gulf War. This group and the group with the desire for a new family structure were the ones most likely to need clinical intervention. Some of these marriages ended in divorce. Within several months of the return of the soldier most families had completed the reunification phase and the families were back to what became their models of normal family structure and operation.

A problem that was prevalent in all phases of the Persian Gulf War was the lack of accurate information. During the predeployment phase families were not aware when their soldiers would be deployed, and there was little information on what agencies would do, due to the agencies changing to new missions. There was also limited and sometimes inaccurate information on how long the soldiers were to be deployed. Once the deployment occurred, families had limited information on the well-being of the soldiers and where the soldiers were in the Gulf due to security issues. They continued to be confused about what agencies could do for them and what they needed to do for themselves. Many families were constant watchers of CNN, in hope of finding the most current information on their soldiers. (After several weeks of constantly watching CNN, to the exclusion of doing other household tasks, some wives made a decision to turn off the TV because it was having a negative effect on their families' lives.) When information was released, in certain situations it was late and sometimes inaccurate. This contributed to family distrust of the military.

When families did not get information, rumors sometimes started. These problems often had a significant negative emotional effect on family members.

All the previously mentioned research and the summary information on the families' reactions to the Persian Gulf War suggest that military and civilian social workers can play a critical role in assisting families and soldiers who are being deployed, are currently deployed, and who have returned from a deployment. The findings indicate that social workers must use their general, clinical, and community organizational skills to meet the needs of these families. The social worker is uniquely trained to meet this mission due to social work's focus and training on the ecological and systems perspective (Hepworth and Larson, 1993). The social worker must step outside of his or her normal "in the office clinical role," be ready to do prevention, be knowledgeable on military and community resources, link families with these resources, be an advocate for families and soldiers, do consultation and education with unit leaders, be able to obtain and provide accurate information to those who need it, and when necessary do clinical interventions. All assessments must have an ecological emphasis to ensure information is gathered not only on the individual but also the environment within which that individual lives.

The prevention work should be initiated prior to any deployment. It should start with command consultation. Commanders must be aware of what they can do to ensure that families and soldiers are prepared for the deployment separation. Commanders can sponsor briefings for families that highlight deployment procedures. Information can be provided on what families need to do to prepare for a deployment, such as getting power of attorney and having single parents create family care plans that certify children can be properly cared for over an extended period of time. Agencies who will provide resources to the families can participate in the briefings and give information on their service and how these services can be obtained. Providing written lists of service agencies with the services they provide and their telephone numbers and addresses would also be helpful for families. Making families aware of unit family support groups and what these groups can and cannot do for their members is very important. Commanders should inform families that the role of the rear detachment will remain at the military post during the deployment and what this unit can do for the families. It is important that units and agencies make the families aware of what services they can realistically expect to be provided and what the families will need to do to take care of them-selves. This information should be provided when there is no indication of a deployment and then again at the time of the deployment. This will help families to develop appropriate expectations as to what help they can expect from the military and various agencies and groups.

Once a deployment is imminent, it is important to determine if it will be a lengthy deployment of six or more months or a shorter deployment. Shorter deployments require fewer significant changes in the family structure and less need for military and nonmilitary services. It could be inappropriate to make changes in family decision making on finances and parenting styles if the soldier is deployed for only a month. It is also less likely the family will need assistance from agencies and rear detachment staff with basic transportation and child care needs. But these short-term deployments can be used to acquaint the family with the role of the rear detachment, the unit family support group, and the use of a limited power of attorney. Families can learn how the rear detachment can assist them in getting information on their soldier, assist them in solving financial problems, and also link them to community and military resources. The military social worker can recommend to the commanders that the preventive efforts listed above be part of the normal unit operations for short-term and long-term deployments.

During a long-term deployment a social worker can provide help to families prior to the deployment, early in the deployment after the soldiers have left, prior to the soldiers returning home, and also during the reunification phase. During predeployment and immediately after the soldier has been deployed, social workers must be ready to link families to resources. It is thus imperative that the social worker knows what agencies are available and what the functions of these military and nonmilitary agencies are. Providing supportive counseling when a family's military paycheck has not been deposited in their checking account will have limited impact. The social worker must be able to link the family to the rear detachment and military finance agencies who are responsible for this issue. If a family is in need of food or a change in housing the social worker must again use the general skills they have been taught to link the family with the appropriate agencies.

The early deployment phase is an appropriate time for social workers to offer lectures and discussion groups to family support groups and other interested organizations on normal reactions to the temporary loss of a spouse, how to deal with stress, appropriate problem-solving strategies, and how to adapt family structures to make them functional while the soldier is deployed. This would be an appropriate time to assist family support groups and others in setting up mentoring programs between the more seasoned and experienced spouse who has past experience with deployments and the younger spouses who have had limited experience.

It is also an appropriate time to offer discussion groups and support sessions with children whose parents have been deployed. These could be single sessions or more if necessary. They could be conducted in schools, family support groups, or other locations and should assist the children in discussing and resolving their fears about a parent being in a hostile environment. Discussions could also occur on what it is like to have a parent gone for an extended time and what they can do to cope with this loss. These interventions with families and children should assume that the families have the basic skills to cope with the deployment and that they only need initial support and ideas on how to adjust to the separation. The families should be considered healthy families going through a stressful adjustment.

For a limited number of families, the social workers should be cognizant that they are at high risk for problems and for the need of a possible clinical intervention. As noted in the previous research, these are the families who had problems prior to the deployment, families with multiple stressors such as a single parent with a career, or families of children who have already had problem. These families may require a more individualized approach and therefore be appropriate candidates for more traditional clinical interventions such as individual therapy, medication, play therapy, and family therapy.

During the final stage of the deployment, often noted as the preunification phase, social workers, chaplains, and others can again provide informational lectures and structured support groups whose focus should be "what families and soldiers can do to make the transition to a family unit again." These services should be provided to the soldiers in the deployment areas and to the families at the home base. Wives are frequently concerned about and want information on how a war or hostile environment will affect the soldier. A soldier may be concerned about the new independence the spouse has developed and how he or she should cope with it. The soldier may be concerned that he or she is no longer needed since the spouse has been able to function without him or her. Soldiers and family members will need recommendations on how soon the returning soldier should assume his or her predeployment family roles. Couples should be encouraged not to make any major changes when they initially reunite, but to take time to become reacquainted again and if possible take time for a vacation. Couples should talk about what has happened to each other during the deployment and what the high points and the low points have been for each. These discussions can help each member understand the challenges the other has faced. It should not be a time to "compare notes" and determine who has had the most difficulty, but a time to understand the feelings and struggles the other member has faced. Couples should be encouraged to share their thoughts and feelings with one another. It should be recommended that the returning soldier affirms what his or her spouse has done to maintain the family during the absence and not to find major faults with the spouse's efforts. It should also be recommended that after a comfortable period of togetherness that couples discuss what roles the returning soldier should assume now that the family is united again. These discussions and support groups need to have an informational focus but should also provide an opportunity for soldiers and family members to address specific questions on their topics of concern. Soldiers and spouses who have had previous experience with deployments and reunification could discuss how they have coped with this in the past, and they could be mentors for the nonexperienced families.

After the soldiers have returned, discussion groups could again be provided to families where the husband and wife can both attend. These groups could provide an opportunity for couples to discuss how their families are readjusting, what the typical patterns have been, how the children have reacted to the returning parent, and what problems they have experienced. The focus of these groups should be on what families have done to adjust positively as well as negatively and that these adjustments have been due to normal challenges associated with an extended separation and not due to pathology and weakness. During this time couples may readjust some of the roles in their relationship based on what they learned about themselves during the deployment.

Individual, family, and marital therapy should be offered to the small group of families who are having significant problems in becoming a functional unit. The sessions should determine if the problems are related to predeployment issues, changes that have occurred during the deployment, or changes following reunification. The focus should be on what procedures the family/couple has tried to solve problems, how effective their communications and problem-solving skills are, and what additional skills the couple could be trained in to solve their current dilemmas.

Once the families have completed the reunification process, time should be taken by social workers and the agencies they have worked with to review the deployment. This activity should be time-sequenced, from the point of alert and deployment to the time when the families are reunited. Discussions could occur on what happened positively and negatively with reference to the agencies' roles in the deployment. It is important to include representatives of the deployed families who were served by these agencies in this process so that they can give their reactions to the assistance that was provided. It is a time for reviewing agency policies and procedures, and if necessary, modifying them to ensure they will meet the needs of future deployments. Finally, information on lessons learned could be generated and shared with other military units and with higher commands so that other units may profit.

As can be seen from this discussion, the deployment of soldiers for peacetime and wartime missions can have a significant impact on military families. This provides an opportunity for the military and civilian social workers who serve these families and soldiers to use multiple skills to assist those involved in the deployments. The social worker must step outside of his or her traditional "in the office" clinical role and become involved in prevention, advocacy, networking, and information provider. These intervention strategies will have to vary based on the deployment phase, the length of the deployment, and the particular needs of the families. It is a unique opportunity for a social worker to employ the varied skills of the generalist, clinician, and community organizer.

REFERENCES

Bey, D. (1972). The returning veteran syndrome. *Medical Insight, 4*(1), 42-49.

Bey, D. and Lange, J. (1974). Waiting wives: Women under stress. *American Journal of Psychiatry, 131*(3), 283-286.

Blount, B., Curry, A., Lubin, G., and Gerald, I. (1992). Family separations in the military. *Military Medicine, 157*(2), 76-80.

Glisson, C., Melton, S., and Roggow, L. (1980). The effects of separation on marital satisfaction, depression, and self-esteem. *Journal of Social Science, 4*(1), 61-76.

Hepworth, D. and Larson, J. (1993). *Direct social work practice*. Pacific Grove, CA: Brooks/Cole.

Hill, R. (1949). *Families under stress: Adjustment to the crises of war separation and reunion.* New York: Harper and Brothers.

Jensen, P., Martin, D., and Watanbe, H. (1996). Children's response to parental separation during Operation Desert Storm. *Journal of the American Academy of Child and Adolescent Psychiatry, 35*(4), 433-441.

Jensen, P., Traylor, J., and Xenakis, S. (1988). Child psychopathology rating scales and interrater agreement: Parents' gender and psychiatric symptoms. *Journal of American Academy of Child and Adolescent Psychiatry, 27*(4), 451-461.

Kashani, J., Beck N., and Burk, J. (1990). Predictors of psychopathology in children of patients with major affective disorders. *Canadian Journal of Psychiatry, 32*(2), 287-290.

Kelly, M. (1994). The effects of military induced separation on family factors and child behavior. *American Journal of Orthopsychiatry, 64*(2), 103-111.

McCubbin, H., Dahl, B., Lester, G., and Ross, B. (1975). The returned prisoner of war: Factors in family reintegration. *Journal of Marriage and the Family, 37*(4), 471-478.

Medway, F., David, K., Cafferty, T., and Chappell, K. (1995). Family disruption and adult attachment correlates of spouse and child reaction to separation and reunion due to Operation Desert Storm. *Journal of Social and Clinical Psychology, 14*(1), 97-118.

Patterson, J. and McCubbin, H. (1984). Gender roles and coping. *Journal of Marriage and the Family, 46*(1), 95-104.

Pearlman, C. (1970). Separation reactions of married women. *American Journal of Psychiatry, 126*(9), 946-950.

Raschmann, J., Patterson, J., and Schofield, G. (1990). A retrospective study of marital discord in pilots: The USAFSAM experience. *Aviation, Space, and Environmental Medicine, 61*(12), 537-546.

Rosen, L., Durand, D., Westhuis, D., and Teitelbaum, J. (1995). Marital adjustment of Army spouses one year after Operation Desert Storm. *Journal of Applied Social Psychology, 25*(7), 677-692.

Rosen, L., Teitelbaum, J., and Westhuis, D. (1993a). Children's reactions to the Desert Storm deployment: Initial findings from a survey of Army families. *Military Medicine, 158*(19), 465-469.

Rosen, L., Teitelbaum, J., and Westhuis, D. (1993b). Stressors, stress mediators, and emotional well-being among spouses of soldiers deployed to the Persian Gulf during Operation Desert Shield/Storm. *Journal of Applied Social Psychology, 23*(1), 1587-1593.

Rosen, L., Westhuis, D., and Teitelbaum, J. (1994). Patterns of adaptation among Army wives during Operation Desert Shield and Desert Storm. *Military Medicine, 159*(8), 43-47.

Segal, M., Kammeyer, K., and Vuozzo, J. (1987). Work-related separation and reunion processes in families: The social construction of marriage and self-perception. Unpublished manuscript, Walter Reed Army Institute of Research, Department Military Psychiatry, Washington, DC.

Teitelbaum, J. (1992). ODS and Post-ODS divorce and child development problems. Unpublished manuscript, Walter Reed Army Institute of Research, Department Military Psychiatry, Washington, DC.

Weissman, M., Leckman, J., Merikangas, K., Gammon, G., and Prusoff, B. (1984). Depression and anxiety disorders in parents and children. *Archives of General Psychiatry, 41,* 845-852.

Wender, P., Kety, S., Rosenthal, D., Schulsinger, F., Ortman, J., and Lunde, I. (1986). Psychiatric disorders in the biological and adoptive families of adopted individuals with affective disorders. *Archives of General Psychiatry, 43,* 923-929.

Chapter 18

Understanding the Military As an Ethnic Identity

James G. Daley

The basic premise of this chapter is that individuals who embrace the military lifestyle develop over time an increasing identification with the military as a core component of who they are, much like an ethnic identity (see also Chapters 13, 14, and 15). The chapter begins by outlining the core components of what constitutes an ethnic identity. Then a general review is given of the distinctness of the military community, especially the family. Third, I advocate that being in the military leads to a military identity. Finally, I suggest areas for exploration and research including basic research on a military identity scale.

WHAT IS AN ETHNIC IDENTITY?

Ethnicity is defined as a common thread of heritage, customs, and values unique to a group of people (Casas, 1984; Queralt, 1996). Distinguished from racial characteristics that are partially based on physical characteristics of genetic origin (Helms, 1990), ethnicity captures a broad range of possible commonalities such as religion, geography, or historical events. These commonalities define and bond its members and produce an ethnic backdrop to everyday life. In fact, "ethnicity patterns our thinking, feeling, and behavior in both obvious and subtle ways, although generally we are not aware of it. It plays a major role in determining what we eat and how we work, relate, celebrate holidays and rituals, and feel about life, death and illness" (McGoldrick, Giordano, and Pearce, 1996, p. viii).

However, as potent as ethnicity can be, an individual's identification with his or her ethnicity is not automatic. In other words, one's ethnic identity stems from the continuum of acceptance of one's ethnicity (Helms, 1990). People embrace or reject their ethnicity by weighing personal identity, reference-group orientation, and ascribed identity (Helms, 1990). Personal identity refers to how one sees oneself. Reference-group orientation indicates the primary support group one turns to for clarity of decisions. Ascribed identity indicates society's value and judgment on the ethnicity. For example, a person from a Hassidic Jewish background might discard expected roles because of a view of himself as pursing a career incompatible with Hassidic principles. He might have developed a group of peers who support his rejection of Hassidic rules. Also, the larger society may encourage his career goals. This example is amply illustrated in the movie *The Jazz Singer* when the main character abandons much of his Hassidic role to pursue a commercial singing career. The main point is that ethnicity is a potent but not automatic influence in a person's life.

MILITARY AS ETHNICITY

People joining the military embrace the full power of its heritage during basic training when they experience carefully designed rituals of entry into the military "family." Whether Army, Navy, Marine, or Air Force, the expectation is that one has entered a new world with set rules and significant consequences for rejection of those rules. Even before beginning the transition, a person is impressed by the gate at the entrance to the base/post ("base" refers to Air Force and Navy and Marine facilities; "post" refers to Army facilities). Armed guards allow only "authorized" personnel onto the base/post, thus ensuring separateness regardless of location worldwide. Status is defined by pieces of cloth (sergeant's stripes) or metal (officer's rank) worn on clothing, which must have components arranged in *exact* locations. Very quickly the recruit looks more quickly for the approaching person's rank than for race or gender. Walking evolves into a special kind of marching in which words called out (e.g., "column left") immediately prompt hundreds of people to move in the same direction. Knowing the rituals of the military becomes the currency most valued, and spontaneity is replaced by discipline. Basic training is designed as a transitional period when ethnicity is infused and the basic principles of military life are begun.

So what do recuits learn? The ethnic standards are straightforward.

Image Is Crucial and Self-Control Expected

A soldier's uniform represents not just himself or herself, but the whole heritage of generations of sacrifice and excellence. Each piece on the uniform has a tradition, from the way the stripes point to whether the "U.S." insignia is embedded in a circle (hint: without a circle means officer, with circle means enlisted). A uniform must be crisp, in good order, and the correct uniform must be worn for the correct setting. A hat is worn only outdoors and *always* worn when outdoors. Each "pretty ribbon" on the uniform has been earned; a lot of ribbons verifies prestige, and the ribbons are placed in a specific order (highest ranking at top, least important at bottom left corner). A nonmilitary person might consider this focus on detail obsessive. But it is no more obsessive than the Hassidic songs sung exactly the same for generations, or the African American stories passed down, or the Japanese emphasis on family honor.

Along with the image of the uniform goes the personal behavior of the soldier. A person is "on duty 24 hours a day, 7 days a week, 365 days a year." In other words, a military member is always accountable regardless of where or when he or she acts. Therefore, the importance of image embraces all aspects of life. A drunk driving incident hundreds of miles from base/post while a person is "off duty" still prompts punitive action by the military authorities. Personal financial ineptness prompts corrective action. Domestic violence leads to military authority involvement. Self-control must be maintained at all times (quite a trick for rebellious adolescents newly absorbed into this very closed society). Corrective action almost always is attempted with the expectation of success. But repeated offenses lead to expulsion from the military society. Jail time is possible for offenses deemed trivial in civilian life.

The impact on the military family is enormous as the military member is held accountable for any behavior by his or her dependents. One child of a military member captured the issue eloquently: "Life in the military is about fronts. Appearances. Masks. The stage persona. That's an important part of military life. Our parents were always obsessively concerned about how things looked. When we were growing up, every aspect of personal and private life was a measure of our fathers' professional competence" (Wertsch, 1991, p. 1). The paradox is how does the importance of image balance with the fact that the military community, like any other community, has its fair share of suicide, family violence, substance abuse, financial crises, acting-out adolescents, and other issues that are hard to fit into a shining image?

The Military Take Care of Their Own

This principle is illustrated by several examples. Nearly every base/post worldwide is designed to provide the basic components of a community: grocery stores, living quarters, department stores, theaters, hospitals (or clinics with an ability to fly patients to the nearest military hospital), schools (elementary and sometimes secondary depending on size of the base/post), post office, community swimming pool, golf course, etc. When soldiers are transferred, the military oversees the moving of household goods, can provide information on the new community, and ensures that adequate health facilities are available for the medical needs of family members. Every military branch has a chain of command with a military officer and senior enlisted person in charge of each soldier, sailor, or airman. The expectation is that the chain of command is responsible to ensure the readiness of each soldier for combat. The commander (officer) and first sergeant (enlisted) are handpicked through rigorous screening procedures and held personally accountable for any misconduct or crisis involing anyone within their command. From the lowest ranking to the highest ranking person, everyone knows who they are accountable for and to. The principle of *taking care of our own* is ingrained within the military. To contrast with the first standard, the military has this oversight expectation only for active duty personnel and will rapidly discharge a person who is "trouble." This seems to create a paradox: help is readily available but you must always be in control and demonstrate a top-notch image.

Mission Is First; Military Needs Take Priority

Whether being called at 3 a.m. to report ready to be deployed worldwide, working *long* hours on the crisis du jour, or attending a military reception, the military person is expected to comply with enthusiasm and provide the best quality work effort. Regardless of family stresses or awkwardness of task, the military person complies. Job changes, added duty responsibility, and increased complexity of demands are all taken in stride with an expectation of resilient competence. In the Navy ships deploy for six months or more, the Army sends whole divisions overseas for many months or on month-long training exercises, and the Air Force sends aircrews on missions of weeks-long rotations many times during the year. Inability to be deployed increases your risk of not being "worldwide qualified" and the possibility of being separated from the service. Devotion to duty ensures continuity in this closed society and reiterates an essential standard. Extensive medical and social services have been established to facilitate family well-being but primarily to reduce barriers to the soldier deploying successfully.

Mobility Within an Unchanging World

Upward mobility dictates geographical relocation, increased responsibility, and taking on new job positions. Every career military person strives for the next level job, usually involving increased command responsibilities. Every step up the success ladder dictates more intensive competition and higher likelihood of failure. Achieving higher rank stems from a highly competitive service folder (personnel folder listing your achievements) in a world where 98 percent of the competitors are also highly competitive. Each promotion has a lower success ratio (e.g., 99 percent get promoted to captain, 70 percent to major, 50 percent to lieutenant colonel, 10 percent to colonel), and therefore only aggressive career management gives a military person any chance of progressing. Mobility to the "right job" is the vital shield against failure. Thus nearly every military person is jockeying throughout his or her whole career to move while demonstrating excellence in the current job. Relocating every two to three years is a standard practice except in the Navy, where the ship deploys every six months but the family might stay at the same port for a sailor's whole career. Thus any base/post has a 33 percent turnover every year and people are constantly coming and going.

The end result is a nomadic lifestyle in which military families and military persons rapidly settle in, make friends whom they might be saying goodbye to within a year, and begin preparing for the next assignment. An internal clock begins ticking upon arrival at the new base/post and, at the two-year mark, the family's anxiety about "Where will we go next?" begins to escalate. In spite of the frequent relocating, the moving has a sameness to it. Moving from Michigan to Mississippi leads to the same community structure. The same rules, expectations, and acceptance stabilize the military family. But the frequent moves do have impact, as Wertsch (1991) describes. "By the time I entered college, I had attended twelve schools and lived in twenty different houses. This kind of mobility seems normal enough as we are undergoing it, but one consequence is that for us, time hardly unfurls in a smooth continuum. . . . When, as children, we were plucked out of one environment and abruptly set down in another, our operating assumption had to be that all our past investments in people outside the family were lost, and that the new people investments we were now rushing to make would in turn be lost when the next inevitable move came about" (p. 352).

Hierarchy Dictates Social Convention

Within the military, there is a constancy of rank status across services but an expectation of socialization dichotomized not by race or ethnicity but by rank. Cordial but distant social interaction occurs between officers and enlisted (see Chapter 16). Even military children awkwardly feel the schism between officer and enlisted, what Wertsch (1991) calls "upstairs/downstairs." "Classes" within the military include officers, noncommissioned officers, and enlisted. Even within classes, there are distinctions such as "the colonel's wife," "the commander," and "the first sergeant." Housing is segregated by rank. Colonels and generals, company-grade officers, field-grade officers, noncommissioned officers, and enlisted all have different housing locations on base. Fraternization is forbidden and intimate relationships between officer and enlisted (even if single, not related by supervisory role) are punishable by military law.

Historically, military spouses, especially of officers and noncommissioned officers, had unspoken expectations to serve as a social conduit for resolving social stressors for families within the organizational structure. Welcoming new families, reaching out to families of military members deployed on a mission, setting up social events, and serving as informal authorities with significant clout were (and some argue still are at times) roles filled by spouses. Feminist advocacy and financial realities (e.g., spouse's own career) have eroded the firmness of the expectation. However, some informal facilitation of social connections and clout remain.

The Medical Field As Exception to the Rule?

Medical officers, including social work officers, travel down a different path of military socialization (the exception is the Navy, which is moving toward social work officers being within the line, not medical career, track). "Line" officers are individuals who join the military and go through a six-week intensive basic training and then further advanced training in a career track (e.g., artillery, pilot, engineering) partially of their choosing. Line officers seek command positions and upward responsibility for more and more military personnel. They pride themselves on being the core disciples of the military ethnicity. Their career and identity is to be a military officer who just happens to have a specialty skill. By contrast, most medical officers (unless they go through the military academy or ROTC) are provided a two-week orientation described jokingly (and by some line officers not as a joke) as "how to not embarrass the military." Medical officers rise in rank by very different competitiveness (see Chapter 12). Their competitiveness is just as intense as the line officers' but centers on the quality of medical care. A colonel line officer would be in charge of a division (thousands of troops) while a colonel medical officer might be in charge of ten people. But the colonel medical officer has achieved the pinnacle of his or her professional standards (board certified, many years of postresidency experience, subspecialty expertise). Medical officers (contrary to the continual indoctrination efforts by military leadership) view themselves as medical professionals first and military officers second role. Therefore, conflict, sibling rivalry, and efforts to create class differences inevitably arise. The military needs the expertise of the medical officer and recognizes that they have to obtain a "ready-made product" (professionally prepared clinician) rather than grow one through military technical schools (though there is one military medical school). But the medical officers accept (and even pride themselves at times) being in the stereotypic stepchild status (part of the family but not completely accepted).

THE EMERGING MILITARY ETHNIC IDENTITY

The previous section painted the broad tapestry of the military as an ethnicity. But, as mentioned, embracing the military as an identity involves more than just being a member. Personal identity is a core component. I once knew a physician who had a two-year service commitment and began counting down his "days left" from the first day. He was an intensely committed physician but rejected any opportunity to be part of the military. By contrast (especially with an all-volunteer force), most newcomers eagerly embrace the new world of the military. Learning the language (e.g., PCS, TDY, OER, BX, commissary), ensuring the proper image, working intensely to achieve the mission, planning for the next assignment, getting to know your military neighbors, and going to the "Club" (restaurant and bar on base) are all acculturation efforts. Family members also meet other families and begin to bond. Welcoming parties for newcomers are common. In sum, the newcomers begin to feel part of a society that has opened just for them.

As the military member and family adapt to their new ethnic identity, their social circle begins to revolve around other military families. Thus, the reference groups become increasingly military linked. Obviously, nonmilitary friends continue, but by the third time the family has transferred, civilian friends seem transitory and the constancy of the military becomes the core support system. Even professional society involvement (e.g., NASW) becomes part of demonstrating military career potential rather than a central source of support. The commonality of experiences makes it easy to talk to other military rather than the "locals." A military child stops trying to explain to a local peer that he has seen Portugal, Paris, and London. He stops talking about fun vacation spots in Japan. But that same military child relates instantly to another military child who is not so intimidated or unsure. Likewise, military peers can increasingly relate to duty stations or co-workers they have in common.

The ascribed identity is defined by the larger society. Vietnam veterans and Desert Storm veterans differ in ascribed identity. Society fluctuates between anxiously building the military and chastising it as a fat cash cow that needs trimming. During my twenty-one-year career, the military has swayed from being viewed as a job, to a combat-ready career, to a way to save money for college, to a deadly force used for firepower. The ascribed identity can prompt "first termers" (people in their initial assignment) to reconsider continuing in a career, but for most "lifers" (people committed to a twenty-plus stint) the ascribed identity is society's problem. The problem only hits home when military children are harassed by locals or fiscal cuts affect choices (e.g., base closings). The primary identity stems from within the military, not beyond the gates.

Ironically, the military has an unwritten code that affects all the lifers. After twenty years of service, you become increasingly vulnerable to retirement. The military needs your expertise and ethnic mentoring skills but also begins any cutbacks with the retirement-eligible personnel. So a lifer begins to feel vulnerable and, when retiring, is dramatically (and quickly) demoted to the nonentity status of "retiree." Your military identification card is changed, medical care becomes space-available, and your role in the military is over. Retirees are social leftovers, and yet many military settle near a military post/base. They settle not just for economic savings but for links with the military. It is part of their heritage, and retirees swap stories with a gleam in their eyes.

AREAS FOR EXPLORATION AND RESEARCH

Very little research has been conducted on military ethnicity (see Chapter 16). Though composed of anecdotal vignettes rather than formal research statistics, Wertsch (1991) is an excellent description of some of the ethnic issues surrounding the military society (or "Fortress" as she calls it). Other descriptive efforts include those of Kaslow and Ridenour (1984), McCubbin, Dahl, and Hunter (1976), and Daley (1983). Most of the psychosocial research has studied ways to enhance war fighting capability (e.g., what type of helmets work best in tanks or the effect of Arctic conditions on teamwork) or the effect of military demands on family functioning (e.g., types of stressors families face when soldiers are deployed or returning from deployment).

No research specifically focuses on military identity assessment or transition during a career. However, there is increasing nonmilitary emphasis on cultural competence training (Ponterotto, 1998; Dunbar, 1997; Phinney, 1996; Green, Jensen, and Jones, 1996), and extensive work is being done to develop scales to measure *ethnic identity,* such as the Personal Dimensions of Difference Scale (Dunbar, 1997), and *racial identity,* such as the White Racial Identity Attitude Scale (WRIAS) (Helms, 1990) and the Racial Identity Scale (RIS) (Resnicow and Ross-Gaddy, 1997). By adapting selected items from the WRAIS and RIS and adding a few items specific to the military, I have developed an untested scale titled the Military Identity Assessment Scale (MIAS) (see Figure 18.1). I advocate that some type of scale, whether MIAS or another scale, should be developed to help gauge military identity. As Helm (1990) has stated, researchers cannot assume that a person identifies with racial (or ethnic) background. Ethnic identity, not just ethnicity, needs to be assessed. Similar empirical research on developing a scale to assess military family identity would be invaluable.

Once such measures are available, essential research questions can be clarified. How long does it take to develop a military identity? Do a military identity and a military family identity develop concurrently or sequentially? Does military identity increase with rank, time in service, type of job, duty assignment, or combat exposure? Does military identity or military family identity decrease as family stressors increase? Does the type of community (mostly military versus mostly civilian) affect military identity development? What type of psychosocial intervention is most effective to enhance military identity? Is a person more likely to develop military identity if he or she also has strong racial identity? These questions and more are feasible directions for research.

Numerous significant societal and military changes conceivably can also affect the degree of military identity. Fiscal cutbacks are prompting some Army posts and Navy bases to remove guards at the front gates or to have civilian guards. More and more health care is being outsourced (see Chapter 5). Military retirement is now possible after sixteen years of service in some instances, thus prompting earlier retirement or separation options. Severe personnel cutbacks have been occurring for several years. Base closings have occurred and are likely to continue. In sum, the societal context surrounding the military has challenged many established military ethnic traditions.

FIGURE 18.1. Military Identity Assessment Scale—Version 1

This questionnaire measures people's views in the military. There are no right or wrong answers. Write the number next to each item that best describes how you feel about each statement. For example if you "agree strongly" with Question 1, you should write "1" on the line preceding the question.

1 = Agree strongly 2 = Agree 3 = Disagree 4 = Disagree strongly

1. ____ It is important to learn more about military history and customs.
2. ____ Most nonmilitary people feel that they are superior to (better than) military people.
3. ____ Military people should give their children names honoring military heroes.
4. ____ I would like to have more nonmilitary friends.
5. ____ I do not really care what happens to the military.
6. ____ I am happy that I am military.
7. ____ I trust military people more than nonmilitary people.
8. ____ Most of my friends are military.
9. ____ The United States government does not care about military people.
10. ____ I would rather people think of me as an American than as a military person.
11. ____ I hardly think about being in the military.
12. ____ I get angry when I think about how nonmilitary people have treated the military.
13. ____ I would rather socialize with military people only.
14. ____ Military and nonmilitary people have much to learn from each other.
15. ____ I have come to believe that military and nonmilitary people are very different.
16. ____ In my family, we never talk about military issues.
17. ____ I go out of my way to avoid associating with military people.
18. ____ I believe that nonmilitary people are inferior to military people.
19. ____ When I am the only military person in a group of nonmilitary people, I feel anxious.
20. ____ I am embarrassed to admit that I am in the military.
21. ____ I believe that military people look and express themselves better than nonmilitary people.
22. ____ I only feel I am "home" when I am on base/post.

FIGURE 18.1 *(continued)*

23. ____ If I had children, I would be very proud if they joined the military.
24. ____ Being in the military is a lifestyle, not just a job.
25. ____ I cannot remember back when I did not feel part of the military.
26. ____ I hope to stay part of the military as long as possible.
27. ____ I regret ever joining the military.
28. ____ When off-duty, I cannot wait to get my uniform off and get away from the base/post.
29. ____ I cannot wait until I finish my service commitment and can leave the military.
30. ____ Joining the military was one of the biggest mistakes of my life.

Note: Scale has adapted some items from the Racial Identity Scale (Resnicow, K. and Ross-Gaddy, D. (1997) "Development of a racial identity scale for low-income African Americans)," *Journal of Black Studies,* 28(2): 239-254; and the White Racial Identity Attitude Scale (Helms, J. E. (Ed.) (1990) *Black and White Racial Identity: Theory, Research, and Practice,* Westport, CT: Praeger, pp. 249-251).

Scale developed by James G. Daley, PhD, School of Social Work, Southwest Missouri State University.

Have these changes eroded military identity making personnel less optimistic about becoming lifers? These issues need careful, longitudinal research to gauge change.

I advocate that military ethnicity is a reality, though not formally measured yet. I further suggest that change is intense around the "Fortress," perhaps eroding its core. And we still know little about what the process of acculturation is or how to best prepare clinicians for working with the military family. What a target-rich environment for research!

REFERENCES

Casas, J.M. (1984). Policy, training, and research in counseling psychology: The racial/ethnic minority perspective. In S.D. Brown and R.W. Lent (Eds.), *Handbook of Counseling Psychology* (pp. 785-831). New York: John Wiley and Sons.

Daley, J.G. (1983, June). Normal transitional points in the life of an Air Force family. Paper presented at the meeting of the Mississippi Association of Marriage and Family Therapy, Long Beach, Mississippi.

Dunbar, E. (1997). The Personal Dimensions of Difference Scale: Measuring multi-group identity with four ethnic groups. *International Journal of Intercultural Relations*, 21(1): 1-28.

Green, G.J., Jensen, C., and Jones, D. (1996). A constructivist perspective on clinical social work practice with ethnically diverse clients. *Social Work*, 41(2): 172-180.

Helms, J.E. (Ed.) (1990). *Black and White Racial Identity: Theory, Research, and Practice.* Westport, CT: Praeger.

Kaslow, F.W. and Ridenour, R.I. (Eds.) (1984). *The Military Family.* New York: Guilford Press.

McCubbin, H.I., Dahl, B.B., and Hunter, E.J. (Eds.) (1976). *Families in the Military System.* Beverly Hills, CA: Sage.

McGoldrick, M., Giordano, J., Pearce, J.K. (Eds.) (1996). *Ethnicity and Family Therapy* (Second Edition). New York: Guilford Press.

Phinney, J.S. (1996). Understanding ethnic diversity: The role of ethnic identity. *American Behavioral Scientist*, 40(2): 143-152.

Ponterotto, J.G. (1998). Charting a course for research in multicultural counseling training. *Counseling Psychologist*, 26(1): 43-68.

Queralt, M. (1996). *The Social Environment and Human Behavior: A Diversity Perspective.* Boston: Allyn and Bacon.

Resnicow, K. and Ross-Gaddy, D. (1997). Development of a racial identity scale for low-income African Americans. *Journal of Black Studies,* 28(2): 239-254.

Wertsch, M.E. (1991). *Military Brats: Legacies of Childhood Inside the Fortress.* New York: Harmony Books.

PART IV: FUTURE DIRECTIONS OF PRACTICE

Chapter 19

The Future of Army Social Work

Griffin David Lockett

This chapter is my vision of Army social work in the future. I could not have written this chapter six months ago when I was selected and appointed as the Social Work Consultant to the Army Surgeon General. It reflects my thinking about the future after almost twenty-four years as an Army social work officer.

Just as the Army has undergone significant downsizing since about 1989, the point in time frequently referred to as the breakup of the Soviet Union, so has Army social work. We have, and continue to experience, many changes that look different for Army social workers who have been active duty officers and Department of Army civilian social workers. Some of the changes are subtle and some seem more profound for those who have served for a number of years. What must look like rather significant changes to some of us are really neither significant nor drastic to professionals just beginning to practice.

At one point, while working through a difficult series of planning meetings and program direction issues, I was reminded of two things. The first is that in five years none of the arguments or resistance to change in our future direction will matter as we recruit and bring new people into Army social work. They will know no other way to proceed. Second, some of the changes may more clearly affect the future of Army social work than others. The more important point is how we will look as a service and what will we be doing in the future, rather than whether we will be a part of the Army in the future.

This chapter consists of the author's opinions and does not reflect the opinions or policies of the U.S. Army.

The future must be viewed in the perspective of our present structure. The current organizational configuration of social work and its place in the U.S. Army Medical Department (AMEDD) is a logical place to begin. We remain a medically based practice, particularly connected by regulation and authority to the AMEDD. The overall leadership and vision of the AMEDD are the responsibilities of the Army Surgeon General. Our base of operations thus clearly falls within the medical realm and medical model. Much of what we do and how we practice social work is within this context. We receive broad guidance and direction within a medical frame of reference, and we operate in a host setting. This context alone has always presented a practice and professional dilemma with its own advantages and disadvantages. We remain a hospital and clinic-based operation straining for full professional recognition and our own professional self-determination. Our mission, practice area, and leadership are also in a medical context. The principal practice domain is medical rather than community based, but this is changing. Our leadership, beyond our social work leaders, are mainly physicians who set organizational and corporate priorities, vision, and mission. We take our rules of operation from a medical reference and fit into that framework. While we are involved in more field (community-based) work, such as Combat Stress Control and Division Mental Health, the majority of our active duty and civilian social work force practice in hospitals or clinics throughout their professional careers. For example, at this writing approximately 90 of our 150 active duty social work officers and almost all of our civilian social workers practice directly in hospitals or clinics or in administrative positions managing social work practice in support of those medical facilities.

The point is that since we are mainly organized and operate under a medical organizational structure, our practice direction and sanction for our purpose, contributions, and scope of practice are defined by it. To a large extent it is within the medical model, leadership, and administration that we are sanctioned, funded, and operate with the leadership's approval and overall direction. The areas that we practice in are determined by the Department of Defense (Health Affairs) and AMEDD to accomplish the Army's mission and support the future plans of the total Army.

Organizationally and functionally, over the past ten years, family advocacy has so dominated social work practice in our medical treatment facilities (MTFs) that it requires special mention. Most of our social work personnel resources are devoted to it, sometimes to the exclusion of other areas of social work practice in the medical setting. This is principally because of important congressional legislation and a protected, fenced source of program funding. This fenced funding ensures that funds reach Social Work Service in individual MTFs to guarantee staff are in place. The advantage is that Family Advocacy Program staff are not susceptible to the same funding reductions as the rest of Social Work Service.

Unlike social work practice in many other areas, military social work exists with the bottom-line function of supporting the readiness of soldiers to fight and win wars for our nation. Our practice begins with that main purpose and everything else we do supports it. Whatever our particular practice area, whether it is family advocacy, discharge planning, substance abuse, mental health, exceptional family members, or something more direct such as support to soldiers in Division Mental Health and Combat Stress Control units, we support the Army's main mission. Some of us allow ourselves to focus on and develop expertise in one or more practice specialty areas, but the main purpose remains the same. Reduced to our most basic purpose, we are here to support soldiers and families with our special skills, knowledge, and experiences. What we bring to the AMEDD is perhaps the most versatile and cost-effective behavior and mental health profession to serve the Army.

It is important to understand that the basis of Army social work is tied closely to the Army's medical mission and to keep this in clear perspective when thinking about the future. This helps explain the future of Army social work and some of the changes we see happening. For example, the reductions in numbers of both active duty and civilian staff is related to the overall reduction in the size of the Department of Defense (DoD) and the Army. The continuing management analyses as we work toward what the leadership sees as the right staff number are principally based on the number needed to support the Army in doing its job. We have participated in analyses with the goal of reaching the right number, mix, and location of social work professionals, and will continue to do so. Make Buy, another staffing analysis, was used to determine the number and location of active duty social workers that could be replaced by civilian social workers. This has not been implemented, but it remains a completed staff reduction tool that may be used in the future to reduce the number of active duty social work officers.

Over the next two years, numbers of active duty officers will be reduced indirectly by the recommendations of the Quadrennial Defense Review, a global look every four years at what is needed to achieve the DoD functions and missions. Additionally, as individual hospital commanders face resource constraints, social workers are very much part of the equation that determines how they will distribute those resources.

Organizationally, the future structure will require less involvement from the social work staff at Medical Command headquarters for operational and clinical control. We will focus our efforts on clinical treatment policy, standards of clinical practice, and continuous quality improvement in all clinical areas. The operative concept is to move operational control down to the Regional Medical Commands (RMCs). Currently there are six: North Atlantic, Southeastern, Great Plains, Western, Pacific, and Europe. Each RMC has a designated social work authorization at the rank of colonel, who is chief of social work for the MTF and for its geographical area. Each RMC Chief of Social Work serves as a consultant and mentor to other social workers in the region. Increasingly in the future, the RMC Chief of Social Work will have more involvement and influence over social work practice in the region. These responsibilities will include consultation to the active duty chiefs and other social workers at the various MTFs in the region. The RMC Chief of Social Work will take on the operational and management role as well as practice issues. These may include credentialing, privileging, and monitoring licensed social workers, quality improvement, and practice standards. The RMC Chief of Social Work may be involved in ensuring training of staff in the region. At this time, full acceptance of this concept is uneven in the regions, but is critical to our future successful operation.

Each RMC Chief of Social Work, along with other senior social work officers, is a member of a council of colonels to help shape policy and direction in social work. They serve as a board of directors in an advisory capacity to the Social Work Consultant to the Army Surgeon General. The council of colonels is becoming more important in conducting program and strategic planning. The headquarters staffing complement for social work, which is already reduced, will be further reduced in the near and midterm. The reduced headquarters staff makes it more difficult to stay abreast of the changes, to embrace them in a positive and constructive way, and, perhaps more important, guide the course for necessary productive changes consistent with solid social work practice and principles.

One of the strengths of Army social work is that we play an active role in defining our course within the constraints of our host medical organization in spite of reductions. Our numbers continue to decline as the Army shrinks, and we have to find new ways to shape our future. Essentially, the direction is determined at a high level and social work determines how it is going to fit within the context of professional standards and scope of practice. In other words, we are given the future direction of the AMEDD, and our job has been to react to those directions by determining our fit and contributions. We work within prescribed parameters. We are not and will not be staffed to the extent necessary to examine the possibilities of directing our practice course, because with the reduction of numbers we cannot keep up with the broad area we are required to, and want to, work in.

Army social workers remain involved in providing services in the MTFs. We less involved in discharge planning as the number of inpatient bed days for most patients is constantly being reduced in a managed care environment. At some of our MTFs, nurses and managed care staff have been assigned discharge planning. The perspective that nurses bring to discharge planning versus social work's perspective, skills, and approach to providing these services has not been studied in our military hospitals to determine advantages or best practices. With the emphasis on case management and reducing the number of inpatient bed days, we simply do not know if there is a difference or if a different perspective is significant. We do not know whether there are benefits if one group or another, or a combination of groups, takes the lead. This area needs more investigation for its implications for social work practice.

Some additional related and interesting questions include: Does one group or the other favor the patient's rights to quality care and services? Also, does one profession meet patient and practice needs as well as those of the institutions, or is there a better model? These issues are clearly in need of future inquiry and study.

We expect that social workers will become more involved in primary care clinics, including family practice, as the Army's focus moves more toward primary care and prevention. We have been slow to institutionalize this philosophy, but we are starting to see real change. We expect and welcome increasing involvement in health and human behavior as a critical part of encouraging individuals to assume responsibility for themselves. A social worker's training for patient and client advocacy, the right to self-determination, and an understanding and working knowledge of systems would suggest the right mix of skills to work in this area. A question that emerges is whether the hospital leadership will accept this as an important and value-added role for social workers.

Another factor that will continue to affect the role and future of hospital social work is TRICARE, which is DoD's managed care system for health care delivery. It is a regionally managed health care program for active duty and retired members of the uniformed services, their families, and survivors. The Army, along with the other services, is of course an active player. Through senior military health care officers, as lead agents with geographical regional responsibility, TRICARE is having far-reaching effects on health care delivery such as we have never seen before. The effects of TRICARE on the delivery of social work services are becoming more apparent in both inpatient and outpatient health.

Today, active duty Army social work officers and civilian social workers continue to practice in a changing variety of ways such as direct clinicians, case managers, service coordinators, program managers, administrators, researchers, and trainers. The following areas are a partial list of the most visible practice areas: medical in- and outpatient services, including limited discharge planning and psychiatric/mental health; exceptional family member program, both direct clinical services and clinical administration; family advocacy program; combat stress control; division mental health; corrections, alcohol and drug abuse prevention and control program; soldier and family support; command consultation; sexual assault; and disaster response team.

In the very near future, Army social workers will continue to expand our use of automation and technology to support our various practice areas. We are moving to establish the Social Work Service Management Information System, including a personal computer, and a server-based system for Social Work Service and Family Advocacy. The automation system will increase efficiency, improve the quality of patient care, and reflect best social work practices. It will link information with several other related automation systems.

The need for active duty social workers to serve on what is commonly considered the "line side" or field will continue. This essentially includes practice settings away from the medical facility. Social workers are increasingly located in units where soldiers train, work, and deploy. It means practicing social work where combat troops are. We must provide mental health consultation to commanders and leaders, provide services to prevent and treat stress reactions at every level, and deal with the effects of exposure to trauma. There is more direct support of soldiers in almost every setting today including combat stress control and division social work. This is a positive trend. I expect that the new social work officer must be exceptionally clinically competent, licensed, and comfortable in delivery services in these expanding settings to be a successful Army social work professional.

In August 1997 and October 1997, two key documents with significant effects on social workers were signed. Those documents are: the DoD Instruction 6490.4, Requirements for Mental Health Evaluations of Members of the Armed Forces, and DoD Directive 6490.1, Mental Health Evaluations of Members of the Armed Forces. In a yet undetermined way, these documents are modifying the requirements for Army social work practice, particularly in the areas of mental health support to soldiers. The new directive and instruction require that social workers who conduct these command-directed evaluations must have a doctoral degree in clinical social work. The directive and instruction limit the role of master's level social workers in assessing the imminent and potential dangerousness of active duty military members. The full effects of this opportunity for clinical doctoral social workers and limitation for master's-prepared social workers remains to be determined. What these directives clearly do is to require doctoral level clinical social workers to be available to fill these practicc areas. Quite simply, social workers will lose out in this critical practice area unless we can recruit doctoral level practitioners. This is an actively debated topic among social workers because of the limitations imposed and its heavy emphasis on mental health and the narrower focus of social work practice.

Most of the sixteen doctoral level social workers currently on active duty are in the senior grades and are more involved in program management and administration. The grades necessary for combat stress control are captains, majors, and lieutenant colonels, not senior lieutenant colonels and colonels. This emphasis on higher level degrees is changing the accession requirements for social workers. It remains to be seen whether we will be able to recruit doctoral level clinical social workers for these jobs and whether the special skills and perspective of master's-prepared social workers are used. Nevertheless, social workers remain important to the Combat Stress Control Units and have demonstrated their worth and provided a valuable contribution to field and combat commanders over and over.

The future of Army social work to some degree still rests with the prevention of dysfunctional coping patterns associated with the stresses of military life across the continuum of a military career. Perhaps one of the more valuable contributions we make now and in the future is the direct support of soldiers wherever they may serve. We have always had a role in making a valued contribution to sustainment, restoration, and enhancement of a soldier's ability to function.

I think Army social workers of the future must become increasingly innovators and entrepreneurs, and find ways to generate programs, services, and revenue for the MTF in which they work, while providing services for patients.

They must be able to market their skills, competencies, and experiences, as much as the profession itself. The future belongs to social workers who can present skills that meet the Army's needs. They must sell medical and nonmedical commanders on their value and contributions. To some extent, this means focusing on marketing skills, not professional titles.

The future of Army social work will also reside with those who can identify new roles and gain recognition and acceptance for social workers. Frequently, when I meet with new Army social workers, I describe opportunities for practice that we were unaware of five to ten years ago. Some of these opportunities were created by social workers who recognized a need and obtained jobs based on their skills and competencies. As the AMEDD has changed, so too have the requirements and new opportunities.

With the emphasis by the Army Surgeon General and especially the Chief of the Medical Service Corps on opening more opportunities to serve outside of one's specialty, parameters are expanding. Social workers and others have the opportunity to work in areas outside of specialty training never before open to us. Opportunities may be considered with significantly fewer limitations. For example, for the first time in the history of Army social work, a social worker has the potential to rise to the general officer rank. It is not likely, but what is more important is that it is not impossible. It could happen, given the right set of circumstances such as diversification in assignments, civilian and military education, and training and an open medical department leadership. Additionally, a senior social worker, because of a variety of skills, could now become a clinic or hospital commander.

The opportunity for expanded specialty assignments does bring with it some special considerations and circumstances. While the number of active duty Army social workers is going down and the opportunity for other jobs is increasing, it creates a dilemma and strain on social work. For example: a young captain is selected to serve as a company commander for an eighteen or twenty-four month tour. This tour effectively removes him or her from the inventory of officers to fill designated authorized social work positions. If we replicate this scenario with other opportunities commensurate with officer grades, our inventory and ability to fill purely social work jobs is affected. To social work's credit, we bring a variety of valuable skills, competencies, and experiences. We offer clinical training and an understanding of human behavior, management, and systems. We provide an attractive set of skills to anyone open enough to use them. I contend that in today's Army, social workers provide a versatility and skill set that adds real value to the organization. Social work officers have always been encouraged to enhance their skills with continuing civilian and military professional education. The AMEDD has not always fully understood or recognized the important and versatile skill set Army social workers offer. It will be some time before the AMEDD fully appreciates this asset. As our numbers continue to decrease so must our opportunities to market ourselves to command for leadership.

The dilemma occurs because we are a small specialty and our numbers do not afford us the flexibility to spread ourselves over the increasing social work practice areas that the Army needs. Our officers are also fully taking advantage of the increasing opportunities to serve in jobs that create promotion potential, diversity, and competitive ability, sometimes away from social work.

The lower and declining number of social work officers is directly tied to the number of military hospitals necessary to support the Army during combat. Our mission must always be tied to the Army's deployments and the AMEDD's support of them. A trend that we expect will continue in the future is the use of contract social work staff. We have seen the increasing use of contract social workers, particularly in the Family Advocacy Program, because the program was given funds to hire staff, not authorizations to support additional permanent clinical staff.

We also expect that some of our social work services in MTFs will be headed by civil service social workers. As we increasingly use the declining number of social work officers in field jobs and a variety of non-social work jobs, we can expect that positions in the MTFs will still need to be filled. Some of our smaller MTFs are already headed by very able and experienced civil service social workers. The main reasons to have active duty social workers in garrison MTFs are for rotational and training assignments and continuous preparation for readiness and peacetime health care. The MTF is our base. A number of social workers report that there is a distinct advantage to having active duty social workers in an MTF, especially in the Family Advocacy Program. The advantages are the identification and relationship with the installation commanders and other military personnel. I think we will compromise that special identification and relationship with the soldiers and commanders as we replace more active duty with civilian social workers.

We must continue to manage and operate programs for families and soldiers that sustain, restore, or enhance functioning, social well-being, and adjustment throughout the career life cycle. We will continue to promote a healthy lifestyle for soldiers and families. We help soldiers and families successfully navigate events throughout the career life cycle. We will continue to work to resolve social system conflicts and challenges that impede mission accomplishment. We must maintain our focus in problem solving. We will continue to perceive and understand people with their needs and problems in a family, social, and Army systems environment.

Chapter 20

The Future of Navy Social Work

David Kennedy

INTRODUCTION

The future of the Navy social work program is tied to its history as a largely volunteer, civilian-run program using relatively few uniformed social workers. The program, with its roots in a variety of informal programs and volunteer organizations, formally developed much later than programs in the other Services. The American Red Cross and other largely volunteer organizations provided a limited number of professionally trained social workers to medical treatment facilities as late as the early 1980s. This reliance on nongovernment support systems enabled the Navy to delay, for years, formalizing a social service delivery system.

Civilian professional social workers were brought into the health care system as early as the 1950s, but the numbers were minuscule. Recognizing a need to formalize the social service delivery system in line with military structure, the Navy Surgeon General outlined a justification for uniformed social workers in a 1979 memo to the Chief of Naval Operations:

> The incumbents of these billets are required to be military for the following reasons: By education and training (Master's degree and certification by the Academy of Certified Social Workers), social workers will perform clinical functions which include case-finding and counseling; coordinating social service activities

This chapter consists of the author's opinions and does not reflect the opinions or policies of the U.S. Navy.

> and maintaining liaison with military and civilian resources. In order to plan for the expeditious and optimum disposition and resolution of beneficiaries' medical/social problems, elements of case-finding may include communication with military personnel at any level in the chain of command, access to confidential or classified material/information, understanding of military order and discipline, and the Uniform Code of Military Justice. With an understanding of Naval organization and culture, mission, policies and the processes of military personnel management gained from officer training and duty experience, the commissioned officer social worker brings a degree of awareness and sensitivity to his or her duties which is essential in gaining rapport and effectively working with others in the military community. In times of national emergency, or other contingencies, the social worker as an officer can fulfill a vital role as may other health professionals in working with military units as well as the families of service personnel. (Navy Bureau of Medicine and Surgery, 1979)

The proposed functions and functional areas he outlined have guided the development of the social work program and provide clues to the future.

The future of the Navy social work program lies in its ability to understand and integrate into the Navy system in wartime as well as in peacetime. The Surgeon General mentions mental health, family advocacy, drug and alcohol programs, contingencies, medical counseling, case finding, liaison, and fleet support. Of interest is that the above concepts and rationale were part of a summary of recommendations developed by civilian social workers who met in 1979 as part of the First Navy Mental Health Professionals Meeting. As illustrated in the memo, the roles for uniformed social workers covered a wide range, and expectations were high for the original twelve social workers commissioned in 1980. By the end of that year there were approximately thirty civilian and twelve military social workers in the medical department.

The primary mission for social work at that time became standardization of discharge planning and medical social work services at major medical treatment facilities (MTFs). The Navy envisioned a cadre of twenty-five to thirty social work officers heading social work departments in MTFs throughout the country. There are currently 300 to 400 civilian and contract and thirty-one military social workers in the Navy Medical Department, Family Advocacy Program, and in Family Service Centers.

The role of active duty and civilian social workers has changed greatly as the Navy's response to health care delivery has evolved and expanded its services to families. A number of changes were occurring in the Navy at the time of the first commissioned officers. The Family Advocacy Program and the Family Service Center system of support came on-line. Social workers, both military and civilian, were newly assigned services in child and spouse abuse and in counseling for individual, marital, and family problems. These programs continue to grow and with them the presence of social workers. Today half of the uniformed social workers are assigned to nonmedical commands as described above.

The Navy social work program will continue to use civil service and contract social workers in large numbers for both hospital-based and Family Service Center programs. The number of active duty social workers is predicted to remain stable at least in the near future.

CAREER TRENDS FOR ACTIVE DUTY

The first cadre of uniformed social workers have been on active duty for eighteen years and are just being considered for O-6. The discipline is young in its development as a specialty within the Medical Service Corps. With few senior officers, social workers have had little opportunity for positions of leadership within the Medical Service Corps and the Navy, which allows little ability to influence programs and policy. There are, also, "growing pains" with such a young discipline.

With a total of thirty-one officers in the social work community, developing a viable career path is particularly challenging. A pyramidal rank and billet structure must develop to support a meaningful career path. That is, there must be sufficient numbers of jobs and personnel at designated ranks to allow a normal career progression. Currently only a few billets are designated at O-4 or higher and none for a doctoral-level person. A shift must occur in the current billet designations that authorize only one commander, two lieutenant commanders, fifteen lieutenants, and eleven lieutenant junior grade officers to more closely match the current grade distribution of Naval officers, which is as follows:

Lieutenant junior grade (O-2)	1
Lieutenant (O-3)	15
Lieutenant commander (O-4)	7
Commander (O-5)	5
Captain (O-6)	1

As currently structured, a billet may be filled with an O-2 who is then replaced by an O-4, and so on. This kind of fluctuation makes it difficult for commanding officers to place our officers in positions of leadership within social service programs. They may instead place civilian staff in those positions to provide continuity, or they may change the requirements of a position, which can have a negative impact on the next assigned officer.

Social workers must compete directly with other specialties for promotion, and so must have positions commensurate with rank. Social work has been able thus far to compete relatively well with other disciplines because many of our billets are at department-head level at entry.

The Navy Family Advocacy Program, once managed by the medical department, is now fully under line control. Realignment was completed in 1997 and included transferring fourteen military and over 180 civilian positions from medical to line commands. Now fully half of all social work billets are attached to line commands. This situation presents both an opportunity and a risk to social work. Operational or line-owned billets are thought of as enhancing a discipline because they are seen as more directly supporting the military mission and can help a well-performing officer get promoted. The line traditionally writes strong fitness reports, so a tour there can enhance promotion opportunity. On the other hand, line commands may place social workers in positions where they are less supported because of a lack of understanding of social work functions.

A few social work officers have requested transfer to other disciplines such as health care administration, hoping to improve their chances for promotion. With a community this small it is nearly impossible to allow someone to transfer because it will negatively affect the rotation pattern. Also, the other disciplines are hesitant to accept those who do not have the desired educational background or experience.

Officers, particularly early in their careers, are given a variety of assignments in terms of setting, duties, and requirements to broaden their experiences. As officers advance and the choices narrow it becomes more difficult to place them in career-enhancing billets. There are only a few senior-level billets as follows:

- Clinical Management and Plans staff officer at the Bureau of Medicine and Surgery
- Sexual Assault Victim Intervention Program manager at the Bureau of Naval Personnel
- Regional Family Advocacy Program managers at San Diego and Naples
- Social work department heads at San Diego and Bethesda

Those jobs are filled with O-5s or senior O-4s. The remainder of the billets are usually filled based on availability rather than seniority. This kind of assignment pattern makes for a less than ideal career path. The Medical Service Corps is developing a career template to assist the various specialties to outline desired career goals for its officers.

OVERSEAS ISSUES

The need for social service support overseas was recognized shortly after the first social workers were commissioned. A number of Stateside billets were shifted to overseas locations in the mid-1980s as it became clear that those locations, without community supports, were vulnerable to problems. Social work leaders welcomed this shift because billets in overseas locations are viewed as "closer to the fleet" and thus more valuable to the Navy.

This shift of billets, however, created problems in the rotation pattern. Overseas tours are shorter, particularly for single individuals, than for persons with families. There must be more Stateside billets than overseas billets to make up for the difference in tour lengths. Currently 50 percent of the active duty billets are located overseas.

Our officers go overseas very quickly (usually after one to one and a half years of a three-year tour). This forced early rotation is extremely difficult because they are adjusting to Navy life, increased responsibilities, and an isolated foreign tour. When they return from an overseas tour, they are faced with another one soon. A number of our officers have voluntarily extended overseas or accepted back-to-back overseas tours, which has been tremendously helpful in alleviating the overseas shortfall.

Under those circumstances quality of life and career issues loom large, particularly for junior officers. Their families must prepare for the demands of overseas life more quickly and more often than most of their MSC counterparts. Rather than beginning their Navy careers with a three-year Stateside tour during which they and their families can adjust to military life, they are moved overseas after one or two years.

Stateside billets at larger commands allow comparison with other officers in fitness reports. This comparison is difficult or impossible in small overseas locations where there are few officers with whom to compare. For midgrade (O-4) officers whose peers are directors for administration or officers in charge of branch clinics, social work functions pale in comparison. The result can be a lower ranking than their peers have at those commands. The need for overseas support continues as strongly as ever. As social workers perform a variety of services in those isolated locations, the demand for their services grows. Without either a shift of billets from overseas to Stateside locations or an increase in Stateside billets to provide the needed balance, the rotation issue will continue to be problematic.

ROLE IN MANAGED CARE/TRICARE

The social work role in managed care remains to be identified. Most clinical social workers are in direct care settings providing a variety of services from counseling to mental health to discharge planning. Many of the billets in managed care are not discipline specific, so they are considered "outfills" and leave gaps within the pool of available officers when filled. Other disciplines, with large cadres of mid- to senior-level officers, such as nursing, have embraced managed care and are better positioned to have an impact.

There is one social work position at the headquarters level in the managed care area. This is the senior billet at the Bureau of Medicine and Surgery (BUMED), which is changing from a position as manager of the BUMED Family Advocacy Program.

Case management is a significant aspect of managed care, but few social workers are involved. Because the Navy is downsizing, TRICARE has arrived, and beneficiaries are able to make choices about their health care, the importance of quality case management is critical. Social work with its unique skills in case management and the concept of the person in the environment should offer meaningful insights into managed care.

The future of social work in this area is also related to the number of senior officers available for assignment in policy positions to "work outside" the community. The Navy social work role in this area should grow as the officer group gains seniority. They will be uniquely qualified to work in this area, which addresses a complex set of interacting systems, both administrative and clinical.

CAREER GROOMING/MENTORING

The Navy Medical Service Corps has embarked on a project to strengthen mentoring, both formally and informally. The Navy Medical Service Corps Executive Steering Committee selected mentoring as a major part of its strategic plan. The introduction to Strategic Goal I of the strategic plan reads as follows:

> The professionalism and experience of the Medical Service Corps officer within the thirty-two disciplines of the Corps is visible throughout the Navy and Marine Corps. Our officers work as part of a multidisciplinary team which inspires innovation and creative thought. Our mentoring program has developed leaders in management, clinical, and technical positions who excel in a dynamic environment and a changing world. Efforts in recruiting, mentoring and retention ensure that only the best provide the foundation of the most diverse, valued component of Navy Medical Department.

> Medical Service Corps Goal 1
>
> The Medical Service Corps will capitalize on its diversity, professionalism, expertise and experience to achieve cohesive teamwork to support Navy and the Military Health Services System missions.
>
> Strategy 1.1: The Medical Service Corps will incorporate mentoring into its culture.
>
> Strategy 1.2: The Medical Service Corps will create a culture where each member feels a sense of belonging and pride.
>
> Strategy 1.3: The Medical Service Corps will assume positions of professional leadership. (Medical Service Corps, 1998, p. 1)

As outlined, mentoring is seen as an essential component of a successful career, both early on as a recipient and later as a mentor. Informal mentoring has always occurred in the Navy. The goal of this plan highlights and provides structure to the mentoring process to encourage its growth.

Social workers, because of their small numbers and isolated duty locations, are at a distinct disadvantage when it comes to mentoring. There are few fellow MSC officers in many locations with which to connect, and the only other social workers are civilians who often have little understanding of the major issues facing military officers. Also, heavy caseloads make it difficult to participate fully in command activities that can enhance mentoring relationships. The Navy Medical Service Corps is based within the Medical Department and many of its activities occur in hospitals and clinics. With the Family Advocacy Program moving out of BUMED, now half of the social work officers are attached to line (nonmedical) commands that afford little opportunity for meaningful interface with MSC colleagues.

Often the mentoring process takes place long-distance and is hampered by communication and technology problems. A lack of readily available senior role models forces social workers to look elsewhere for mentors. Social work officers report using officers in other disciplines such as administrators, civilians, and so on as mentors, which is encouraged but not as effective as mentoring from another social worker. As the mentoring project continues to develop it is critical that social workers take full advantage of the opportunities it presents. The future looks bright as more and more social workers are moving into the senior ranks and will function in positions of leadership, both within the social work community and in the Navy Medical Department. Any medical department officer selected for O-6 may elect to screen for command positions and possibly become an executive officer or commanding officer of an MTF. The Deputy Surgeon General of the Navy is a Medical Service Corps officer, and it is possible for a Medical Service Corps officer to be selected as the Surgeon General of the Navy.

MILITARY-CIVILIAN INTERFACE

The organized Navy social work program began with civilian practitioners in medical treatment facilities in the 1950s doing medical social work, discharge planning, and counseling. In the early 1970s eight social workers were hired by the Navy to help to assist in the repatriation of prisoners of war and their families and to assist families of service members listed as missing in action. These social workers remained in the system long after the programs ended and performed a variety of functions in hospitals and clinics. Many added staff as the demand for services increased, and some created departments of social work. They also were instrumental in providing a justification for uniformed social workers as outlined earlier.

Uniformed social work officers have had to integrate into civilian-run programs such as hospital social work departments and Family Service Centers. They report feeling isolated because their duties keep them apart from their fellow Medical Service Corps officers, and their civilian counterparts cannot identify with the needs of a military officer.

There have been conflicts as commands embraced the uniformed officers, leaving the civilian staff feeling ignored. On the other hand, line commands, in particular, are often unfamiliar with social work functioning and do not offer the kind of support and understanding needed, or they may place a very junior officer in a position of leadership, much to the chagrin of civilian colleagues. If the officer is not up to the challenge of managing a department of unhappy civilians the result can be disastrous.

Most civilian staff members, however, welcome their military counterparts and see them as a bridge to the command structure, interpreting policies and carrying social work principles to the command by participation in the uniformed Navy community.

The Bureau of Naval Personnel now has two billets at the headquarters level, which will enable senior officers to assist those in the field with the issues mentioned above. With a ratio of greater than 10 to 1 civilian social workers to military officers, civilian staff will continue to provide the vast majority of services. The military-civilian interface will continue to develop, with the uniformed officers providing liaison with commands and identification with the military chain of command as envisioned by the Surgeon General, and with civilian staff providing continuity and the bulk of clinical, supervisory, and administrative services.

LICENSE/CREDENTIALING

The Navy uniformed social work program, at inception, required its officers to have a state license or certification by the National Association of Social Workers' Academy of Certified Social Workers (ACSW), which requires two years post-master's experience as a condition of commissioning. A license or certification was seen as essential because most of the billets were "lone wolf" and required the individual to function independently. The social work program, with limits in size, could not afford to bring in inexperienced officers and "grow its own." The license/certification allowed the officer to enter with credentials in hand. The hope was that the credential would enhance credibility in MTFs where most other providers were licensed or credentialed in their disciplines. Only twenty-three states had established licensing procedures at the time, so possession of an ACSW was recognized as the most widely accepted certification.

The situation has changed, and now every state has a licensing/certification process in place. BUMED uses the civilian standard for privileging an individual, regardless of discipline, which means that all independent practitioners must have a state license or certification. Most social workers in the Navy system do possess a state license; however, a few individuals possess only the ACSW and will have to obtain a state license to remain in the Navy.

This change in practice relates to the shift in the mission of social work. Originally medical social work was the primary mission and social workers functioned in the context of the hospital system, but that has shifted to outpatient counseling and mental health-related services where more independent functioning occurs. The credentialing/privileging system will continue to develop in a manner similar to the civilian sector and licensure regulation will become more stringent. Risk management issues are a key driving force in determining the level of certification required for independent practice. Social work, like other clinical disciplines, will continue to mirror the standards in the civilian community, which are becoming more stringent in terms of requirements for experience, education, and supervision.

DEPLOYMENT SUBSTITUTABILITY IN MENTAL HEALTH/CONTINGENCY

The need to become an integral part of the mental health team responding to contingency operations has been an ongoing theme. Social work substitutability for psychiatry and psychology in the theater of operations has received recent emphasis as all disciplines are faced with possible downsizing or elimination. The fact that now social workers are licensed/certified in every state to practice independent mental health therapy clarifies the issue.

The survival of Navy social work will depend, in part, on its ability to provide mental health services in contingency operations, which means substituting for psychiatrists and psychologists. This has been a longstanding issue for social work, from the early days of trying to establish separate social work departments in MTFs and battling psychiatry's attempts to annex social workers into their departments. The profession claimed that social workers offered different services than psychiatry or psychology and fiercely defended the need to remain separate from them. At the same time, social work maintained an identity with the mental health profession and proudly boasted of its mental health skills.

Combat stress centers are geared as nonmedical operations to get sailors and marines back in action are currently staffed with psychiatrists and psychologists. The model calls for realistic, goal-oriented intervention without medications for the most part. Experience has shown that the number of sailors and marines incapacitated because of family-centered concerns is high. The social work model of intervention fits well into this concept, and there is work to be done to regain a foothold in this critical area.

Navy contingency plans call for psychiatric and psychological services in the theater of operations, and now social work is struggling to become a mental health "team member." Our fleet hospitals, combat stress centers, and hospital ships deleted social work as a required specialty due to space limitations and other personnel cuts. Social work will need to regain billets in these critical areas if the discipline is to remain a viable part of the Medical Service Corps.

Social work faces threats from many areas including small size, late development, ability to function in many roles which diffuses identity, downsizing, and the move to managed care. Historically, Navy social work has done well given the obstacles and has continued to evolve to meet ever-changing needs. It must remain flexible, anticipate changes, and seize opportunities, such as the move to managed care, to display skills and take a leadership role. As more officers gain seniority, hold positions of leadership, and contribute to the mission of the Navy, the Surgeon General's 1979 vision of a multitalented, essential cadre of officers who contribute greatly to the Navy will continue to be realized.

REFERENCES

Medical Service Corps (1998). *Strategic Plan* (brochure). Washington, DC: Department of the Navy.

Navy Bureau of Medicine and Surgery (1979, April 26). NOBC/Subspecialty Code for Social Worker: Justification For. Memo from Chief, Navy Bureau of Medicine and Surgery to Chief of Naval Operations. Washington, DC: Department of the Navy.

Chapter 21

The Future of Air Force Social Work

Alice A. Tarpley

I find it a daunting proposition to be writing about the future of Air Force social work. In the years to come, readers can look at what I have written and know how well I "foresaw" the future. (It reminds me of the rumors in the late 1970s that soon all of the military services would combine in creating one "purple" Department of Defense [DoD] Medical Service and that the Air Force Medical Service [AFMS] as we knew it would disappear. Today, the AFMS remains a strong institution and its personnel continue the tradition of the "blue-suiter." And those who predicted one consolidated DoD Medical Service still wait.) So, while I will not pretend to know where AF social work will be in twenty years, I can state unequivocally that we are in a very dynamic period as the AF social work system faces fantastic challenges and opportunities.

Currently 215 active duty and over 225 civil service and contract social workers are working for the Department of the Air Force (DAF). The vast majority of the civil service and virtually all of the contract social workers are employed under the auspices of the Air Force Family Advocacy Program (AF FAP). Because that system has been addressed elsewhere in this book, the following thoughts are confined to a discussion of the future of AF active duty social work. This is in no way meant to discount the importance of the contribution of the DAF's civilian social workers, but rather to recognize that they operate under different personnel and program planning systems.

Opinions expressed in this chapter are the author's and do not reflect any policy or opinions of the U.S. Air Force.

All active duty social workers belong to the AFMS and are commissioned as medical officers in the Biomedical Science Corps (BSC). Active duty social workers fall under the medical Air Force Specialty Code (AFSC) designated specifically for clinical social workers. While social workers can be assigned to selected positions that are typically line officer authorizations, they remain AFMS assets unless they officially cross-train into a different AFSC. Because social workers are members of the BSC, all facets of personnel actions, such as determination of the number of new clinical social workers accessed each year, the total number of social work authorizations in any given year, promotion and assignment opportunities, and requirements for advanced academic degrees (PhD, DSW, or postdoctoral fellowships) are controlled by the AFMS.

The current AFMS is built upon the concept that four strategic pillars form the backbone of the medical system. All efforts of personnel assigned to the AFMS (no matter what their AFSC might be) are designed to support one or more of these strategic pillars. These pillars are:

1. Medical readiness
2. Building healthy communities
3. Rightsizing
4. Deploying TRICARE

Senior leadership within the AFMS met in 1997 to build upon these pillars, mission support plans, and initiatives of installation medical facilities to reengineer the AFMS. The Surgeon General of the Air Force, Lieutenant General Charles Roadman, challenged senior leadership to be vigilant to the many opportunities that accompany change in order to develop a leaner health care system that is even more efficient, productive, and responsive (Roadman, 1997).

To understand the direction of AF social work in the future, it is essential to understand the mission of the AFMS, because to the extent that any discipline stops contributing to the mission, it becomes frivolous. The AFMS's mission is reflected in the strategic pillars identified above. The mission is to:

1. Expand, mobilize, and deploy medical support for contingency operations worldwide
2. Develop and operate a comprehensive and cost-effective community health care system
3. Promote health, safety, and morale of Air Force people
4. Provide or arrange timely, high-quality health care. (Department of the Air Force, 1998)

This mission provides a framework around which future directions of AF social work can be organized for discussion.

MEDICAL READINESS

Historical analyses of this century's conflicts suggest that somewhere between 9 and 46 percent of casualties suffer from combat stress or other psychiatric ailments during wartime. If these troops were all evacuated out of a theater of operations during a war, the mission of combat units would degrade significantly. Because of this potential degradation, the value of mental health services is increasingly recognized.

During Operations Desert Shield and Desert Storm (1990-1991), two-thirds of AF mental health personnel sent to Southwest Asia were clinical social workers. These individuals were tasked with: (1) providing prevention efforts to help ameliorate the effect of the sudden deployment, (2) offering clinical intervention with those at risk for having to be returned home due to mental health-related issues, (3) assessing and triaging those who displayed symptoms of a significant psychiatric disturbance, and (4) setting up combat stress units for the thousands of casualties expected in the event of full scale, prolonged fighting.

While the activation of the AF Combat Stress Units never became fully necessary, recognition of the importance of mental health assets in such a theater of operations became increasingly entrenched. In the years following ODS, the AFMS began the process of reengineering the way medical services deploy and provide care in war and "operations other than war" (OOTW) scenarios. (OOTW refers to peacekeeping and humanitarian operations such as responses to natural or manmade disasters.) Social workers have played a key role in helping to design the way mental health assets will deploy in the future.

This recently introduced concept calls for a building block approach in which medical planners can design a response package that is tailored for the type of operation at hand. Two types of mental health packages have been proposed that can be available to deploy with Air Transportable Hospitals (ATHs) and Theater Hospitals established in the area of responsibility (AOR) or as stand-alone units at designated military sites.

The first proposed unit (referred to as a UTC or Unit Type Code) would be the Rapid Response Team, which would generally be composed of one psychiatrist, one psychologist, one clinical social worker, one mental health nurse, and one technician. This team will be prepared to depart home station with less than twenty-four hours notice, taking the supplies they need in military backpacks. This team's mission would be to (1) perform in-theater prevention and outreach services, including command consultation, critical incident stress management, and education; (2) operate an outpatient mental health clinic; (3) further deploy within theater, as needed; (4) provide assistance to the ATH when mental health patients are hospitalized on general medical wards; and (5) operate a Combat Stress Facility when joined by the Mental Health Augmentation Team (MHAT).

This second team would include two mental health nurses and one technician. With the availability of the MHAT team and their equipment package, the two teams together could establish a Combat Stress Unit, as well as manage more serious psychiatric patients on an inpatient unit in the ATH or Theater Hospital.

Social workers bring invaluable expertise to these teams. Through the combination of clinical skills and the "person in environment" perspective, they are equipped to address the unique stressors of a wartime or OOTW situation. This background helps them provide effective prevention, intervention, and leadership consultation services.

Prevention and intervention efforts in the field are designed to prevent, identify, and manage adverse combat stress responses in units; optimize mission performance; conserve fighting strength; prevent or minimize adverse effects of combat stress on military members' physical and psychological health; and return units or service members to duty as quickly as possible. Leadership consultation is an area in which social workers have worked informally for years. Through programs such as Family Advocacy and Family Support, they have advised commanders on the problems and needs of their respective communities and possible solutions. Social workers will be expected to hone their consultation skills and translate these processes to the deployment situation.

To be successful in a contingency operation, it will be vital for social workers to de-emphasize the traditional mental health practitioner role and get out of their humble "office in a tent." They will have to spend time around the troops, both to offer a presence and to be attentive to issues that may begin to fester. Social workers deployed to SWA both during and after ODS describe these efforts as the backbone of the work they did there. Troops who were reluctant to seek out an unknown clinician at a designated mental health tent readily approached the workers who spent time with them at their ammo dumps and security outposts. Usually the conversations on these occasions centered on issues such as missing families, spouses, and fiancees. Sometimes more serious concerns would be identified, such as thoughts the person was entertaining about hurting himself or herself, or someone else. In both situations, the outreach efforts provided an opportunity to defuse issues that could have become problematic or life-threatening. As in ODS, social workers who successfully perform outreach efforts in future operations will repeatedly be in a position of hearing rumors or issues that have started to fester among the deployed community. They will need to have developed access to the senior leaders who have the ability to address and implement solutions for these problems.

Readiness activities are not solely limited to the actual deployment. They begin prior to the development of a contingency situation with the preparation of the community and its members for this possibility. Likewise, the process continues after the troops return home and try to reintegrate into their families, units, and communities. These areas provide rich opportunities for social workers to further collaborate with other helping agencies to maximize the effectiveness of readiness programs.

After ODS, returning AF troops identified their key stressors as including: inequities in homecoming celebrations, inequities in time off, readjustment to marital relationships, and difficulties in relationships with children (Caliber Associates, 1992). Many individuals may have intuitive ideas regarding how to ameliorate these concerns. However, the reality is that we still do not empirically know which interventions work best at the individual, family, unit, and community level to successfully reduce problems that occur during deployment and subsequent reunion. Through collaboration with other helping agencies, tremendous potential exists for developing, implementing, and assessing effectiveness of prevention and intervention strategies.

I believe that it is vital for clinical social workers to remain fully engaged in the entire spectrum of the readiness mission. Efforts to recruit social workers will have to include screening to identify applicants who truly appreciate the warfighting mission of the AF and who are willing to fully support it. Ratings of applicants for active duty social work positions will have to include assessment of their willingness to deploy on short notice to austere conditions and their willingness to work in the field with combatants and support personnel. Once clinical social workers are on active duty, they will need to increasingly focus attention on acquiring ongoing training and education necessary to practice in a field environment. Intensive training on topics such as leadership consultation will be vital.

BUILDING HEALTHY COMMUNITIES

Social workers have a long history of solid contributions to building healthy AF communities. They lead the Family Advocacy Programs in efforts to minimize the occurrence and effect of family violence. They are key members of mental health clinics, providing assessment and intervention with active duty members, families, and retirees. They teach family practice residents how to integrate biopsychosocial factors in the medical treatment of patients. Social workers manage inpatient, outpatient, and partial hospitalization substance abuse units. They lead prevention efforts to combat a wide spectrum of issues such as suicide, violence in the workplace, sexual assaults, and gang involvement.

Although there will be ongoing efforts within the AFMS to review ways that these vital services can continue to be provided in the future in the most cost-effective fashion, I expect that active duty social workers will continue to have a presence in performing all of these roles.

Several new initiatives are underway that should also offer exciting opportunities. These include the Integrated Service Delivery System, Primary Care Demonstration Project, and the budding interest in the area of community adaptation.

Integrated Delivery System (IDS)

The IDS is a multidisciplinary team of helping professionals collaborating to "provide synergistic preventive services to the AF community that promote spiritual growth, mental and physical health, and strong individuals and families" (Moorman, 1997, p. 1). The mission of the IDS is to "draw together expertise and resources of helping agencies to provide the optimal collaboration of services intended to enhance the spiritual, emotional, mental and physical dimensions of AF members, their families and communities" (p. 1).

The concept of the IDS is not new, but the timing seems right for its reintroduction in a new package. In today's culture of needing to do more with less, it just makes sense to work smartly and collaboratively with others who have similar missions and goals.

The IDS provides an opportunity for clinical social workers to draw on their roots as community organizers. The teams are free to be innovative in designing services that help meet the specific needs of a community. The members of the team are able to draw on one another's expertise and energies to create a synergy of effort.

It has been clear within mental health circles that prevention efforts absolutely must be part of any mission plan. Resources are simply too scarce to handle every crisis that arises without accompanying efforts to ward off those which can be prevented. Just as in the deployed environment, clinicians who become "office bound" lose their ability to identify opportunities for prevention and early intervention. Likewise, they miss opportunities to network with other agencies and community personnel whose spirit of volunteerism can make these efforts a success. Involvement in the IDS will be vital to social work practice.

Primary Care Demonstration Project

Primary care providers (physicians, physician assistants, and nurse practitioners) have historically seen a large number of patients whose primary problems are psychosocial or mental health related. These problems have frequently gone undiagnosed, resulting in large expenditures of resources to treat only the symptoms and not the underlying cause of the patient's complaints. A three-year demonstration project was initiated in the Family Practice Clinic at Tinker AFB in late 1997 to assess a new model for integrating mental health care with the medical care of patients. This project placed a full-time social worker, a psychologist, and a part-time psychiatrist in the Family Practice Clinic to demonstrate the impact of utilizing mental health providers on the primary care team and to develop and validate a service delivery model for use in AF primary care clinics.

The protocol calls for the use of a biopsychosocial model rather than the traditional medical model. In the latter, the physician's almost exclusive area of interest and treatment are the biological causes of the condition for which the patient sought an appointment. Under this model, patients are typically referred to a geographically separate mental health clinic for treatment of mental health concerns, if any are identified. In the former model, the biopsychosocial needs of the patient drive case conceptualization and treatment for both the primary care and mental health providers. The demonstration project requires new patients to complete a patient questionnaire that includes mental health problem screening. The primary care provider then involves the mental health provider if he or she believes there is a problem, if the patient questionnaire suggests a problem, if medical compliance with care is a problem, if the patient requires an unusually high frequency of contacts, or if the patient requests a mental health provider. The mental health provider in this project may provide brief therapeutic intervention or simply serve as a consultant to the primary care provider.

If successful, this model has the potential to dramatically change the way in which mental health care is provided in the AF. If this model is shown to reduce health care costs for primary care patients and decrease demand for traditional mental health clinic appointments, clinical social workers may increasingly be assigned outside of mental health clinics. In the future, this format for testing the effectiveness and efficiency of mental health service delivery through nontraditional forums may further be tested through placement of mental health providers in other settings, such as military units. Such demonstration projects would create exciting opportunities, as well as challenges, to social workers in the future.

Community Adaptation

This area is just beginning to bud through the joint efforts of Dr. Gary Bowen of the University of North Carolina and the AF Family Advocacy Program office (AF FAP), under the guidance of Colonel John Nelson. The AF FAP is leading the way in developing a research roadmap to address the concept of community adaptation.

Top Air Force leaders recognize that one of the AF's most important attributes is a sense of community among its members and families. This sense of community is one of the foundations that drives motivational identity and commitment, which in turn are key to the core values, career decisions, and combat capability of AF members. Leaders have begun to rededicate efforts to maintain and build this sense of community.

At a time when the value of sense of community is increasingly recognized, however, there appears to be a sense that AF members and their families feel less bonded with the AF community than in the past. Bowen identifies several realities that may contribute to this: "dramatic shifts in the mission and structure of the AF and its community support mechanisms, a smaller and more deployable force, an increasing concentration of members and families in CONUS, greater integration of its Reserve components, and the increased privatization and outsourcing of non-operational support functions" (Bowen, 1998, p. 2).

Bowen notes that the concepts of both community adaptation and community resiliency have been neglected in research done by the AF. He defines community adaptation as "the outcomes of efforts by community members to manage the demands of military life and to work together in meeting military expectations and achieving individual and collective goals"; while community resiliency is "the ability of a community facing normative or non-normative adversity or the consequences of adversity to establish, maintain or regain an 'expected' or 'satisfactory' range of functioning that is equal to or is better than prestressor functioning" (p. 6).

The AF FAP has formed a research group composed of military and civilian consultants to begin to explore the science of community practice in the AF. These efforts are likely to lead to opportunities for clinical social workers to participate in the design, implementation, and assessment of efforts to increase both community adaptation and resiliency.

RIGHTSIZING

Rightsizing involves the Department of the Air Force's attempts to make sure that the correct number of personnel with the right level of rank and experience are maintained on active duty. The AFMS is currently undergoing a bottom-up review of the required staffing necessary in each medical discipline to adequately meet mission requirements.

Current projections suggest that AD social work staffing will level off somewhere between 188 and 202 social workers by the year 2003. This represents a reduction of approximately 10 to 15 percent of current authorizations. The final number of authorizations is determined through a complex integration of numbers of personnel needed for wartime roles and day-to-day operations.

The process through which these reductions will be made will largely involve normal attrition (retirements and separations) as well as a limited number of separations through special incentive programs (early retirement, waiver of time in grade requirements).

As social work enters the rightsizing era, it will be imperative to ensure that an appropriate balance is maintained in the level of experience in its group. Large numbers of clinical social workers were accessed in the late 1970s and early 1980s as the substance abuse and family advocacy programs mushroomed and drove a need for increased numbers. As these groups now attain retirement eligibility, and turnover rates (rates at which individuals enter the service for only one or two tours of three to six years duration) increase, we are left with high recruiting goals for the next several years. This will result in a fairly dramatic change in the composition of AF social work. Currently, nearly half of all AF social workers hold the rank of major or above. However, in the near future, due to the retirement of many senior AF social workers, the majority will be junior in rank.

This trend will reduce the number of more senior social workers available to act as experienced mentors. It will be increasingly important for newly accessed social workers to enter active duty already holding the credentials needed to practice clinical social work independently. While it is not considered desirable to send new social workers to bases where they are likely to be the only social workers present, this will likely be increasingly necessary until the force becomes less junior.

To build a force of more seasoned individuals, it will be increasingly necessary to make concentrated efforts to keep quality performers beyond their initial tour of duty. Efforts in this area will need to include:

1. assurance that new accessions are aware of the lifestyle they will be likely to lead;
2. increased efforts to mentor new accessions who currently may feel overwhelmed by the need to adjust to a new career field, the military culture, and demanding workloads simultaneously;
3. increased opportunities for social workers to broaden their professional experiences; and
4. clearly defined career paths.

DEPLOYMENT OF TRICARE

The deployment of the TRICARE system has been addressed elsewhere in this book and will not be repeated here, except to emphasize briefly some of the primary effects of this system on the practice of social work. Due to a shortage of resources, the TRICARE system requires that health care be offered in a cost-effective manner. Under the managed care concept, clinical interventions offered by social workers in their role as mental health clinicians will most likely become more time limited and focused. Treatment goals will be focused on achieving of an appropriate level of functioning, rather than more lofty, self-actualizing goals. Along with specific treatment goals, measures to assess both a patient's status related to a given problem and progress toward achieving treatment goals will become essential. These trends will require paradigm shifts for many, and there will be a need to adjust to the increased involvement by others in the management of individual patients. Concentrated efforts on the part of senior social workers will be essential to ensure that social workers continue to have opportunities to launch innovative programs, test new service delivery platforms, and research the efficacy of treatment interventions.

OTHER THOUGHTS

Training Needs

The many facets of opportunities for clinical social workers to support the AFMS and AF missions require them to be multitalented. They need to have strong expertise in numerous areas of clinical practice, possess keen community organization skills, and be capable in the role of consultant, as well as demonstrate exemplary supervisory and leadership skills. The social worker who can be successful in all of these arenas must have a solid understanding of the military, its mission, and its procedures. This is a tall order for entry-level social workers.

Currently the majority of psychologists and psychiatrists enter active duty through AF residency programs that offer a course of military-specific training. This training is designed to help residents employ their knowledge and skills in a unique military system. Social workers currently have no such training. They have been intimately involved in development of standardized military-specific training for the psychology and psychiatry residencies. A future goal for AF social work should be the development of a forum to offer this training to social workers and any other mental health professionals who enter the AF through channels other than the AF residency programs.

Career Paths

Several career paths for social workers appear to be emerging. One involves acquisition of a PhD and movement into jobs that are designated advanced academic degree jobs. These include positions at headquarters Air Force in family advocacy and family support, major command headquarters jobs at several of the larger commands, faculty positions at family practice residencies and senior social work positions at the military treatment facilities. there are a total of nineteen designated advanced academic degree positions that range from captain through colonel authorizations. the majority of the senior positions that deal specifically with social work issues are among these nineteen positions. This makes the acquisition of a PhD increasingly important for those interested in this career path.

Another career path that is becoming increasingly defined is the command route. There are no longer requirements for flight commanders, squadron commanders, or even medical group commanders to be members of certain corps (i.e., physicians, dentists). All AFMS officers can compete for these positions. Social workers have been appointed to commanding officer positions at each of these levels. Opportunities will continue for social workers to demonstrate potential for command positions and acceptance of these opportunities, when offered, will be essential for career progression.

Still other paths are beginning to emerge in specialty areas such as readiness and psychological operations. Increasing opportunities are likely to open up in these and other nontraditional social work roles.

Closing Thoughts

The pace of change is dynamic within the AF as is the pace at which opportunities arise. Social workers have a history of developing opportunities through grassroots efforts to identify a need and a means to meet it. Several of social work's key roles developed after individuals implemented model programs to meet local needs. As these efforts gained visibility and recognition, leadership at other bases demanded similar services until such programs became the norm.

I believe that this process will continue with issues that are not yet widely recognized. With social work's current roles and those yet to be developed, clinical social work as a discipline will continue to be a vital component of the AFMS and overall AF mission.

REFERENCES

Bowen, Gary L. (1998). Community resiliency: A research roadmap. Unpublished AF Research Planning Seminar Report.

Caliber Associates. (1992). A study of effectiveness of family assistance programs in the AF during Operation Desert Shield/Storm, executive summary." In Department of Defense (Ed.), *Family Policy and Programs: Persian Gulf Conflict.* Washington, DC: Department of Defense.

Department of the Air Force. (1998). Air Force Medical Service Strategic Plan Roadmap to the Year 2000. (On the Internet: www.sam.brooks.af.mil/html/sggoats.htm.)

Moorman, T.S. (1997, June 3). Guidance for base-level human services integrated delivery system. Attachment to a letter from Air Force Vice Chief of Staff to all Air Force installation commanders. Washington, DC: Department of the Air Force.

Roadman, Charles. (1997). Opening Remarks to Air Force Medical Service Senior Leadership Symposium, Leesburg, VA.

Chapter 22

Military Social Work Practice: Putting It All Together

James G. Daley

As promised, I have captured much of the rich tapestry of military social work practice. This exciting, demanding, potent arena of practice is having an impact at micro, mezzo, and macro levels with a myriad of clients. Military social workers have embraced the potential for organizational change with an aggressive passion for success and produced programs that are worthy of dissemination both within the military and to our civilian colleagues. In fact, the toughest challenge is for military social workers to make such a dissemination a priority.

SURVIVING TODAY'S HIGH-RISK SCENARIO

Military social work practice is at a pivotal point in its history. It is simultaneously eroding and expanding. First, the military is downsizing its force, prompting a sometimes irrational privatization and outsourcing of military personnel. Military social work leaders are being confronted with the Solomon-like decision as to which positions must remain military and which can become civilian. Military readiness and deployment-linked positions are the golden fleece around which retention of military personnel slots is being justified. Second, the mechanisms to achieve a PhD or DSW within one's career (Air Force Institute of Technology-sponsored PhD programs for the Air Force, the combined Walter Reed fellowship and DSW at Catholic University for the Army) are decreasing. This reduction has the potential to underprepare tomorrow's military social work leaders, reduce possible scholarship, and eliminate a significant target for career enhancement. Third, the clinical autonomy of military social workers has been directly challenged with changes in Department of Defense directives (see Chapter 19).

But while erosion is occurring, the opportunities for advancement are increasing. Positions are opening up to military social workers as never before. Jobs historically reserved for line officers (e.g., squadron commander) or physicians (e.g., clinic commander) can now be competed for by all disciplines. Military social workers, as they have become more savvy about navigating a military career, have carved out an increasing range of jobs. With the broadening span of possibilities, military social workers have less identification as mental health officers and more identification as social change advocates. For the newly commissioned social worker, these changes can produce career confusion or an unfortunate distance from senior social workers. For senior military social work leadership, these expanded horizons produce a paucity of senior social workers to place within traditional leadership slots. Positions historically held by field grade officers are being filled by junior captains as senior social workers move to nontraditional positions that enhance career potential. Unfortunately, an alarming number of military social workers are not continuing beyond their first enlistment. The delicate balance is not being maintained between expanding the potential influence of social work within the military and ensuring that adequate supervisory and mentoring infrastructure remains.

So what are the solutions? First, military social workers must continue their highly successful rise in the ranks, maximizing every opportunity to demonstrate their value as military officers. The higher the rank, the more access to the potent decision makers who seek (naively or purposefully) to erode this practice arena. Without continued success stories, military social work's forward progress will stop. But junior officers need careful attention. Aggressive efforts to facilitate mentoring are being implemented (see Chapters 19-21).

These mentoring efforts will only prove effective with baseline and trend analysis surveys to track the retention history of military social workers, exit interview surveys of social workers departing the military, and periodic career satisfaction surveys of current military social workers. This data had not been collected when I served on a command surgeon staff and an Air Force staff-level task force. The lack of such data leaves military social work leadership with anecdotal information and speculation as their only pulse beat of progress. Most significantly, the surveys should be standardized across the three services (a herculean feat, as anyone familiar with tri-service efforts knows).

Besides enhancing career retention and better assessing the reasons for a suspected hemorrhage of departing junior officers, social workers need a mechanism to communicate their significant achievements. There should be effective tri-service task forces on combat stress teams, family assistance during deployment, family violence prevention strategies, partnerships with academicians, and management skill building. Particular attention should be paid to justifying the longitudinal benefits of training PhD/DSW-level social workers. The doctoral-level social workers have contributed immensely to scholarship, enhanced critical thinking on policy issues, and acted as conduits to effective targeted use of academicians (e.g., the partnership looking at community wellness described in Chapter 21).

An annual white paper on a key topic should be developed. The paper, sponsored by the three service chiefs, should utilize expertise within military ranks, civilian settings, and academic circles. I suggest that an excellent initial topic would be the application of doctoral-level social workers within the military. Such a paper would directly challenge the ludicrous notion that doctoral-level social workers are needed to conduct clinical evaluations and refocus their utility on policy development, scholarship, and critical evaluation of partnerships between contractors and the military. Other topics for white papers might include building wellness across the military career (building on Parker, Call, and Barko's work in Chapter 16); social service linkages between the military, TRICARE, the Veterans Administration, and civilian agencies; ethical dilemmas in the provision of military social work; or military human service agencies from a social work perspective. The main point is to target key issues and develop comprehensive documents that cover them. These documents would allow enhanced communication between services and between the military and civilian social work leadership.

Cross-fertilization of program ideas and solutions between the three services is essential to demonstrate overall effectiveness and accumulate success stories to use as fodder for the cannons of advocacy. Military social workers tend to become service-myopic, failing to systematically communicate across services. For example, each social work service chief sends out to all military social workers in that service a quarterly (or annual) short update on what is happening along with a personnel roster. I received the updates throughout my career. The update never mentioned any events occurring in the other services. I strongly suspect that the service chiefs (Colonel Tarpley, Colonel Lockett, Captain Kennedy) do not routinely send courtesy copies of their updates to their counterparts. Further, I suspect that the three service chiefs rarely get together and that coordinated advocacy between the three services is rare. Each service chief is already overwhelmed by demands on his or her time. But their battles are often about the same issues. Linking service with combat readiness, applying fenced family advocacy funds, reacting to damaging DoD directives, developing mentoring and training initiatives, balancing staffing needs with career-broadening opportunities, seeking the best balance of civilian to military resources, and enhancing line opportunities are issues common to all three services. Dialogue between chiefs (e-mail, meetings, etc.) could lead to better overall solutions. Besides communication between chiefs, I suggest an expansion of Colonel Lockett's concept of the "council of colonels" to allow a council of colonels consisting of tri-service representatives (including reserve colonels). Seasoned leaders offer expertise, and a tri-service task force would facilitate a better understanding of common versus service-unique solutions. I compliment Colonel (retired) Harris and Captain Kennedy for their efforts at creating the Uniformed Services Social Work Conference, which has occurred for several years in conjunction with the annual conference of the National Association of Social Workers. This conference has been a wonderful, albeit underattended, opportunity for cross-fertilization of ideas.

EXPANDING THE COMMUNICATION HORIZON

As essential as cross-service communication is, a larger solution is needed. Military social workers are bound by military law to speak only through their chain of command, and public statements must be cleared through the public affairs office. The reader will notice that every chapter which has a military author has a disclaimer at the bottom of the first page of the chapter. These chapters had to be reviewed and cleared by public affairs. The reason is simple. Every statement might cause a firestorm of controversy that will have to be doused by someone within the military. However, there are issues that need to be bluntly challenged, such as the restriction of military social workers from conducting mental health evaluations (see Chapter 19). Military psychologists have long bypassed the restriction by having a military psychology section within the American Psychological Association. This section can voice concerns or confront issues without military law boundaries. We have no such vehicle within military social work. A military social work section of the National Association of Social Workers or a separate military social work association should be created to allow an avenue of advocacy on issues affecting military social work. It is essential that the section include retired military social workers and civilian social workers who are not bound by military law. In this era of personnel and policy changes, we need a voice that challenges the illogic or damage of some decisions.

Besides defending and advocating, this section or association can be a vehicle for disseminating trends and interesting projects, and helping our civilian colleagues better appreciate the top-quality efforts occurring within the military. In fact, this section or association could seek the development of a specialty journal, the *Journal of Military Social Work Practice*, which is long overdue. This journal, akin to the existing *Military Psychology* journal, could offer a scholarly outlet for research and practice issues. Finally, this section or association could offer a mechanism for cross-fertilization between new and retired military social workers (a surprisingly rare event). Such cross-fertilization can help clarify and embrace the rich heritage of military social work. Too often, military social workers (especially newly commissioned officers) have little understanding of the historical or current context of their practice setting. This book will help that issue immensely. However, a section or association allows a vibrant and ongoing mechanism of communication.

BETTER UNDERSTANDING OF INTERNATIONAL MILITARY SOCIAL WORK

Communication efforts need to expand beyond just the U.S. military social work cadre. There are social workers within other countries' military. How do they function and what is their history? There is no published literature which contrasts the military social work programs of other countries and U.S. programs. How do Israeli military social workers function compared to Canadian social workers? What proportion of other countries have a designated military position for a social worker? We are slowly becoming more knowledgeable about the historical context and current directions of U.S. military social work. However, little is known about our larger global context and scant between-country dialogue seems to occur. It is difficult to predict the potential benefits of enhanced multiple-country interaction. But I advocate that a better collaboration facilitates new ideas, helps put U.S. military social work policies and program initiatives into a broader context, and expands the opportunities for clarity of history, policy, and clinical services.

As I conclude this book, I recognize that the next step is to collate information on the different international military social work programs. The path to achieve this goal is unclear at this moment. But by the time you read this chapter, I hope to be well into the journey!

Index